Headache

Series Editor

Paolo Martelletti
Roma, Italy

The purpose of this Series, endorsed by the European Headache Federation (EHF), is to describe in detail all aspects of headache disorders that are of importance in primary care and the hospital setting, including pathophysiology, diagnosis, management, comorbidities, and issues in particular patient groups. A key feature of the Series is its multidisciplinary approach, and it will have wide appeal to internists, rheumatologists, neurologists, pain doctors, general practitioners, primary care givers, and pediatricians. Readers will find that the Series assists not only in understanding, recognizing, and treating the primary headache disorders, but also in identifying the potentially dangerous underlying causes of secondary headache disorders and avoiding mismanagement and overuse of medications for acute headache, which are major risk factors for disease aggravation. Each volume is designed to meet the needs of both more experienced professionals and medical students, residents, and trainees.

More information about this series at http://www.springer.com/series/11801

Timothy J. Steiner • Lars Jacob Stovner
Editors

Societal Impact of Headache

Burden, Costs and Response

Springer

EUROPEAN HEADACHE FEDERATION
EHF

Editors
Timothy J. Steiner
Department of Neuromedicine
and Movement Science
NTNU Norwegian University of Science
and Technology
Trondheim
Norway

Division of Brain Sciences
Imperial College London
London
UK

Lars Jacob Stovner
Department of Neuromedicine
and Movement Science
NTNU Norwegian University of Science
and Technology
Trondheim
Norway

Norwegian Advisory Unit on Headaches
Department of Neurology and Clinical
Neurophysiology
St Olavs University Hospital
Trondheim
Norway

ISSN 2197-652X ISSN 2197-6538 (electronic)
Headache
ISBN 978-3-030-24726-3 ISBN 978-3-030-24728-7 (eBook)
https://doi.org/10.1007/978-3-030-24728-7

This Springer imprint is published by the registered company Springer Nature Switzerland AG
The registered company address is: Gewerbestrasse 11, 6330 Cham, Switzerland

Foreword

Headache disorders are ubiquitous, highly prevalent and disabling. In the Global Burden of Disease Study 2010, tension-type headache and migraine were recognized as the second and third most prevalent disorders in the world. Headache is experienced by nearly everybody at some time or times in their lives. At any one time, at least 40% of the world's adults have personal experience of one or more headache disorders, while recent surveys suggest the proportion of adults with headache on any particular day exceeds 1 in 20. In the Global Burden of Disease Study 2016, migraine was ranked as the second highest cause of disability overall and first in young adults (aged 15–49 years).

The high prevalence of headache disorders gives rise to ill health and disability on a very substantial scale, which is being increasingly acknowledged. This monograph considers the public health perspective, and societal impact, of these conditions. While our understanding of the global burden attributable to headache disorders is still incomplete and our knowledge of healthcare resource allocation to headache is scant, there is good evidence to indicate that very large numbers of people disabled by headache do not receive effective healthcare. The barriers responsible for this vary throughout the world, but poor awareness in a context of limited resources generally—and for healthcare in particular—is undoubtedly high among them.

The World Health Organization's *Atlas of Headache Disorders and Resources in the World 2011* had this message for health planners and policy-makers:

> The facts and figures presented [in the *Atlas*] illuminate the worldwide neglect of a major cause of public ill-health and reveal the inadequacies of responses to it in countries throughout the world.

Moreover:

> Given the very high indirect costs of headache, greater investment in health care that treats headache effectively, through well-organized health services and supported by education, may well be cost-saving overall.

This, therefore, is a monograph not so much about headache, or headache disorders, but rather about public health. In particular, the book provides a detailed analysis of the epidemiological and socioeconomic consequences of headache disorders, together with proposed and ongoing institutional and societal responses over the life course and across health and other sectors.

Dan Chisholm
Programme Manager for Mental Health
Division of NCDs and Promoting Health Through the Life-Course
World Health Organization Regional Office for Europe
Copenhagen, Denmark

Contents

Contributors

Dan Chisholm Programme Manager for Mental Health, Division of NCDs and Promoting Health Through the Life-Course, World Health Organization Regional Office for Europe, Copenhagen, Denmark

Raquel Gil-Gouveia Hospital da Luz Headache Center, Lisbon, Portugal

Lara Gitto CEIS Economic Evaluation and HTA (EEHTA), Faculty of Economics, University "Tor Vergata", Rome, Italy

Knut Hagen Department of Neuromedicine and Movement Science, NTNU Norwegian University of Science and Technology, Trondheim, Norway

Norwegian Advisory Unit on Headache, Department of Neurology and Clinical Neurophysiology, St Olavs University Hospital, Trondheim, Norway

Nelly Huynh Research Centre of the Sainte-Justine University Hospital, Montreal, QC, Canada

Rigmor Jensen Department of Neurology, Danish Headache Centre, University of Copenhagen, Rigshospitalet Glostrup, Glostrup, Denmark

Zaza Katsarava Evangelical Hospital Unna, Unna, Germany

Department of Neurology, University of Duisburg-Essen, Essen, Germany

EVEX Medical Corporation, Tbilisi, Georgia

IM Sechenov First Moscow State Medical University (Sechenov University), Moscow, Russian Federation

Paolo Martelletti Department of Clinical and Molecular Medicine, Sapienza University, Rome, Italy

Regional Referral Headache Centre, Sant'Andrea Hospital, Rome, Italy

Francesco Saverio Mennini CEIS Economic Evaluation and HTA (EEHTA), and IGF Department, Faculty of Economics, University "Tor Vergata", Rome, Italy

Institute for Leadership and Management in Health, Kingston University, Kingston, UK

Emma Nichols Institute for Health Metrics and Evaluation (IHME), University of Washington, Seattle, WA, USA

Jes Olesen Department of Neurology, Danish Headache Centre, University of Copenhagen, Rigshospitalet Glostrup, Glostrup, Denmark

Timothy J. Steiner Department of Neuromedicine and Movement Science, NTNU Norwegian University of Science and Technology, Trondheim, Norway

Division of Brain Sciences, Imperial College London, London, UK

Lars Jacob Stovner Department of Neuromedicine and Movement Science, NTNU Norwegian University of Science and Technology, Trondheim, Norway

Norwegian Advisory Unit on Headaches, Department of Neurology and Clinical Neurophysiology, St Olavs University Hospital, Trondheim, Norway

Hallie Thomas Department of Neuromedicine and Movement Science, NTNU Norwegian University of Science and Technology, Trondheim, Norway

Michela Tinelli Personal Social Services Research Unit, The London School of Economics and Political Science, London, UK

Derya Uluduz Neurology Department, Cerrahpaşa School of Medicine, Istanbul University, Istanbul, Turkey

Theo Vos Institute for Health Metrics and Evaluation (IHME), University of Washington, Seattle, WA, USA

Abbreviations

BASH	British Association for the Study of Headache
BMI	Body mass index
CATI	Computer-assisted telephone interview
CG	Condition group (in ICF)
CH	Cluster headache
CI	Confidence interval
CM	Chronic migraine
CMSCs	Chronic musculoskeletal complaints
COI	Cost of illness
CSF	Cerebrospinal fluid
CT	Computer tomography
DALY	Disability-adjusted life year
DW	Disability weight (applied to a health state in GBD)
EBC	European Brain Council
EC	European Commission
EEM	Equal effects model
EHF	European Headache Federation
EM	Episodic migraine
ENT	Ear, nose and throat
ERB	Ethics review board
EU	European Union
GBD	Global Burden of Disease (study)
GCA	Giant cell arteritis
GDP	Gross domestic product
GP	General (medical) practitioner
GPAC	Global Patient Advocacy Coalition
HADS	Hospital Anxiety and Depression Scale
HALT	Headache-attributed lost time (index)
HARDSHIP	Headache-attributed restriction, disability, social handicap and impaired participation (questionnaire)
HCP	Healthcare provider

HOH	Headache on the (Capitol) Hill
HUNT	Helseundersøkelsen i Nord-Trøndelag (The Nord-Trøndelag Health Study)
HURT	Headache under-response to treatment (questionnaire)
IBMS	International Burden of Migraine Study
ICD	International Classification of Diseases
ICF	International Classification of Functioning, Disability and Health
ICHD	International Classification of Headache Disorders
IHS	International Headache Society
LTB	*Lifting The Burden*
LWDE	Lost workday equivalent
MIDAS	Migraine Disability Assessment
MOH	Medication-overuse headache
MRI	Magnetic resonance imaging
NIH	National Institutes of Health
NTNU	Norwegian University of Science and Technology
NWDM	Number of workdays with migraine
OR	Odds ratio
OTC	Over the counter (medication)
OUCH	Organization for Understanding Cluster Headache
PDSA	Plan-do-study-act (cycles)
PIFP	Primary idiopathic facial pain
pMOH	Probable medication-overuse headache
PPP	Purchasing power parity
QVM	Qualité de vie et migraine (QoL instrument)
RR	Relative risk
SAH	Subarachnoid headache
SD	Standard deviation
SES	Socioeconomic status
SF	Short form (QoL instrument)
SQE	Service quality evaluation
STROBE	Strengthening the Reporting of Observational studies in Epidemiology
TELM	Total employment lost (due to) migraine
TMWD	Total (number of) migraine-related missed workdays
TN	Trigeminal neuralgia
TTH	Tension-type headache
UdH	Undifferentiated headache
UI	Uncertainty interval
UK	United Kingdom
UK-ONS	UK Office for National Statistics (survey)
US(A)	United States (of America)
USSR	Union of Soviet Socialist Republics
VO_2	Peak oxygen uptake
WG	Working group (in ICF)

WHA	World Headache Alliance
WHO	World Health Organization
WHOQoL	WHO quality of life (questionnaire)
WTP	Willingness to pay
YLD	Year lived with disability
YLL	Year of life lost (to early mortality)

Part I
Headache and Public Ill Health

Chapter 1
Introduction

Timothy J. Steiner and Lars Jacob Stovner

Tension-type headache (TTH) and migraine are very common: the Global Burden of Disease (GBD) study 2010 (GBD2010) found them to be the second and third most prevalent disorders in the world, after dental caries [1]. Prevalence of disease, however, is not on its own a signal of disease impact, and it is certainly not a measure of it. Impact is made by the *loss of health* that disease in one or more ways imposes on people, a loss commonly referred to as "burden". It is the purpose of this monograph to say something about the burden attributable to headache disorders.

There is a background story of evidence accruing but ignored, or at least given inadequate weight, over many years. GBD1990, the first of the GBD studies and conducted by the World Health Organization (WHO), had nothing at all to say about headache disorders in general or any one of them specifically: they were not thought to be of any importance to global public health [2]. In the years leading up to GBD2000, and especially during 1996–1999, much lobbying was taking place at WHO: headache disorders, ubiquitous, prevalent, disabling and treatable, met each one of their criteria for priority. While we collated the published *prevalence* data for migraine, at that time with a global estimated mean of about 11%, WHO methodology transformed these into *disability* estimates. GBD2000 duly attributed to migraine 1.4% of all years of life lived with disability (YLDs), and ranked this

T. J. Steiner (✉)
Department of Neuromedicine and Movement Science, NTNU Norwegian University of Science and Technology, Trondheim, Norway

Division of Brain Sciences, Imperial College London, London, UK
e-mail: t.steiner@imperial.ac.uk

L. J. Stovner
Department of Neuromedicine and Movement Science, NTNU Norwegian University of Science and Technology, Trondheim, Norway

Norwegian Advisory Unit on Headaches, Department of Neurology and Clinical Neurophysiology, St Olavs University Hospital, Trondheim, Norway
e-mail: lars.stovner@ntnu.no

T. J. Steiner, L. J. Stovner (eds.), *Societal Impact of Headache*, Headache,
https://doi.org/10.1007/978-3-030-24728-7_1

disorder 19th among all causes of disability worldwide [3]. Largely because of this "discovery", WHO recognized the priority claims of headache [4–6].

Ten years later, GBD2010 found migraine to be the *seventh* highest specific cause of disability, accounting for 2.9% of all YLDs worldwide [1], a revelation so significant that all three major headache journals recorded it by carrying the same editorial simultaneously [7–9]. Of course, migraine had not grown in these 10 years. Simply, the evidence submitted to GBD2000 had been seriously deficient, and in the meantime it had improved. A key agent in achieving this was *Lifting The Burden* (LTB), the UK-registered charity conducting the Global Campaign against Headache [4, 10, 11] in official relations with WHO [12] and working with the GBD project [13]. LTB had two objectives for GBD2010: to secure inclusion of the other headache disorders of public health importance—TTH and medication-overuse headache (MOH)—and to show, as was then believed, that headache disorders collectively were among the top ten causes of disability worldwide. TTH was indeed included, but the low disability weight (DW) attributed to it added little impact—relative to that of migraine—despite the higher prevalence of TTH. MOH was also initially included but, in the end, not reported because the prevalence data were not good enough to support regional estimates of burden attributable to this disorder. This had changed by the time of GBD2013: migraine, again on better evidence, was now the *sixth* highest cause of disability worldwide; MOH, reported for the first time, was also in the top 20 (18th) of the disability league table [14]. GBD2013 ranked headache disorders collectively as *third* among the worldwide causes of YLDs [14, 15]. Better informed still, GBD2016 ranked migraine *second*, responsible for 5.6% of YLDs [16]. In young adults—an important group because of their contribution to production—it was *top* (8.2%) [16, 17]. GBD2017 [18], the most recently published at the time of writing, also ranked migraine second (behind low back pain), costing the world over 47 million YLDs, again 5.6% of the total.

This story relates a part of the continuing endeavour—sometimes amounting to a struggle—to keep headache disorders above the public-health horizon and fully visible in their scope and scale. To understand the global disability burden, which the GBD studies endeavour to capture [13], it is first necessary to explore individual burden, because it is on *people* that headache burden falls directly. Disability during migraine attacks, for example, is attributable to pain and the associated symptoms of nausea, photophobia and phonophobia. These are easily recognized; much less so is an *interictal* disability, arising because people, fearful of the next attack, avoid potential triggers and compromise their lifestyles in this pursuit. Also poorly recognized are the less tangible burdens: for example, those arising from opportunities missed as a consequence of recurrent illness, which build cumulatively over a lifetime. Surveys such as GBD, focusing on descriptive health states such as "ictal migraine" or "interictal migraine", cannot of course capture all these aspects of burden.

Nevertheless, despite giving a still incomplete account of the societal impact of headache disorders, GBD has, finally, put them—and not just migraine—firmly on the public-health agenda. This monograph aims to add some of the missing elements to that account.

Very little in the book is new. It collates the published work of its many authors into a monograph in a way we hope will be useful. The chapters follow a theme, and in sequence tell a story, but, so that they better stand alone, there is some repetition. The book is published under the auspices of the European Headache Federation, so its focus is Europe, but many parts have much wider relevance.

References

1. Vos T, Flaxman AD, Naghavi M, Lozano R, Michaud C, Ezzati M, Shibuya K, Salomon JA, Abdalla S, Aboyans V, Abraham J, Ackerman I, Aggarwal R, Ahn SY, Ali MK, Alvarado M, Anderson HR, Anderson LM, Andrews KG, Atkinson C, Baddour LM, Bahalim AN, Barker-Collo S, Barrero LH, Bartels DH, Basáñez MG, Baxter A, Bell ML, Benjamin EJ, Bennett D, Bernabé E, Bhalla K, Bhandari B, Bikbov B, Bin Abdulhak A, et al. Years lived with disability (YLD) for 1160 sequelae of 289 diseases and injuries 1990-2010: a systematic analysis for the Global Burden of Disease Study 2010. Lancet. 2012;380:2163–96.
2. World Health Organization. WHO global burden of disease publications. http://www.who.int/healthinfo/global_burden_disease/publications/en/.
3. World Health Organization. World health report 2001. Geneva: WHO; 2001.
4. Steiner TJ. *Lifting The Burden*: the global campaign against headache. Lancet Neurol. 2004;3:204–5.
5. World Health Organization, *Lifting The Burden*. Atlas of headache disorders and resources in the world 2011. Geneva: WHO; 2011.
6. Steiner TJ, Stovner LJ, Dua T, Birbeck GL, Jensen R, Katsarava Z, Martelletti P, Saxena S. Time to act on headache disorders. J Headache Pain. 2011;12:501–3.
7. Steiner TJ, Stovner LJ, Birbeck GL. Migraine: the seventh disabler. J Headache Pain. 2013;14:1.
8. Steiner TJ, Stovner LJ, Birbeck GL. Migraine: the seventh disabler. Headache. 2013;53:227–9.
9. Steiner TJ, Stovner LJ, Birbeck GL. Migraine: the seventh disabler. Cephalalgia. 2013;33:289–90.
10. Steiner TJ. *Lifting The Burden*: the global campaign to reduce the burden of headache worldwide. J Headache Pain. 2005;6:373–7.
11. Steiner TJ, Birbeck GL, Jensen R, Katsarava Z, Martelletti P, Stovner LJ. *Lifting The Burden*: the first 7 years. J Headache Pain. 2010;11:451–5.
12. Steiner TJ, Birbeck GL, Jensen R, Katsarava Z, Martelletti P, Stovner LJ. The global campaign, World Health Organization and *Lifting The Burden*: collaboration in action. J Headache Pain. 2011;12:273–4.
13. Institute for Health Metrics and Evaluation. Global burden of disease (GBD). http://www.healthdata.org/gbd.
14. Vos T, Barber RM, Bell B, Bertozzi-Villa A, Biryukov S, Bolliger I, Charlson F, Davis A, Degenhardt L, Dicker D, Duan L, Erskine H, Feigin VL, Ferrari AJ, Fitzmaurice C, Fleming T, Graetz N, Guinovart C, Haagsma J, Hansen GM, Hanson SW, Heuton KR, Higashi H, Kassebaum N, Kyu H, Laurie E, Liang X, Lofgren K, Lozano R, MacIntyre MF, Moradi-Lakeh M, Naghavi M, Nguyen G, Odell S, Ortblad K, et al. Global, regional, and national incidence, prevalence, and years lived with disability for 301 acute and chronic diseases and injuries in 188 countries, 1990-2013: a systematic analysis for the Global Burden of Disease Study 2013. Lancet. 2015;386:743–800.
15. Steiner TJ, Stovner LJ, Vos T. GBD 2015: migraine is the third cause of disability in under 50s. J Headache Pain. 2016;17:104.
16. Vos T, Abajobir AA, Abate KH, Abbafati C, Abbas KM, Abd-Allah F, Abdulkader RS, Abdulle AM, Abebo TA, Abera SF, Aboyans V, Abu-Raddad LJ, Ackerman IN, Adamu AA,

Adetokunboh O, Afarideh M, Afshin A, Agarwal SK, Aggarwal R, Agrawal A, Agrawal S, Ahmadieh H, Ahmed MB, Aichour MTE, Aichour AN, Aichour I, Aiyar S, Akinyemi RO, Akseer N, Al Lami FH, Alahdab F, Al-Aly Z, Alam K, Alam N, Alam T, et al. Global, regional, and national incidence, prevalence, and years lived with disability for 328 diseases and injuries for 195 countries, 1990–2016: a systematic analysis for the Global Burden of Disease Study 2016. Lancet. 2017;390:1211–59.

17. Steiner TJ, Stovner LJ, Vos T, Jensen R, Katsarava Z. Migraine is *first* cause of disability in under 50s: will health politicians now take notice? J Headache Pain. 2018;19:17.
18. GBD 2017 Disease and Injury Incidence and Prevalence Collaborators. Global, regional, and national incidence, prevalence, and years lived with disability for 354 diseases and injuries for 195 countries and territories, 1990–2017: a systematic analysis for the Global Burden of Disease Study 2017. Lancet. 2018;392:1789–858.

Chapter 2
The Meaning of "Headache" in the Context of Society

Timothy J. Steiner

2.1 Introduction

Headache is common—one of the most frequently experienced symptoms of mankind [1]. Almost everybody has experience of it. It is also one of the most common medical complaints, which is not the same thing. To put some numbers to these statements, at least 40% of adults in all countries report headache as a recurring nuisance, 10–30% are at least sometimes disabled by it and 2–10% bear it, with varying levels of incapacity, on more days than not [2, 3].

This very attribute somehow, perversely, works against it. Headache is so common that people often regard it as "normal", a perception that fosters a marked societal ambivalence towards it: while it renders some people almost helpless, others look upon all manifestations of headache with scorn or derision. Headache is the most frequent cause of consultation in both primary care and neurological practice [3]. It prompts many visits to internists, ENT specialists (otorhinolaryngologists), ophthalmologists, dentists, orthopaedic surgeons, psychologists and the proponents of a wide variety of complementary and alternative medical practices [3]. Headache is far from unknown as a presenting symptom in emergency departments, although it rarely signals serious underlying illness.

Headache may be mostly benign, but it hurts, and with pain comes disability. When headache is recurrent, repeated episodes of disability diminish quality of life, while impaired productivity leads to financial loss—each a personal burden. The public-health and *societal* importance of headache lies in these causal associations expressed in large numbers of people.

T. J. Steiner (✉)
Department of Neuromedicine and Movement Science, NTNU Norwegian University of Science and Technology, Trondheim, Norway

Division of Brain Sciences, Imperial College London, London, UK
e-mail: t.steiner@imperial.ac.uk

T. J. Steiner, L. J. Stovner (eds.), *Societal Impact of Headache*, Headache,
https://doi.org/10.1007/978-3-030-24728-7_2

2.2 Headache Disorders

Headache itself is a feature, often characteristic, of a very large number of disorders. The International Classification of Headache Disorders (ICHD) describes more than 200 headache types, subtypes or subforms [1]. As Table 2.1 shows, ICHD distinguishes between *primary headaches*, which have no other underlying causative disorder, and *secondary headaches*, attributed to some other disorder. The third section of ICHD covers painful cranial neuropathies and other facial pain [1].

Tables 2.2, 2.3 and 2.4 briefly describe the relatively few of these disorders that are common or, for other reasons, important. These are the headaches of which all healthcare providers, including and especially those in primary care, should have knowledge and some understanding in order to meet the very substantial need they generate for professional care. The secondary headaches in Table 2.3 must never be missed. As for the primary headaches (Table 2.2), effective management of these is often achievable without recourse to professional care, by lifestyle adaptation and appropriate use of over-the-counter (OTC) medications. But equally often this is not the case, and the need for professional care arising from these disorders places a substantial demand on health services. Recognition of where this demand comes from, and an understanding based on empirical evidence of the people and the disorders that most contribute to it, are key to the design and implementation of headache services, and to the delivery, within these, of effective, efficient and equitable headache care.

Table 2.1 International classification of headache disorders, 3rd edition (ICHD-3) [1]

Chapter	Part One: The Primary Headaches
1	Migraine
2	Tension-type headache
3	Trigeminal autonomic cephalalgias
4	Other primary headache disorders
	Part Two: The Secondary Headaches
5	Headache attributed to trauma or injury to the head and/or neck
6	Headache attributed to cranial and/or cervical vascular disorder
7	Headache attributed to non-vascular intracranial disorder
8	Headache attributed to a substance or its withdrawal
9	Headache attributed to infection
10	Headache attributed to disorder of homoeostasis
11	Headache or facial pain attributed to disorder of the cranium, neck, eyes, ears, nose, sinuses, teeth, mouth or other facial or cervical structure
12	Headache attributed to psychiatric disorder
	Part Three: Painful Cranial Neuropathies, Other Facial Pain and Other Headaches
13	Painful lesions of the cranial nerves and other facial pain
14	Other headache disorders

Table 2.2 Important primary headaches in ICHD-3 [1]

1. Migraine
1.1 *Migraine without aura*
Recurrent headache attacks lasting 4–72 h. Typically, the headache is unilateral, pulsating, moderate or severe, aggravated by routine physical activity and associated with nausea and/or photophobia and phonophobia.
1.2 *Migraine with aura*
Recurrent attacks, lasting minutes, of unilateral fully reversible visual, sensory or other central nervous system symptoms that usually develop gradually and are usually followed by headache and associated migraine symptoms.
1.3 *Chronic migraine*
Headache occurring on $\geq$15 days/month for >3 months, which, on $\geq$8 days/month, has the features of migraine headache.
2. Tension-type headache (TTH)
2.2 *Frequent episodic tension-type headache*
Frequent episodes of headache lasting minutes to days. Typically, it is bilateral, pressing or tightening and mild or moderate. It lacks the specific characteristics of migraine: neither aggravated by routine physical activity nor associated with nausea (either photophobia or phonophobia may be present).
2.3 *Chronic tension-type headache*
A disorder evolving from frequent episodic TTH, with daily or very frequent headache lasting hours to days, or unremitting, typically bilateral, pressing or tightening and mild or moderate. The pain does not worsen with routine physical activity, but may be associated with mild nausea, photophobia or phonophobia.
3. Trigeminal autonomic cephalalgias
This group of uncommon disorders shares the clinical features of short-duration headache and prominent cranial parasympathetic autonomic features.
3.1 *Cluster headache*
Attacks of severe, strictly unilateral, orbital, supraorbital and/or temporal pain lasting 15–180 min and occurring from once every other day to eight times a day. The pain is associated with ipsilateral conjunctival injection, lacrimation, nasal congestion, rhinorrhoea, forehead and facial sweating, miosis, ptosis and/or eyelid oedema, and/or with restlessness or agitation.
3.1.1 *Episodic cluster headache*
Cluster headache attacks occurring in periods lasting from 7 days to 1 year, separated by pain-free periods lasting at least 3 months.
3.1.2 *Chronic cluster headache*
Cluster headache attacks occurring for 1 year or longer without remission, or with remission periods lasting <3 months.

Two primary headache disorders—migraine and tension-type headache (TTH)—are widespread, prevalent and often lifelong conditions. These are subjects of this monograph; secondary headache disorders, with the single exception of medication-overuse headache (MOH), are not—even those listed in Table 2.3. Collectively, migraine, TTH and MOH affect at least 40% of most populations [4] and are the cause of much disability throughout the world [4, 5]. Other headache disorders, such as cluster headache, may be highly disabling at individual level, but they are too uncommon to signify at societal level.[1]

[1] The meaning here is that they add insignificantly to societal burden, not that no provision should be made for healthcare for such disorders. Headache services set up adequately to manage headache disorders (see Chap. 15) would take these and rarer disorders into account.

Table 2.3 Important secondary headaches in ICHD-3 [1]

5. Headache attributed to trauma or injury to the head and/or neck
5.2 ***Persistent headache attributed to traumatic injury to the head***
Headache of >3 months' duration caused by traumatic injury to the head. It is often part of the post-traumatic syndrome, which includes symptoms such as equilibrium disturbance, poor concentration, decreased work ability, irritability, depressive mood and sleep disturbances.
6. Headache attributed to cranial and/or cervical vascular disorder
6.2.2 ***Acute headache attributed to non-traumatic subarachnoid haemorrhage (SAH)***
Headache caused by non-traumatic SAH, typically severe and sudden in onset, peaking in seconds (thunderclap headache) or minutes. Non-traumatic SAH is one of the most common causes of thunderclap headache. It is serious: delayed diagnosis often has a catastrophic outcome.
6.4.1 ***Headache attributed to giant cell arteritis (GCA)***
Headache, with variable features, caused by and symptomatic of GCA. Conspicuously associated with headache, GCA must be recognised: any persisting headache with recent onset in a patient >60 years of age should suggest it. Blindness is a major risk, preventable by immediate steroid treatment.
7. Headache attributed to non-vascular intracranial disorder
7.2 ***Headache attributed to low cerebrospinal fluid (CSF) pressure***
Headache caused by low CSF pressure, usually orthostatic and accompanied by neck pain, tinnitus, changes in hearing, photophobia and/or nausea. It remits after normalization of CSF pressure. Three subtypes are distinguished by aetiology: following recent dural puncture, attributed to persistent CSF leakage (CSF fistula) or spontaneous.
7.4.1 ***Headache attributed to intracranial neoplasm***
Headache caused by one or more space-occupying intracranial tumours. Headache is a common symptom of intracranial tumours, more so in young patients (including children), but it rarely remains the only symptom: neurological deficits and seizures are common.
8. Headache attributed to a substance or its withdrawal
8.1.3 ***Carbon monoxide (CO)-induced headache***
Headache caused by exposure to CO, resolving within 72 h after its elimination. Dependent on carboxyhaemoglobin level, headache ranges from mild without other symptoms to severe with nausea, vomiting, blurred vision and, ultimately, impaired consciousness.
8.2 ***Medication-overuse headache (MOH)***
Headache on ≥15 days/month in a patient with a pre-existing primary headache (usually migraine or TTH), developing as a consequence of regular overuse for >3 months of acute or symptomatic medication for headache. Usually, it resolves after the overuse is stopped. Correct diagnosis of MOH is important because patients will not improve without withdrawal of the offending medication.
9. Headache attributed to infection
9.1.1 ***Headache attributed to bacterial meningitis or meningoencephalitis***
Headache of variable duration caused by bacterial meningitis or meningoencephalitis. It may develop with mild flu-like symptoms and is typically acute and associated with neck stiffness, nausea, fever and changes in mental state and/or other neurological symptoms and/or signs. In most cases, headache resolves with resolution of the infection.
11. Headache or facial pain attributed to disorder of the cranium, neck, eyes, ears, nose, sinuses, teeth, mouth or other facial or cervical structure
11.3.1 ***Headache attributed to acute angle-closure glaucoma***
Headache, usually unilateral, caused by acute angle-closure glaucoma and associated with other symptoms and clinical signs of this disorder (eye and/or periorbital pain, visual acuity loss (blurring), conjunctival injection and oedema, nausea and vomiting). Early diagnosis is essential: as intraocular pressure rises, so does the risk of permanent visual loss.

Table 2.4 Important painful cranial neuropathies and other facial pain in ICHD-3 [1]

13. Painful lesions of the cranial nerves and other facial pain
13.1.1 ***Trigeminal neuralgia (TN)***
A disorder characterized by recurrent unilateral brief electric shock-like pains, abrupt in onset and termination, limited to the distribution(s) of one or more divisions of the trigeminal nerve and triggered by innocuous stimuli. Additionally, there may be concomitant continuous pain of moderate intensity within the same nerve distribution(s). TN may develop without apparent cause or be a result of another disorder.
13.12 ***Persistent idiopathic facial pain (PIFP)***
Persistent facial and/or oral pain, with varying presentations but recurring daily for >2 h/day over >3 months, in the absence of clinical neurological deficit. PIFP presents with high levels of psychiatric comorbidity and psychosocial disability and may be comorbid with other pain conditions such as chronic widespread pain and irritable bowel syndrome.

2.2.1 Migraine

At the societal level, migraine far outweighs all other headache disorders in its deleterious effect on health. It is second only to low back pain among all causes of disability [4, 5], responsible for almost half the financial cost of headache [6], and the principal progenitor of MOH, which is responsible for another third [6].

Migraine is the most recognized and best studied of the headache disorders [1]. It is a familial disorder, with a genetic component not yet fully understood. Its prevalence among adults varies worldwide, from 9.3% in China [7] to over 30% in Nepal [8] according to studies conducted with similar methods, and therefore comparable [9, 10]. The global mean is almost certainly higher than the current estimate of about 15% [5, 6]. The Global Burden of Disease study 2010 (GBD2010) ranked migraine as the third most prevalent disorder in the world [11]. Women are 1.5–3 times more likely to be affected than men [2] because of hormonal influences [1].

Migraine is an unpleasant illness. In the great majority of cases, it is a recurrent episodic disorder starting in childhood or adolescence (in girls, in particular, it may start at puberty) and in many cases lasting throughout life. Attack frequency is subject to lifestyle and environmental factors and varies widely between and within individuals, averaging once or twice a month. Headache and nausea (with or without vomiting) are the most characteristic attack features; photophobia and phonophobia are common and relatively specific symptoms [1]. The headache, lasting for hours to 2–3 days, is typically moderate or severe and likely to be unilateral, pulsating and aggravated by routine physical activity [1].

Migraine has two major types. *Migraine without aura* is a clinical syndrome characterized by these features, most of which are captured in the diagnostic criteria of ICHD [1] (Table 2.5). About 10% of migraine attacks overall are *migraine with aura*, experienced only by a third of people with migraine and distinguished by the transient focal neurological symptoms that usually precede but sometimes accompany the headache [1] (Table 2.5). Some people, with either type of migraine, also experience a prodromal phase, occurring hours or days before the headache, and/or

Table 2.5 ICHD-3 diagnostic criteria for migraine with and without aura [1]

1.1 ***Migraine without aura***	**1.2** ***Migraine with aura***
A. At least five attacks fulfilling criteria B–D B. Headache attacks lasting 4–72 h (when untreated)[1] C. Headache has at least two of the following four characteristics: 1. Unilateral location 2. Pulsating quality 3. Moderate or severe pain intensity 4. Aggravation by or causing avoidance of routine physical activity (e.g., walking or climbing stairs) D. During headache at least one of the following: 1. Nausea and/or vomiting 2. Photophobia and phonophobia E. Not better accounted for by another ICHD-3 diagnosis. *Note:* 1. In children and adolescents (aged under 18 years), attacks may last 2–72 h.	A. At least two attacks fulfilling criteria B and C B. One or more of the following fully reversible aura symptoms: 1. Visual 2. Sensory 3. Speech and/or language 4. Motor, brainstem and/or retinal[1] C. At least three of the following six characteristics: 1. At least one aura symptom spreads gradually over ≥5 min 2. Two or more aura symptoms occur in succession 3. Each individual aura symptom lasts 5–60 min 4. At least one aura symptom is unilateral[2] 5. At least one aura symptom is positive[3] 6. The aura is accompanied, or followed within 60 min, by headache[4] D. Not better accounted for by another ICHD-3 diagnosis. *Notes:* 1. Motor, brainstem and retinal symptoms are atypical, occurring in specific subtypes of migraine with aura, and should lead to referral. 2. Aphasia is regarded as a unilateral symptom. 3. Scintillations and pins and needles are positive symptoms of aura. 4. *Typical aura without headache* is a recognised subtype.

a postdromal phase following headache resolution. Common prodromal symptoms include fatigue, elated or depressed mood, unusual hunger and cravings for certain foods; postdromal symptoms include fatigue, elated or depressed mood and cognitive difficulties. Together, this array of symptoms, not surprisingly, are disabling: GBD2016 [4] and GBD2017 [5] ranked migraine as the second-highest cause of disability worldwide.

Between attacks, most people with either of these migraine types are completely well. However, for many, attacks tend to be unpredictable: they can start at any time, and some people are more prone to attacks than are others. So-called trigger factors play a part in this. While this calls for their avoidance as a sensible management tactic, avoidance itself, involving lifestyle compromise, can be a factor relevant to burden (Chap. 4).

A third type, *chronic migraine*, is specifically characterized by very frequent attacks and/or loss of episodicity. Headache occurs on 15 or more days per month, but not always with the features of migraine headache (for the diagnosis, these are required only on 8 or more days per month [1]). Chronic migraine is very highly disabling, but it still lacks a universally accepted definition. The criteria of ICHD-3

Table 2.6 ICHD-3 diagnostic criteria for chronic migraine [1]

1.3 *Chronic migraine*

A. Headache (migraine-like or tension-type-like[1]) on ≥15 days/month for >3 months, and fulfilling criteria B and C
B. Occurring in a patient who has had at least five attacks fulfilling criteria B–D for 1.1 *Migraine without aura* and/or criteria B and C for 1.2 *Migraine with aura*
C. On ≥8 days/month for >3 months, fulfilling any of the following:
   1. Criteria C and D for 1.1 *Migraine without aura*
   2. Criteria B and C for 1.2 *Migraine with aura*
   3. Believed by the patient to be migraine at onset and relieved by a triptan or ergot derivative
D. Not better accounted for by another ICHD-3 diagnosis[2].

Notes:

1. Because it is impossible to distinguish the individual episodes of headache in patients with such frequent or continuous headaches, attacks with and those without aura are both counted in diagnosing 1.3 *Chronic migraine*, as are both migraine-like and tension-type-like headaches.
2. The most common cause of symptoms suggestive of chronic migraine is medication overuse. Around 50% of patients apparently with chronic migraine revert to an episodic migraine type after drug withdrawal.

[1] (Table 2.6) may appear to be authoritative but are regularly modified by researchers and authors, so that the disorder is confusingly conflated with MOH (e.g., [12, 13]). Therefore, the prevalence of chronic migraine has not been reliably established. By the best working definition, it is rare [14], and, like cluster headache, not itself of great public-health importance.[2]

2.2.2 *Tension-Type Headache (TTH)*

TTH is the most prevalent of all the headache disorders, but highly variable in its expression and uncommonly a cause of serious disability. It has some societal importance, but much less than that of migraine.

TTH is the common sort of headache that nearly everyone has occasionally, so that many people refer to it as "normal" or "ordinary" headache, terms that deny its status as a headache disorder. While GBD2010 ranked it as the second most prevalent disorder in the world (behind dental caries) [10], its reported prevalence is nonetheless hugely variable [2]. This, probably, is due in most part to under-reporting of mild cases. The true prevalence probably exceeds 50% [2], but only when infrequent episodic TTH is included (less than 1 episode per month), which may indeed fall outside the definition of headache disorder [1]. In most but not all populations, TTH affects rather more women than men; children report it also, but to a lesser extent.

[2] As before, this means it does not add significantly to societal burden, not that no healthcare provision should be made for it. Headache services set up adequately to manage headache disorders (see Chap. 15) would take adequate account of it.

Table 2.7 ICHD-3 diagnostic criteria for the important types of tension-type headache [1]

2.2 *Frequent episodic tension-type headache*	2.3 *Chronic tension-type headache*
A. At least 10 episodes of headache occurring on 1–14 days/month on average for >3 months and fulfilling criteria B–D B. Lasting from 30 min to 7 days C. At least two of the following four characteristics: 1. Bilateral location 2. Pressing or tightening (non-pulsating) quality 3. Mild or moderate intensity 4. Not aggravated by routine physical activity such as walking or climbing stairs D. Both of the following: 1. No nausea or vomiting 2. No more than one of photophobia or phonophobia E. Not better accounted for by another ICHD-3 diagnosis.	A. Headache on ≥15 days/month on average for >3 months, fulfilling criteria B–D B. Lasting hours to days, or unremitting C. At least two of the following four characteristics: 1. Bilateral location 2. Pressing or tightening (non-pulsating) quality 3. Mild or moderate intensity 4. Not aggravated by routine physical activity such as walking or climbing stairs D. Both of the following: 1. No more than one of photophobia, phonophobia or mild nausea 2. Neither moderate or severe nausea nor vomiting E. Not better accounted for by another ICHD-3 diagnosis[1,2]. *Notes:* 1. Both 2.3 *Chronic TTH* and 1.3 *Chronic migraine* require headache on ≥15 days/month. For 2.3 *Chronic TTH*, headache must on ≥15 days meet criteria B–D above; for 1.3 *Chronic migraine*, headache must on ≥8 days meet criteria B–D for 1.1 *Migraine without aura*. A patient can fulfil criteria for both, for example, with headache on 25 days/month meeting migraine criteria on 8 days and TTH criteria on 17. Only 1.3 *Chronic migraine* is then diagnosed. 2. In many uncertain cases, there is overuse of medication. After withdrawal, there may be reversion to episodic TTH.

TTH episodes vary greatly in duration, from minutes to several days, but usually last a few hours. Their frequency also varies widely, both between people and in individual people over time. The pain of TTH lacks the specific characteristics of migraine, as is reflected in the diagnostic criteria of ICHD [1] (Table 2.7): it neither worsens with routine physical activity nor is associated with nausea (although either photophobia or phonophobia may be present). Further, it is usually bilateral or generalized; people describe it as a squeezing or pressure, like a tight band around the head—the opposites of descriptions of migraine headache. TTH often spreads down to or up from the neck. Although mostly moderate or mild, this headache can be bad enough to make it difficult to carry on entirely as normal [15].

TTH pursues a highly variable course, commonly beginning in the teenage years and reaching peak levels in the 30s. Although never serious, in a few people TTH becomes bothersome enough to need medical attention, usually because it has become frequent. There are distinct types although, in any individual, one may give way to another. Two are important (Table 2.7). Frequent episodic TTH occurs, like migraine, in attack-like episodes. Chronic TTH, which has a prevalence of up to 3% in adults [2], is a disorder evolving from frequent episodic TTH, with daily or very frequent episodes of similarly described headache, lasting hours to days and sometimes unremitting over long periods. This headache may be associated with mild nausea [1]. It can be quite disabling and distressing.

2.2.3 Medication-Overuse Headache (MOH)

MOH may top the list in terms of societal importance, not because it is the most prevalent headache disorder but for two other reasons: at individual level it is the most disabling and by far the most costly of the common headaches [6], and, unlike migraine and TTH, it is wholly avoidable.

ICHD defines MOH as a secondary headache [1], but it occurs only in patients with a prior headache disorder. The cause is chronic excessive use of medication(s) taken to treat that headache. MOH is therefore better considered as a *sequela* of a primary headache disorder, more usually migraine than TTH. This was recognized in GBD2016 [4], and again in GBD2017 [5], which, instead of reporting MOH separately, attributed its disability burden proportionately to these primary headaches (see Chap. 9).

All medications used to treat acute headache are associated with this problem, although the mechanism through which MOH develops undoubtedly varies between different drug classes. Wherever they are available, opioids such as codeine tend especially to be implicated, but this probably is a consequence of selection by patients who erroneously believe the solution lies in "stronger" medications, coupled with the exhortative messages by which codeine-containing medications are generally promoted to the public (Fig. 2.1). The risk of MOH escalates with medication frequency regardless of the drug, and is high whenever these treatments are taken regularly on more than 2–3 days a week. In individual patients, an evolutionary course can often be retrospectively charted: the usual start is that occasional headache attacks increase in frequency, through natural variation or because an additional headache has developed. Medication use follows, also becoming more frequent, and this is encouraged initially by its apparent efficacy. Over time, weeks or sometimes very much longer, as headache episodes and medication intake become ever more frequent, efficacy wanes. Natural responses then are to switch to medications perceived to be stronger, and to increase doses. While these behaviours lead inexorably to worsening in the long term, attempts at withdrawal induce

THERE ARE 8 MILLION MIGRAINE SUFFERERS IN THE UK.

Approximately **1 in 5 women and 1 in 15 men** will develop migraine at some time in their life, so it's really important that there's a migraine treatment you can trust.

Fig. 2.1 Promotional message, aimed at the public and typical of many, for a branded over-the-counter codeine-containing acute migraine therapy

Table 2.8 ICHD-3 diagnostic criteria for medication-overuse headache [1]

8.2 *Medication-overuse headache*
A. Headache occurring on ≥15 days/month in a patient with a pre-existing headache disorder
B. Regular overuse for >3 months of one or more drugs that can be taken for acute and/or symptomatic treatment of headache[1,2]
C. Not better accounted for by another ICHD-3 diagnosis.
Notes:
1. Drugs may be ergotamine, one or more triptans, non-opioid analgesics including paracetamol (acetaminophen), acetyl salicylic acid and other non-steroidal anti-inflammatory drugs (NSAIDs), opioids, combination analgesics (typically containing simple analgesics plus opioids, butalbital and/or caffeine) or any combination of these.
2. Overuse is defined as intake on ≥15 days/month for non-opioid analgesics alone and in all other cases as intake on ≥10 days/month.

immediate—and highly discouraging—aggravation of symptoms. In the end-stage, if this process is not interrupted, MOH is unremitting, only fluctuating with medication use repeated every few hours.

Correct diagnosis is important for these reasons, and more so because patients will not improve without withdrawal of the offending medication(s), which are often multiple. On the other hand, most patients with MOH improve within 2 months after withdrawal, as does their responsiveness to preventative treatment.

The ICHD diagnostic criteria [1] for MOH are in Table 2.8. It is an oppressive headache, obviously persistent, and highly disabling.

MOH has a highly variable prevalence worldwide, and estimates are uncertain [16]; while the average is 1.5–2% in adults [17], some national estimates exceed 7% with reasonable certainty [18, 19]. Factors contributing are high prevalences of the progenitor headaches (putting more people at risk) and, probably, easy access to OTC medications coupled with poor access to healthcare and lack of public health-education [18, 19].

2.3 Concluding Remarks

Although more than 200 headache disorders are clearly defined by their distinct characteristics and clinical features [1], and several of these disorders are described here, just three contribute significantly to the societal impact of headache. Migraine, TTH and MOH overwhelm all others in their shares of the total population ill health that is attributable to headache. Furthermore, MOH may properly be regarded as a *sequela* of migraine and TTH; its burdens in reality belong to these two primary headache disorders [4, 5].

It is essentially for these few conditions that society must make provision, if it wishes to lessen the impact. This fact makes the task (described in Chap. 15) a great deal easier.

References

1. Headache Classification Committee of the International Headache Society. The international classification of headache disorders, 3rd edition. Cephalalgia. 2018;38:1–211.
2. Stovner LJ, Hagen K, Jensen R, Katsarava Z, Lipton R, Scher A, Steiner TJ, Zwart JA. The global burden of headache: a documentation of headache prevalence and disability worldwide. Cephalalgia. 2007;27:193–210.
3. World Health Organization. *Lifting The Burden*. Atlas of headache disorders and resources in the world 2011. Geneva: WHO; 2011.
4. Vos T, Abajobir AA, Abate KH, Abbafati C, Abbas KM, Abd-Allah F, Abdulkader RS, Abdulle AM, Abebo TA, Abera SF, Aboyans V, Abu-Raddad LJ, Ackerman IN, Adamu AA, Adetokunboh O, Afarideh M, Afshin A, Agarwal SK, Aggarwal R, Agrawal A, Agrawal S, Ahmadieh H, Ahmed MB, Aichour MTE, Aichour AN, Aichour I, Aiyar S, Akinyemi RO, Akseer N, Al Lami FH, Alahdab F, Al-Aly Z, Alam K, Alam N, Alam T, et al. Global, regional, and national incidence, prevalence, and years lived with disability for 328 diseases and injuries for 195 countries, 1990–2016: a systematic analysis for the Global Burden of Disease Study 2016. Lancet. 2017;390:1211–59.
5. GBD 2017 Disease and Injury Incidence and Prevalence Collaborators. Global, regional, and national incidence, prevalence, and years lived with disability for 354 diseases and injuries for 195 countries and territories, 1990–2017: a systematic analysis for the Global Burden of Disease Study 2017. Lancet. 2018;392:1789–858.
6. Linde M, Gustavsson A, Stovner LJ, Steiner TJ, Barré J, Katsarava Z, Lainez JM, Lampl C, Lantéri-Minet M, Rastenyte D, Ruiz de la Torre E, Tassorelli C, Andrée C. The cost of headache disorders in Europe: the Eurolight project. Eur J Neurol. 2012;19:703–11.
7. Yu S, Liu R, Zhao G, Yang X, Qiao X, Feng J, Fang Y, Cao X, He M, Steiner T. The prevalence and burden of primary headaches in China: a population-based door-to-door survey. Headache. 2012;52:582–91.
8. Manandhar K, Risal A, Steiner TJ, Holen A, Linde M. The prevalence of primary headache disorders in Nepal: a nationwide population-based study. J Headache Pain. 2015;16:95.
9. Stovner LJ, Al Jumah M, Birbeck GL, Gururaj G, Jensen R, Katsarava Z, Queiroz LP, Scher AI, Tekle-Haimanot R, Wang SJ, Steiner TJ. The methodology of population surveys of headache prevalence, burden and cost: principles and recommendations from the global campaign against headache. J Headache Pain. 2014;15:5.
10. Steiner TJ, Gururaj G, Andrée C, Katsarava Z, Ayzenberg I, Yu SY, Al Jumah M, Tekle-Haimanot R, Birbeck GL, Herekar A, Linde M, Mbewe E, Manandhar K, Risal A, Jensen R, Queiroz LP, Scher AI, Wang SJ, Stovner LJ. Diagnosis, prevalence estimation and burden measurement in population surveys of headache: presenting the HARDSHIP questionnaire. J Headache Pain. 2014;15:3.
11. Vos T, Flaxman AD, Naghavi M, Lozano R, Michaud C, Ezzati M, Shibuya K, Salomon JA, Abdalla S, Aboyans V, Abraham J, Ackerman I, Aggarwal R, Ahn SY, Ali MK, Alvarado M, Anderson HR, Anderson LM, Andrews KG, Atkinson C, Baddour LM, Bahalim AN, Barker-Collo S, Barrero LH, Bartels DH, Basáñez MG, Baxter A, Bell ML, Benjamin EJ, Bennett D, Bernabé E, Bhalla K, Bhandari B, Bikbov B, Bin Abdulhak A, et al. Years lived with disability (YLD) for 1160 sequelae of 289 diseases and injuries 1990–2010: a systematic analysis for the Global Burden of Disease Study 2010. Lancet. 2012;380:2163–96.
12. Castillo J, Munoz P, Guitera V, Pascual J. Epidemiology of chronic daily headache in the general population. Headache. 1999;39:190–6.
13. Adams AM, Serrano D, Buse DC, Reed ML, Marske V, Fanning KM, Lipton RB. The impact of chronic migraine: The Chronic Migraine Epidemiology and Outcomes (CaMEO) Study methods and baseline results. Cephalalgia. 2015;35:563–78.
14. Natoli JL, Manack A, Dean B, Butler Q, Turkel CC, Stovner L, Lipton RB. Global prevalence of chronic migraine: a systematic review. Cephalalgia. 2012;30:599–609.

15. Steiner T, Lange R, Voelker M. Episodic tension-type headache (ETTH): evidence of prolonged disability from a placebo-controlled comparison of aspirin and paracetamol. Cephalalgia. 2003;23:630.
16. Steiner TJ. Can we know the prevalence of MOH? Cephalalgia. 2014;34:403–4.
17. Westergaard ML, Hansen EH, Glumer C, Olesen J, Jensen RH. Definitions of medication-overuse headache in population-based studies and their implications on prevalence estimates: a systematic review. Cephalalgia. 2014;34:409–25.
18. Ayzenberg I, Katsarava Z, Sborowski A, Chernysh M, Osipova V, Tabeeva G, Yakhno N, Steiner TJ. The prevalence of primary headache disorders in Russia: a countrywide survey. Cephalalgia. 2012;32:373–81.
19. Mbewe E, Zairemthiama P, Yeh H-H, Paul R, Birbeck GL, Steiner TJ. The epidemiology of primary headache disorders in Zambia: a population-based door-to-door survey. J Headache Pain. 2015;16:30.

Chapter 3
Headache in Children and Adolescents: A Broader Approach Is Needed than in Adults

Timothy J. Steiner and Derya Uluduz

3.1 Introduction

Chapter 2 explains the meaning of "headache" in the context of society. It concludes that, while more than 200 headache disorders are clearly defined by their distinct characteristics, just three—migraine, tension-type headache (TTH) and medication-overuse headache (MOH)—contribute significantly to the societal impact of headache. In the Global Burden of Disease study 2010 (GBD2010) [1], TTH and migraine were revealed as second and third most prevalent disorders in the world. In GBD2013, headache disorders collectively were third among the leading causes of disability [2]. In GBD2016, migraine came top—the single most disabling disorder—in the age group 15–49 years [3].

It is a very important proviso that the data underpinning these statistics were derived in the main from studies in adults aged 18–65 years ([4]; also Chap. 9). Extrapolations to children (6–11 years) and adolescents (12–17 years) in the GBD studies put migraine among the top 10 global causes of years lived with disability (YLDs) in the 50 most populous countries [5]. Nevertheless, in these age groups, the prevalence of headache disorders is not so well established, from relatively limited data. Accordingly, the burdens attributed to them are only unreliably estimated.

There is no complete explanation for this, but multiple contributory factors can be identified. With regard to the paucity of data, first there are relatively few published epidemiological studies among these age groups ([4]; also Chap. 8)

T. J. Steiner (✉)
Department of Neuromedicine and Movement Science, NTNU Norwegian University of Science and Technology, Trondheim, Norway

Division of Brain Sciences, Imperial College London, London, UK
e-mail: t.steiner@imperial.ac.uk

D. Uluduz
Neurology Department, Cerrahpaşa School of Medicine, Istanbul University, Istanbul, Turkey

T. J. Steiner, L. J. Stovner (eds.), *Societal Impact of Headache*, Headache,
https://doi.org/10.1007/978-3-030-24728-7_3

(which itself lacks a good explanation). Second, most of these have been conducted in middle- or high-income Western countries, leaving very large geographical gaps. This was true of adult studies also, until relatively recently [4]. Third, substantial methodological differences between the published studies limit their comparability. Apart from these is a fourth factor, with perhaps the most important implications for addressing this issue: it arises from the operational diagnostic criteria set out in the universally accepted International Classification of Headache Disorders (ICHD), now in its third edition (ICHD-3) [6].

3.1.1 Is Headache in These Age Groups Different?

This key question cannot be answered only with regard to *prevalence*. Primary headaches may be less common in children [4] but, with an incidence peak around puberty, they catch up in adolescents. Are they different in *character*?

As noted in Chap. 2, while ICHD recognizes more than 200 headache disorders [6], only migraine and TTH among the primary headaches have public-health importance [1–4]. The ICHD diagnostic criteria for migraine in *adults* specify recurrent, moderate-to-severe headache of 4–72 h duration, together with a range of specific characteristics (unilaterality, pulsating quality, aggravation by physical activity) and accompanying symptoms (photophobia *and* phonophobia; nausea and/or vomiting) ([6]; also Chap. 2). In *children*, it is noted that the headache may be of shorter duration (2–72 h). The criteria for TTH specify mild-to-moderate headache lasting from 30 min to 7 days, with neither the specific characteristics nor the accompanying symptoms of migraine [6]. But in a pilot school-based prevalence survey conducted in Turkey and Austria, mild headache of less than 1 h duration, often with migraine-like features, was reported by more than a third (37.2%) of participants aged 6–17 years [7].

Such headache could not be given a definite diagnosis of migraine or, when there were migraine-like features, of TTH. Furthermore, although ICHD criteria for TTH allow a duration lower-limit of 30 min, the authors of this study later questioned whether TTH really existed in a form in which headache was *typically* (rather than occasionally) of less than 1 h duration [8]. In the context of their continuing epidemiological studies in Turkey, undertaken as a project within the Global Campaign against Headache, they found themselves in doubt as to how this evidently common presentation of headache should be labelled [8].

3.2 Undifferentiated Headache

The problem was not new: it had been recognized previously, but, surprisingly, apparently ignored. The most recent survey of headache in children and adolescents [9], together with a Medline search, found 59 relevant studies. Over half (54%)

reported selected diagnoses only, usually definite migraine, crucially failing to specify the proportions of headaches that were unclassifiable. But in five studies that did report them [10–14], unclassifiable headaches ranged in prevalence from 2.9% to 35.5% (mean 18.3%) [8]—almost one in five participants!

An adequate account of the burden of headache in these age groups clearly requires a broader approach than ICHD allows. The characteristics of adult migraine (and perhaps TTH) may be undeveloped in 6–17-year-olds. An additional diagnostic category is needed, which has been termed *undifferentiated headache* (UdH), defined by duration of less than 1 h and mild intensity [8].

3.2.1 Clinical Features of UdH

The survey in Turkey referred to above was a nationwide cross-sectional study, school-based, with data gathered in 31 schools [8]. Conducted under the auspices of the Global Campaign against Headache [15, 16], it applied the methods developed and tested in the earlier pilot studies in Istanbul and Vienna [7]. It compared the clinical features of UdH with those of migraine and TTH, and the burdens attributable to each [8]. Of the 7889 invited pupils, 7068 (89.6%) self-completed a structured questionnaire [17] administered by a mediator to entire classes [8]. The following evidence emerged.

First and foremost, UdH is common. Headache of any type during the preceding year was reported by 73.7% of participants. UdH, reported by 29.2%, led all other types: migraine 26.7% (7.3% definite, 19.4% probable), TTH 12.9% (definite 6.7%, probable 6.2%), MOH 0.9% (always probable, because no evidence could be gathered of causation), other headaches on 15 or more days per month 3.4% and still unclassifiable headache 0.5% [8]. Sub-classified according to frequency in the same manner as TTH [6], 26.7% of cases were infrequent episodic UdH, 72.0% were frequent episodic UdH and 1.3% were chronic UdH [8].

Comparisons with migraine and TTH, combining definite and probable cases as recommended [18], showed that UdH differed from both with respect to almost all headache features and associated symptoms, generally falling between the two (Table 3.1) [8]. UdH was less likely to be pulsating than migraine, but more than TTH. It was less associated with nausea, vomiting and photophobia than migraine, but, for all of these, more than TTH. Headache days were fewer in UdH than in migraine or TTH; accordingly, UdH was less likely to be reported on the preceding day ("headache yesterday") (Table 3.2) [8]. Intensity of headache yesterday was lower in UdH, but, of course, UdH is defined by mild intensity. Nonetheless, 16.3% of pupils with the diagnosis of UdH rated headache yesterday as moderate or severe (Table 3.2) [8]. Although pupils with UdH took acute medication less frequently than those with migraine or TTH, large proportions nonetheless did so: 38.9% in the previous week and 43.2% in the previous 4 weeks.

Table 3.1 Headache features in undifferentiated headache, migraine and tension-type headache [9]

	Undifferentiated headache (N = 2066)		Migraine[a] (N = 1888)		Tension-type headache[a] (N = 911)		Undifferentiated headache vs. migraine[a]		Undifferentiated headache vs. tension-type headache[a]	
	n	%	n	%	n	%	OR [95% CI]	p[b]	OR [95% CI]	p[b]
Headache in previous week	2036		1864		899					
No	949	46.6	417	22.4	322	35.8	Reference		Reference	
≥1 day	1087	53.4	1447	77.6	577	64.2	0.33 [0.29–0.38]	<0.001	0.64 [0.54–0.75]	<0.001
Headache in previous 4 weeks	2050		1880		898					
No	548	26.7	207	11.0	161	17.9	Reference		Reference	
≥1 day	1502	73.3	1673	89.0	737	82.1	0.34 [0.29–0.40]	<0.001	0.60 [0.49–0.73]	<0.001
Quality	2044		1885		908					
Pulsating	1437	70.3	1478	78.4	555	61.1	Reference		Reference	
Pressing	607	29.7	407	21.6	353	38.9	1.5 [1.3–1.8]	<0.001	0.66 [0.56–0.78]	<0.001
Localization	2048		1887		906					
Unilateral	645	31.5	463	24.5	158	17.4	0.90 [0.76–1.07]	NS	1.7 [1.4–2.1]	<0.001
Middle	652	31.8	421	22.3	269	29.7	Reference		Reference	
Bilateral	751	36.7	1003	53.2	479	52.9	0.48 [0.41–0.56]	<0.001	0.65 [0.54–0.78]	<0.001
Aggravation by physical activity	2059		1886		910					
No	1356	65.9	596	31.6	509	55.9	Reference		Reference	
Yes	703	34.1	1290	68.4	401	44.1	0.24 [0.21–0.27]	<0.001	0.66 [0.56–0.77]	<0.001
Avoidance of physical activity	2060		1888		911					
No	1009	49.0	319	16.9	408	44.8	Reference		Reference	
Yes	1051	51.0	1569	83.1	503	55.2	0.21 [0.18–0.25]	<0.001	0.85 [0.72–0.99]	0.04

Nausea	2053		1887		909					
No	1381	67.3	578	30.6	751	82.6	Reference		Reference	
Yes	672	32.7	1309	69.4	158	17.4	0.22 [0.19–0.25]	<0.001	2.3 [1.9–2.8]	<0.001
Vomiting	2054		1887		902					
No	1842	89.7	1364	72.3	845	93.7	Reference		Reference	
Yes	212	10.3	523	27.7	57	6.3	0.30 [0.25–0.36]	<0.001	1.7 [1.3–2.3]	<0.001
Photophobia	2058		1883		908					
No	1385	67.3	622	33.0	752	82.8	Reference		Reference	
Yes	673	32.7	1261	67.0	156	17.2	0.24 [0.21–0.24]	<0.001	2.3 [1.9–2.9]	<0.001
Phonophobia	2062		1887		909					
No	257	12.5	72	3.8	125	13.8	Reference		Reference	
Yes	1805	87.5	1815	96.2	784	86.2	0.28 [0.21–0.37]	<0.001	1.1 [0.89–1.4]	0.3

[a]Including definite and probable
[b]Chi-squared test

Table 3.2 Headache yesterday in undifferentiated headache, migraine and tension-type headache [8]

Headache yesterday	Undifferentiated headache N = 2066		Migraine[a] N = 1888		Tension-type headache[a] N = 911		Undifferentiated headache vs. migraine[a]		Undifferentiated headache vs. tension-type headache[a]	
	n	%	*n*	%	*n*	%	OR [95% CI]	*p*[b]	OR [95% CI]	*p*[b]
Present	2027		1872		895					
No	1624	80.1	1053	56.3	645	72.1	Reference			
Yes	403	19.9	819	43.7	250	29.9	0.32 [0.28–0.37]	<0.001	0.64 [0.56–0.77]	<0.001
Intensity	403		819		250					
Mild	328	83.7	408	50.6	151	62.7	3.9 [2.8–5.4]	<0.001	2.8 [1.9–4.2]	<0.001
Moderate	55	14.0	265	32.9	72	29.9	Reference		Reference	
Severe	9	2.3	133	1.5	18	7.4	0.33 [0.16–0.68]	0.002	0.66 [0.27–1.6]	0.3
Lost lessons at school	403		819		250					
No	360	90.2	693	87.3	217	89.7	Reference		Reference	
Yes	39	9.8	101	12.7	25	10.3	0.74 [0.50–1.1]	0.1	0.94 [0.55–1.6]	0.8

[a]Including definite and probable
[b]Chi-squared test

3.2.2 *Burden of UdH*

As a short-duration mild headache, UdH might not be the most burdensome headache, but one fifth (21.3%) of those with UdH in the survey (6.1% of all pupils) lost school time in the preceding 4 weeks because of it (Table 3.3) [8]. Impact on school attendance and leisure-time activities was lower in UdH than in migraine or TTH, and UdH was less likely than migraine, but not TTH, to cause a parent to leave work [8]. Table 3.3 shows, very clearly, that these were burdens that ought not to have been ignored simply because the headache had no label.

3.2.3 *Implications of UdH*

Longitudinal studies suggest that a considerable proportion (8.3–71%) of children and adolescents with migraine evolve to TTH or vice versa [19], with, as might be expected, higher diagnostic stability in definite migraine and definite TTH than in probable migraine or probable TTH [20]. This supports the concept of *undifferentiated* headache, and the use of this diagnostic label as an appropriate term among these age groups.

The implications are quite far reaching. ICHD, of course, needs to take note of this diagnostic gap. More pertinent here are the implications for future epidemiological studies and burden estimates in these age groups—indeed, for accounts of the societal impact of headache generally. While children and adolescents make up

Table 3.3 Burden of undifferentiated headache, migraine and tension-type headache (preceding 4 weeks) [9]

Burden measure	Undifferentiated headache N = 2066		Migraine[a] N = 1888		Tension-type headache[a] N = 911		Undifferentiated headache vs. migraine[a]		Undifferentiated headache vs. tension-type headache[a]	
	n	%	*n*	%	*n*	%	OR [95% CI]	*p*[b]	OR [95% CI]	*p*[b]
School absence	2046		1866		900					
No	1792	87.6	1439	76.2	753	83.7	Reference		Reference	
≥1 day	254	12.4	427	23.8	147	16.3	0.48 [0.40–0.57]	<0.001	0.73 [0.59–0.91]	0.004
School left early	1997		1818		884					
No	1819	91.1	1479	81.4	766	86.7	Reference		Reference	
≥1 day	177	8.9	339	18.6	118	13.3	0.43 [0.35–0.52]	<0.001	0.64 [0.50–0.81]	<0.001
Impact on activity	2015		1800		887					
No	1261	62.6	582	32.3	459	51.7	Reference		Reference	
≥1 day	754	37.4	1218	67.7	428	48.3	0.29 [0.25–0.33]	<0.001	0.64 [0.55–0.75]	<0.001
Parent took work leave	2044		1880		902					
No	1906	93.2	1607	85.5	832	92.2	Reference		Reference	
≥1 day	138	6.8	273	14.5	70	7.8	0.43 [0.34–0.53]	<0.001	0.86 [0.64–1.2]	0.3

[a]Including definite and probable
[b]Chi-squared test

a large proportion of the population, UdH, their most common headache, appears not to have been in the reckoning. Most previously published surveys would not have reported these cases; burden estimates, if made, would have taken no account of them. There are clinical implications too, also with a societal dimension, if UdH, while clearly distinct from migraine, is in fact a precursor or immature form of it. Can its evolution be halted, or will it inevitably transform into the highly burdensome disorder that is migraine?

3.3 Concluding Remarks

Headache-attributed burden is not well estimated among children and adolescents, but undoubtedly high. GBD estimates fill the large data gaps by extrapolation, putting migraine among the top 10 global causes of YLDs in the 50 most populous countries [5]. Undifferentiated headache, characterized by mild headaches lasting less than 1 h, differing measurably in most respects from both migraine and TTH, and defying labelling within ICHD, has not been included. It is common in both age groups and associated with burden sufficient to cause lost school time in over 6% of pupils. Accounts of headache in these age groups have been seriously deficient on this account.

Future longitudinal studies will show whether UdH represents those headaches that are in a shifting state between migraine and TTH before maturing by adulthood into one or the other. Meanwhile, differentiating UdH from migraine and TTH has important implications for needs assessment, health policy and healthcare provision. The first and most important need is to recognize its existence.

References

1. Vos T, Flaxman AD, Naghavi M, Lozano R, Michaud C, Ezzati M, Shibuya K, Salomon JA, Abdalla S, Aboyans V, Abraham J, Ackerman I, Aggarwal R, Ahn SY, Ali MK, Alvarado M, Anderson HR, Anderson LM, Andrews KG, Atkinson C, Baddour LM, Bahalim AN, Barker-Collo S, Barrero LH, Bartels DH, Basáñez MG, Baxter A, Bell ML, Benjamin EJ, Bennett D, Bernabé E, Bhalla K, Bhandari B, Bikbov B, Bin Abdulhak A, et al. Years lived with disability (YLD) for 1160 sequelae of 289 diseases and injuries 1990–2010: a systematic analysis for the Global Burden of Disease Study 2010. Lancet. 2012;380:2163–96.
2. Vos T, Barber RM, Bell B, Bertozzi-Villa A, Biryukov S, Bolliger I, Charlson F, Davis A, Degenhardt L, Dicker D, Duan L, Erskine H, Feigin VL, Ferrari AJ, Fitzmaurice C, Fleming T, Graetz N, Guinovart C, Haagsma J, Hansen GM, Hanson SW, Heuton KR, Higashi H, Kassebaum N, Kyu H, Laurie E, Liang X, Lofgren K, Lozano R, MacIntyre MF, Moradi-Lakeh M, Naghavi M, Nguyen G, Odell S, Ortblad K, et al. Global, regional, and national incidence, prevalence, and years lived with disability for 301 acute and chronic diseases and injuries in 188 countries, 1990–2013: a systematic analysis for the Global Burden of Disease Study 2013. Lancet. 2015;386:743–800.
3. Vos T, Abajobir AA, Abate KH, Abbafati C, Abbas KM, Abd-Allah F, Abdulkader RS, Abdulle AM, Abebo TA, Abera SF, Aboyans V, Abu-Raddad LJ, Ackerman IN, Adamu AA, Adetokunboh O, Afarideh M, Afshin A, Agarwal SK, Aggarwal R, Agrawal A, Agrawal S, Ahmadieh H, Ahmed MB, Aichour MTE, Aichour AN, Aichour I, Aiyar S, Akinyemi RO, Akseer N, Al Lami FH, Alahdab F, Al-Aly Z, Alam K, Alam N, Alam T, et al. Global, regional, and national incidence, prevalence, and years lived with disability for 328 diseases and injuries for 195 countries, 1990–2016: a systematic analysis for the Global Burden of Disease Study 2016. Lancet. 2017;390:1211–59.
4. Stovner LJ, Hagen K, Jensen R, Katsarava Z, Lipton R, Scher A, Steiner TJ, Zwart JA. The global burden of headache: a documentation of headache prevalence and disability worldwide. Cephalalgia. 2007;27:193–210.
5. Kyu HH, Pinho C, Wagner JA, Brown JC, Bertozzi-Villa A, Charlson FJ, Coffeng LE, Dandona L, Erskine HE, Ferrari AJ, Fitzmaurice C, Fleming TD, Forouzanfar MH, Graetz N, Guinovart C, Haagsma J, Higashi H, Kassebaum NJ, Larson HJ, Lim SS, Mokdad AH, Moradi-Lakeh M, Odell SV, Roth GA, Serina PT, Stanaway JD, Misganaw A, Whiteford HA, Wolock TM, Wulf Hanson S, Abd-Allah F, Abera SF, Abu-Raddad LJ, AlBuhairan FS, Amare AT, et al. Global and national burden of diseases and injuries among children and adolescents between 1990 and 2013: findings from the Global Burden of Disease 2013 Study. JAMA Pediatr. 2016;170:267–87.

6. Headache Classification Committee of the International Headache Society. The international classification of headache disorders, 3rd edition. Cephalalgia. 2018;38:1–211.
7. Wöber-Bingöl C, Wöber C, Uluduz D, Uygunoğlu U, Aslan TS, Kernmayer M, Zesch H-E, Gerges NTA, Wagner G, Siva A, Steiner TJ. The global burden of headache in children and adolescent—developing a questionnaire and methodology for a global study. J Headache Pain. 2014;15:86.
8. Wöber C, Wöber-Bingöl C, Uluduz D, Aslan TS, Uygunoglu U, Tüfekçi A, Alp SI, Duman T, Sürgün F, Emir GK, Demir CF, Balgetir F, Özdemir YB, Auer T, Siva A, Steiner TJ. Undifferentiated headache: broadening the approach to headache in children and adolescents, with supporting evidence from a nationwide school-based cross-sectional survey in Turkey. J Headache Pain. 2018;19:18.
9. Wöber-Bingöl Ç. Epidemiology of migraine and headache in children and adolescents. Curr Pain Headache Rep. 2013;17:341.
10. Krogh AB, Larsson B, Linde M. Prevalence and disability of headache among Norwegian adolescents: a cross-sectional school-based study. Cephalalgia. 2015;35:1181–91.
11. Chong SC, Chan YH, Ong HT, Low PS, Tay SK. Headache diagnosis, disability and co-morbidities in a multi-ethnic, heterogeneous paediatric Asian population. Cephalalgia. 2010;30:953–61.
12. Heinrich M, Morris L, Kröner-Herwig B. Self-report of headache in children and adolescents in Germany: possibilities and confines of questionnaire data for headache classification. Cephalalgia. 2009;29:864–72.
13. Kong CK, Cheng WW, Wong LY. Epidemiology of headache in Hong Kong primary-level schoolchildren: questionnaire study. Hong Kong Med J. 2001;7:29–33.
14. Rho YI, Chung HJ, Lee KH, Eun BL, Eun SH, Nam SO, Kim WS, Kim YO, Park HJ, Kim HS. Prevalence and clinical characteristics of primary headaches among school children in South Korea: a nationwide survey. Headache. 2012;52:592–9.
15. Steiner TJ. *Lifting The Burden*: the global campaign against headache. Lancet Neurol. 2004;3:204–5.
16. Steiner TJ. *Lifting The Burden*: the global campaign to reduce the burden of headache worldwide. J Headache Pain. 2005;6:373–7.
17. Steiner TJ, Gururaj G, Andrée C, Katsarava Z, Ayzenberg I, Yu SY, Al Jumah M, Tekle-Haimanot R, Birbeck GL, Herekar A, Linde M, Mbewe E, Manandhar K, Risal A, Jensen R, Queiroz LP, Scher AI, Wang SJ, Stovner LJ. Diagnosis, prevalence estimation and burden measurement in population surveys of headache: presenting the HARDSHIP questionnaire. J Headache Pain. 2014;15:3.
18. Stovner LJ, Al Jumah M, Birbeck GL, Gururaj G, Jensen R, Katsarava Z, Queiroz LP, Scher AI, Tekle-Haimanot R, Wang SJ, Steiner TJ. The methodology of population surveys of headache prevalence, burden and cost: principles and recommendations from the global campaign against headache. J Headache Pain. 2014;15:5.
19. Antonaci F, Voiticovschi-Iosob C, Di Stefano AL, Galli F, Özge A, Balottin U. The evolution of headache from childhood to adulthood: a review of the literature. J Headache Pain. 2014;15:15.
20. Albers L, Straube A, Landgraf MN, Heinen F, von Kries R. High diagnostic stability of confirmed migraine and confirmed tension-type headache according to the ICHD-3 beta in adolescents. J Headache Pain. 2014;15:36.

Chapter 4
Headache-Attributed Burden: Its Qualitative Components

Timothy J. Steiner and Lars Jacob Stovner

4.1 Introduction

"Burden of disease" at a population level is the sum of all the negative effects a disease has on the individuals within that population, together with any societal burden. It is a complex construct.

When the Global Burden of Disease (GBD) studies measure "burden", they value health states associated with the included diseases by attaching to each a *disability weight* (DW), derived through a global consultation exercise from a brief description of the "average" condition ([1]; also Chap. 9). The product of DW and time in that health state provides an estimate of lost health, which slightly confusingly is referred to as *disability* and quantified in *years lived with disability* (YLDs). A complete account adds *years of life lost* (YLLs) due to early mortality, when this occurs. YLLs and YLDs have equal value, each representing the equivalent of 1 year's total loss of health. Their sum yields the composite metric, *disability-adjusted life years* (DALYs) ([1]; also Chap. 9).

People with primary headache disorders do not die. Or, more correctly, they are no more likely to die than people without headache. The burden of headache is expressed "only" in the impairments of pain and associated symptoms, the disability

T. J. Steiner (✉)
Department of Neuromedicine and Movement Science, NTNU Norwegian University of Science and Technology, Trondheim, Norway

Division of Brain Sciences, Imperial College London, London, UK
e-mail: t.steiner@imperial.ac.uk

L. J. Stovner
Department of Neuromedicine and Movement Science, NTNU Norwegian University of Science and Technology, Trondheim, Norway

Norwegian Advisory Unit on Headaches, Department of Neurology and Clinical Neurophysiology, St Olavs University Hospital, Trondheim, Norway
e-mail: lars.stovner@ntnu.no

T. J. Steiner, L. J. Stovner (eds.), *Societal Impact of Headache*, Headache,
https://doi.org/10.1007/978-3-030-24728-7_4

and lost productivity these cause, and the diminished quality of life and reduced wellbeing that result. In GBD, it is expressed only in YLDs. As will be seen, the sum of these may be substantial at individual level, while it is very large indeed at population (societal) level. But the fact that no mortality is associated with the common headache disorders probably explains to a large extent why, historically, they have been so poorly acknowledged [2–4].

This chapter provides a qualitative account of the many elements of headache-attributed burden. A quantitative account is in Chap. 8.

4.2 The Burden of Headache: Scope and Scale

As noted in Chap. 2, only migraine, tension-type headache [TTH] and medication-overuse headache [MOH] contribute significantly to the public-health impact of headache disorders. Even so, little was known of this impact until quite recently. It was not known how, or how much, they affected many of the populations of the world, or how healthcare and other resources were utilized to mitigate their effects. The global survey conducted jointly by *Lifting The Burden* (LTB) and the World Health Organization (WHO) for the *Atlas of Headache Disorders and Resources in the World 2011* ([2]; also, Chaps. 5 and 13) was the first to enquire into these matters, finding "worldwide neglect of major causes of public ill-health".

Clearly evident now, through a concerted programme of information gathering [5–13], is that "burden of disease" in relation to headache is very substantial in scale. It also has a very broad scope, composed of many different elements, with impact extending beyond those who actually have the disease. These are described below.

4.2.1 Burdens Within the Attack

Symptom burden is readily recognizable: pain especially, but also the accompanying symptoms of nausea, vomiting, photophobia and phonophobia, which while present cause debility, sometimes to the extent of prostration. Pain can be quantified at individual level as a product of frequency, duration and intensity, although the last of these is purely subjective. At population level, it is quantified as the product of the average among individuals and prevalence [14]. Nausea, photophobia and phonophobia are almost impossible to quantify, not only because they are subjective but also because there are no units or yardsticks by which to measure them. Their occurrence can at least be recorded, and frequencies expressed.

Above all, headache disorders are disabling [15–18]. Each of the symptoms mentioned may contribute to a secondary *disability burden* within the attack. "Disability" here means limited ability to engage in certain tasks or actions, or to participate in usual daily activities, its correct sense rather than that used in GBD

[1]. Disability attributed to headache is also difficult to quantify completely, but lost productive time is a common proxy for which well-validated instruments exist [19, 20]. Inability to work because of headache, and reduced effectiveness when work is continued despite headache, have magnified importance because headache is most common in people between their teens and 50–60 years of age—the productive years, during which people build families, careers and the capital on which their later lives will depend. To the *lost-productivity burden* is attached a *personal financial burden* from lost pay.

These are all elements of *ictal burden*.

4.2.2 Burdens Beyond the Attack

All the components of ictal burden are readily appreciated. Other burdens, less obvious, are still important [14].

Direct treatment costs supplement the indirect financial costs from lost productivity. Consultations with physicians occupy time, and all lost time has a cost. So do medications. These expenditures, part of the *personal financial burden*, are generally incurred outside attacks, as investments to prevent or mitigate ictal burden. In theory they are cost-saving, but empirical evidence of this is lacking (Chap. 15).

Apart from this, because headache attacks are unpleasant, simple awareness that they will recur, and the expectation that results, are often sufficient to diminish quality of life. It cannot be surprising if people who experience them frequently worry about when the next may occur, and there is good evidence that they do [21]. Neither can it be surprising if this provokes anxiety, and avoidance behaviour, for which again there is good evidence [21]. People with migraine in particular may, rightly or wrongly, identify triggers that they then endeavour to eliminate by lifestyle compromise, not always in ways that they would otherwise wish. Leisure activities may be cancelled or curtailed because of headache; when this has happened often, social events are likely not to be planned in the first place. Social life may simply cease. These are elements of *interictal burden*.

The huge importance of interictal burden lies in the fact that it is *continuous*, rather than present only during attacks that occur perhaps on only one or a few days per month. Interictal burden affects wellbeing and quality of life and is perhaps adequately, if not specifically, quantified by measures of these [14]. Few quantitative studies exist, but the Eurolight project conducted in ten countries of the EU established that interictal burden is considerable [21].

A consequence of recurring inability to work may be a reputation for poor reliability, or inability to cope. Decreased probability of promotion follows, with failure to develop full career potential; in egregious cases, early retirement may be a forced result of persistent ill health. A consequence of lost school-time, negatively affecting education, may be reduced career opportunities later. In both cases, the result is lower pay and impaired financial security. Accruing over a lifetime, the *cumulative burden* of these losses can be substantial, albeit very hard to measure [14].

4.2.3 Burdens Beyond the Person with Headache

People with headache bear much of these burdens, but not all. *Burden on others* who are themselves unaffected by headache is invariably difficult to measure and coloured by subjective interpretation, but it unquestionably exists, arising in several ways.

Failed or abdicated social roles during attacks affect partnership and parenthood. Family and friends lose the companionship they reasonably expect, but which is not given by a person shut away in a dark room. Children may not always be looked after. Partners and other family members may inherit increased shares of chores and responsibilities. They may acquire a *carer burden*, called to look after the person with headache. Carers, as well as the person with headache, can lose time from work.

Similarly, employers and work colleagues carry part of the burden of headache when paid work is not done. Either the employer pays for nothing, or colleagues must take on extra duties to make up.

4.2.4 Societal Burdens

Healthcare resource consumption must be paid for by someone. Often, at least in part, this is the person with headache, but, when treatment costs for a group of conditions affecting up to 40% of the population are reimbursed by a State-funded health system, the *direct societal financial burden* is likely to be substantial. Nevertheless, as a contributor to societal burden, these costs are dwarfed, ten-fold, by the *indirect societal financial burden* that falls on national economies from absenteeism, reduced effectiveness at work (presenteeism) and lost gross domestic product (GDP) [22, 23]. The financial cost of headache is the subject of Chap. 12.

It is worth a comment that financial costs to society may not be so dominant in resource-poor countries where labour costs are lower, but the consequences to individuals of being unable to work or care for children can nevertheless be severe, and they are particularly unforgiving in resource-poor countries [14].

4.3 Burden of Headache in GBD

This is the subject of Chap. 9. This present chapter is about the qualitative components of headache-attributed burden, while GBD is essentially concerned with measurement. It is mentioned here only with the purpose of noting its limitations, despite which headache disorders are ranked second among all causes of YLDs [12, 13].

The scope of GBD is heroic [1], and there are no better means than are offered by GBD for comparing diseases according to their impact on health. For headache disorders, population estimates are arrived at by multiplying prevalence, mean proportion of time in the ictal state (i.e., with headache) and the DW for the ictal state. The limitations are obvious. GBD cannot and does not take account of the less tangible components of burden, it takes little if any note of interictal burden, and it ignores cumulative burden.

It is also absolutely dependent on data. The first iteration, GBD1990, conducted by WHO on behalf of the World Bank, found nothing to say about headache. The first International Classification of Headache Disorders had only recently been published [24], and epidemiological studies prior to this lacked diagnostic validity. Even at the time of GBD2000, and still in 2007, the published data included no studies of acceptable quality from Eastern Europe, the entire Eastern Mediterranean Region, most of the African Region, all of South-East Asia and most of the Western Pacific Region [19]. In these parts of the world were living more than half the people of the world.

GBD2010, commencing in 2007 and accepting data until 2010, was conducted not by WHO but by the Institute for Health Metrics and Evaluation, Seattle, Washington, supported by the Bill and Melinda Gates Foundation [1]. During these years, the Global Campaign against Headache was filling in the major knowledge gaps with new population-based studies, beginning in Russia, China and India, countries occupied by 2.6 billion people [4–6]. With better data, the estimated global mean 1-year prevalence of migraine rose from 11.2% [25] to 14.7% [8, 9]. GBD2010 reported TTH as the second most prevalent disorder in the world (after dental caries), and migraine third [8, 9], but despite this, and because of a very low DW, TTH had little impact compared with that of migraine on estimated global disability burden. MOH was not included until the next iteration, GBD2013 [10, 11]. In the interim, further Global Campaign studies had filled other knowledge gaps. By GBD2016 [12], these studies included India and Nepal in South East Asia, Saudi Arabia, Pakistan and Morocco in Eastern Mediterranean, Zambia and Ethiopia in African Region, China and Mongolia in Western Pacific and Russia, Georgia and Lithuania in Eastern Europe. Considerably better informed than their predecessors, GBD2016 [12] and GBD2017, the most recently published [13], both ranked migraine as the second-highest cause of disability worldwide.

4.4 The Burden of Insouciance

Of course, headache has not grown in these 27 years of the GBD programme so far. Rather, the evidence has greatly improved, is now fully assimilated and is given due weight by GBD. Sadly, this is not the case more generally: headache as a cause of ill health is still poorly acknowledged [2–4].

These various burdens, arising from a set of disorders that are very common, inevitably generate a large healthcare demand: even decades ago, headache was noted to be high among causes of consulting both general practitioners and neurologists [26, 27]. They might also be expected to engender a robust healthcare response, but this is emphatically not the case. Very large numbers of people who need it do not receive effective healthcare for headache [2, 28]. Direct evidence shows this to be so in developed countries [29–33], and it cannot be anticipated that people with headache fare any better in countries where resources are more limited [34].

Poor healthcare for headache is a feature of society's insouciance (about which more is said in Chap. 13): despite all the evidence of its impact, manifested in public ill health and disability, lost production and financial cost, society disdains headache and fails abjectly to respond to it [2]. People with headache, not unreasonably, feel this as an additional burden.

4.5 Concluding Remarks

The burden of headache is complex in scope and substantial in scale, and composed of many different elements, some not quantifiable but amenable only to qualitative (descriptive) analysis. Its impact extends to people not directly affected, and to society as a whole. The GBD studies may rank headache among the top causes of disability, but they do not capture its burden in full.

References

1. Institute for Health Metrics and Evaluation. About GBD. http://www.healthdata.org/gbd/about.
2. World Health Organization, *Lifting The Burden*. Atlas of headache disorders and resources in the world 2011. Geneva: WHO; 2011.
3. Steiner TJ. Headache in the world: public health and research priorities. Expert Rev Pharmacoecon Outcomes Res. 2013;13:51–7.
4. Katsarava Z, Steiner TJ. Neglected headache: ignorance, arrogance or insouciance? Cephalalgia. 2012;32:1019–20.
5. Steiner TJ. *Lifting The Burden*: the global campaign against headache. Lancet Neurol. 2004;3:204–5.
6. Steiner TJ. *Lifting The Burden*: the global campaign to reduce the burden of headache worldwide. J Headache Pain. 2005;6:373–7.
7. Steiner TJ, Birbeck GL, Jensen R, Katsarava Z, Martelletti P, Stovner LJ. *Lifting The Burden*: the first 7 years. J Headache Pain. 2010;11:451–5.
8. Vos T, Flaxman AD, Naghavi M, Lozano R, Michaud C, Ezzati M, Shibuya K, Salomon JA, Abdalla S, Aboyans V, Abraham J, Ackerman I, Aggarwal R, Ahn SY, Ali MK, Alvarado M, Anderson HR, Anderson LM, Andrews KG, Atkinson C, Baddour LM, Bahalim AN, Barker-Collo S, Barrero LH, Bartels DH, Basáñez MG, Baxter A, Bell ML, Benjamin EJ, Bennett D, Bernabé E, Bhalla K, Bhandari B, Bikbov B, Bin Abdulhak A, et al. Years lived with disability (YLD) for 1160 sequelae of 289 diseases and injuries 1990–2010: a systematic analysis for the Global Burden of Disease Study 2010. Lancet. 2012;380:2163–96.
9. Steiner TJ, Stovner LJ, Birbeck GL. Migraine: the seventh disabler. J Headache Pain. 2013;14:1.
10. Vos T, Barber RM, Bell B, Bertozzi-Villa A, Biryukov S, Bolliger I, Charlson F, Davis A, Degenhardt L, Dicker D, Duan L, Erskine H, Feigin VL, Ferrari AJ, Fitzmaurice C, Fleming

T, Graetz N, Guinovart C, Haagsma J, Hansen GM, Hanson SW, Heuton KR, Higashi H, Kassebaum N, Kyu H, Laurie E, Liang X, Lofgren K, Lozano R, MacIntyre MF, Moradi-Lakeh M, Naghavi M, Nguyen G, Odell S, Ortblad K, et al. Global, regional, and national incidence, prevalence, and years lived with disability for 301 acute and chronic diseases and injuries in 188 countries, 1990–2013: a systematic analysis for the Global Burden of Disease Study 2013. Lancet. 2015;386:743–800.

11. Steiner TJ, Birbeck GL, Jensen RH, Katsarava Z, Stovner LJ, Martelletti P. Headache disorders are third cause of disability worldwide. J Headache Pain. 2015;16:58.
12. Vos T, Abajobir AA, Abate KH, Abbafati C, Abbas KM, Abd-Allah F, Abdulkader RS, Abdulle AM, Abebo TA, Abera SF, Aboyans V, Abu-Raddad LJ, Ackerman IN, Adamu AA, Adetokunboh O, Afarideh M, Afshin A, Agarwal SK, Aggarwal R, Agrawal A, Agrawal S, Ahmadieh H, Ahmed MB, Aichour MTE, Aichour AN, Aichour I, Aiyar S, Akinyemi RO, Akseer N, Al Lami FH, Alahdab F, Al-Aly Z, Alam K, Alam N, Alam T, et al. Global, regional, and national incidence, prevalence, and years lived with disability for 328 diseases and injuries for 195 countries, 1990–2016: a systematic analysis for the Global Burden of Disease Study 2016. Lancet. 2017;390:1211–59.
13. GBD 2017 Disease and Injury Incidence and Prevalence Collaborators. Global, regional, and national incidence, prevalence, and years lived with disability for 354 diseases and injuries for 195 countries and territories, 1990–2017: a systematic analysis for the Global Burden of Disease Study 2017. Lancet. 2018;392:1789–858.
14. Steiner TJ, Gururaj G, Andrée C, Katsarava Z, Ayzenberg I, Yu SY, Al Jumah M, Tekle-Haimanot R, Birbeck GL, Herekar A, Linde M, Mbewe E, Manandhar K, Risal A, Jensen R, Queiroz LP, Scher AI, Wang SJ, Stovner LJ. Diagnosis, prevalence estimation and burden measurement in population surveys of headache: presenting the HARDSHIP questionnaire. J Headache Pain. 2014;15:3.
15. Stewart WF, Lipton RB, Kolodner K, Sawyer J, Lee C, Liberman JN. Validity of the Migraine Disability Assessment (MIDAS) score in comparison to a diary-based measure in a population sample of migraine sufferers. Pain. 2000;88:41–52.
16. Steiner TJ, Lipton RB on behalf of *Lifting The Burden*: The Global Campaign against Headache. The Headache-Attributed Lost Time (HALT) Indices: measures of burden for clinical management and population-based research. J Headache Pain. 2018;19:12.
17. Schwartz BS, Stewart WF, Lipton RB. Lost workdays and decreased work effectiveness associated with headache in the workplace. J Occup Environ Med. 1997;39:320–7.
18. Steiner TJ, Scher AI, Stewart WF, Kolodner K, Liberman J, Lipton RB. The prevalence and disability burden of adult migraine in England and their relationships to age, gender and ethnicity. Cephalalgia. 2003;23:519–27.
19. Stovner LJ, Hagen K, Jensen R, Katsarava Z, Lipton R, Scher A, Steiner TJ, Zwart JA. The global burden of headache: a documentation of headache prevalence and disability worldwide. Cephalalgia. 2007;27:193–210.
20. Selekler MH, Gökmen G, Steiner TJ. Productivity impact of headache on a heavy-manufacturing workforce in Turkey. J Headache Pain. 2013;14:88.
21. Lampl C, Thomas H, Stovner LJ, Tassorelli C, Katsarava Z, Laínez JMA, Lantéri-Minet M, Rastenyte D, Ruiz de la Torre E, Andrée C, Steiner TJ. Interictal burden attributable to episodic headache: findings from the Eurolight project. J Headache Pain. 2016;17:9.
22. Hu XH, Markson LE, Lipton RB, Stewart WF, Berger ML. Burden of migraine in the United States: disability and economic costs. Arch Intern Med. 1999;159:813–8.
23. Linde M, Gustavsson A, Stovner LJ, Steiner TJ, Barré J, Katsarava Z, Lainez JM, Lampl C, Lantéri-Minet M, Rastenyte D, Ruiz de la Torre E, Tassorelli C, Andrée C. The cost of headache disorders in Europe: the Eurolight project. Eur J Neurol. 2012;19:703–11.
24. International Headache Society. Classification and diagnostic criteria for headache disorders, cranial neuralgias and facial pain. Cephalalgia. 1988;8:1–96.
25. World Health Organization. World health report 2001. Geneva: WHO; 2001.
26. Hopkins A, Menken M, DeFriese G. A record of patient encounters in neurological practice in the United Kingdom. J Neurol Neurosurg Psychiatry. 1989;52:436–8.

27. Wiles CM, Lindsay M. General practice referrals to a department of neurology. J Roy Coll Phys Lond. 1996;30:426–31.
28. American Association for the Study of Headache, International Headache Society. Consensus statement on improving migraine management. Headache. 1998;38:736.
29. Rasmussen BK, Jensen R, Olesen J. Impact of headache on sickness absence and utilisation of medical services: a Danish population study. J Epidemiol Community Health. 1992;46:443–6.
30. Dowson A, Jagger S. The UK migraine patient survey: quality of life and treatment. Curr Med Res Opin. 1999;15:241–53.
31. Lipton RB, Scher AI, Steiner TJ, Kolodner K, Liberman J, Stewart WF. Patterns of health care utilization for migraine in England and in the United States. Neurology. 2003;60:441–8.
32. Takeshima T, Ishizaki K, Fukuhara Y, Ijiri T, Kusumi M, Wakutani Y, Mori M, Kawashima M, Kowa H, Adachi Y, Urakami K, Nakashima K. Population-based door-to-door survey of migraine in Japan: the Daisen study. Headache. 2004;44:8–19.
33. Katsarava Z, Mania M, Lampl C, Herberhold J, Steiner TJ. Poor medical care for people with migraine in Europe—evidence from the Eurolight study. J Headache Pain. 2018;19:10.
34. Manandhar K, Risal A, Linde M, Steiner TJ. Health-care utilization for headache disorders in Nepal: a population-based door-to-door survey. J Headache Pain. 2018;19:116.

Chapter 5
Headache Disorders and the World Health Organization

Timothy J. Steiner, Nelly Huynh, and Lars Jacob Stovner

5.1 Introduction

The Global Burden of Disease study 1990 (GBD1990), the first such study, conducted by the World Health Organization (WHO), had nothing at all to say about headache disorders in general or any one of them specifically. They were not thought to be of any importance in global public health. The reason was lack of evidence. WHO's perfectly correct criteria for priority gave importance to diseases that were ubiquitous, prevalent, disabling and treatable. In 1990, headache did not *evidentially* meet these.

Ten years later, GBD2000 was also conducted by WHO, with collaborators intent on the inclusion at least of migraine. At that time, the published *prevalence* data for migraine, coming mostly from Western Europe and North America, yielded an estimated global mean of about 11%. WHO transformed these into *disability* data using their metric of years of life lost to disability (YLDs). The outcome was a

T. J. Steiner (✉)
Department of Neuromedicine and Movement Science, NTNU Norwegian University of Science and Technology, Trondheim, Norway

Division of Brain Sciences, Imperial College London, London, UK
e-mail: t.steiner@imperial.ac.uk

N. Huynh
Research Centre of the Sainte-Justine University Hospital, Montreal, QC, Canada
e-mail: nelly.huynh@umontreal.ca

L. J. Stovner
Department of Neuromedicine and Movement Science, NTNU Norwegian University of Science and Technology, Trondheim, Norway

Norwegian Advisory Unit on Headaches, Department of Neurology and Clinical Neurophysiology, St Olavs University Hospital, Trondheim, Norway
e-mail: lars.stovner@ntnu.no

T. J. Steiner, L. J. Stovner (eds.), *Societal Impact of Headache*, Headache,
https://doi.org/10.1007/978-3-030-24728-7_5

revelation: migraine was among the top 20 causes of disability (19th), accounting for 1.4% of all YLDs worldwide [1].

Sceptical questions were raised about how exact this disability estimate was, and later estimates in fact revised it substantially upwards ([2, 3]; also, Chaps. 4 and 9), but it nonetheless changed perceptions of migraine permanently. It could never again be doubted that its public-health impact was substantial.

5.2 The Global Campaign Against Headache

WHO's response was to recognize headache disorders as a global public-health priority, which they did first in an internal publication coming out of an expert technical consensus meeting in Geneva [4] and then by crystallizing discussions, which had been ongoing throughout this period, into action. The outcome, after a period of planning, was the launch of the Global Campaign against Headache ([5]; also, Chap. 14), followed by its diligent pursuit [6–10].

5.2.1 Knowledge for Action

In order to address the problem of headache, the ultimate purpose of the Global Campaign, it was necessary first to know much more of its nature, scope and scale—that is, the burden of headache—everywhere in the world. *Knowledge for action* was therefore the first of the three originally conceived objectives of the Global Campaign [5, 6]. In 2003, when it launched, very little was known of this burden for more than half the people of the world. Most of the Western Pacific, including China, all of South East Asia, including India, all of Eastern Europe, including Russia, most of Eastern Mediterranean and most of Africa were data-free [11].

The Global Campaign filled the major knowledge gaps by undertaking new population-based studies, in Georgia, Russia, Lithuania, Turkey, China, Mongolia, Nepal, India, Pakistan, Iran, Saudi Arabia, Morocco, Ethiopia, Zambia, Cameroon, Benin and Peru so far, an action programme still in progress [10]. This enquiry, focused first on adults but now extending to children and adolescents, assesses both prevalence and burden and informs the ongoing Global Burden of Disease studies (Chap. 9).

5.2.2 Awareness

Knowledge informs policy by creating *awareness*: recognition that change is needed, and the second of the three originally conceived objectives of the Global Campaign [5, 6]. Awareness is the prerequisite for *action to make change happen* (the third and ultimate objective [5, 6]), implementing solutions proposed on the basis of knowledge.

To complete the picture of the public-health problem that action must address, global enquiry, complementary to formal epidemiological studies, was also needed into how, if at all, healthcare systems were responding to headache. WHO had initiated its *Project Atlas* for this very purpose: to collect, compile and disseminate information on healthcare resources in countries, for various domains of mental and neurological services and conditions of public-health priority. The *Atlas of Headache Disorders and Resources in the World 2011* [12], an important addition to this series, presenting information from more than 100 countries, was undertaken by WHO and *Lifting The Burden* jointly as a project within the Global Campaign.

Most of the information was collected through a questionnaire survey of neurologists, general practitioners and patients' representatives, performed from October 2006 until March 2009. Only epidemiological data of sound provenance were included: those supported by peer-reviewed publication, comprehensively compiled by systematic review [11], and those of verifiably high quality gathered in population-based studies undertaken within the Global Campaign but not all published at the time [10].

5.3 Messages from WHO's Atlas of Headache

5.3.1 The "Neglected" Public-Health Problem

Prevalence studies included in the *Atlas* estimated that half to three quarters of adults in the world reported headache at least once in the preceding year [12]. This may have reflected interest bias, but the 10% reporting migraine is now known to be a substantial underestimate [2, 3]. Extrapolation from estimates of migraine prevalence and attack incidence suggested that 3000 migraine attacks occurred *every day* for each million of the general population [13]. Episodic tension-type headache (TTH) was the most common headache disorder; over 70% prevalence was reported in some populations (probably an overestimate, inflated by inclusion of infrequent episodic TTH [11]). Worldwide, its 1-year prevalence appeared to vary greatly, with an average of 42% in adults [11, 12]. Between 1.7 and 4% of adults were affected by headache on 15 or more days every month; medication-overuse headache (MOH), the most prevalent secondary headache, was reported in more than 1% of some populations [14].

Headache disorders were most prevalent during the productive years of adulthood (30s–50s). Their estimated financial cost to society—principally from lost working hours and reduced productivity due to impaired working effectiveness [15]—was therefore enormous (see Chaps. 4 and 12). In the UK it was noted, for example, some 25 million working or school days were lost every year because of migraine alone [13].

The *Atlas* concluded [12]:

> "Headache disorders are ubiquitous, prevalent, disabling and largely treatable, but under-recognized, under-diagnosed and under-treated. Illness that could be relieved is not, and burdens, both individual and societal, persist. Financial costs to society through lost productivity are enormous—far greater than the health-care expenditure on headache in any country."

5.3.2 The "Inadequate" Healthcare Response

Against this background of obvious burden and healthcare need, only 18% of countries that responded undertook any evaluation, for health policy, of the societal impact of headache [12]. Only 12% included headache disorders in an annual health-reporting system, and even fewer, 7%, included them in national expenditure surveys [12].

Worldwide, headache management reportedly depended on self-treatment by 50% of those with headache, without consultation with any health professional [12]. This is not in apparent conflict with ideal healthcare provision, since more than 50% should be able to self-manage perfectly well ([16]; also, Chap. 15), but almost certainly it reflects biased reporting by professionals who see *patients* (usually at the bad end of the spectrum) rather than *people with headache*. Up to 10% were treated by neurologists, although fewer in the African Region and South East Asia [12]. The top three causes of consultation for headache, in both primary and specialist care, were migraine, TTH and these in combination. MOH as a cause of specialist consultation increased in frequency (1–10%) with country income [12], but this might reflect ease of access to care rather than prevalence. Overall, a minority of people with headache disorders were professionally diagnosed: the estimated proportions were 40% for migraine and TTH and only 10% for MOH [12]. If these were reflective of quality and reach of headache services, they indicated much room for improvement in all regions. They might in fact be overestimates, but the last is anyway a major cause for concern since MOH cannot effectively be self-managed or brought under control if not diagnosed.

Specialists used International Headache Society diagnostic criteria (at that time, the International Classification of Headache Disorders, 2nd edition [17]) to support diagnosis in 56% of countries that responded: usage was lower in African and Eastern Mediterranean Regions and South East Asia, and lowest in low-income countries [12]. Investigation rates, mainly for diagnostic purposes, were high, despite that investigations are usually not needed to support diagnosis. Instruments to assess impact of headache were used routinely in only 24% of countries that responded, and very little in lower-middle- or low-income countries [12]. Management guidelines were in routine use in 55% of responding countries, but much less commonly in low-income countries. Despite there being a range of drugs with efficacy against headache, countries in all income categories identified non-availability of appropriate medication (probably referring to limited reimbursement) as a barrier to best management [12]. Among specific antimigraine drugs, ergotamine—cheaper, but less effective, more toxic, liable to accumulate and with greater overuse potential—was more widely available than triptans. Among alternative and complementary therapies, physical therapy, acupuncture and naturopathy were clear preferences, at least one of these being in the top three such therapies in all regions and all income categories [12].

The Global Campaign has advocated structured headache services as a key component of good healthcare, and the only effective, efficient and equitable means of delivering it ([16]; also, Chap. 15). A third of responding countries recommended, as a proposal for change, improved organization and delivery of healthcare for headache [12].

The *Atlas* concluded [12]:

> "Health care for headache must be improved, and education is required at multiple levels to achieve this. Most importantly, health-care providers need better knowledge of how to diagnose and treat the small number of headache disorders that contribute substantially to public ill-health.
>
> Given the very high indirect costs of headache, greater investment in health care that treats headache effectively, through well-organized health services and supported by education, may well be cost-saving overall."

5.3.3 Education: The Underlying Deficiency

Worldwide, the survey found, headache disorders were taught during only 4 h of formal undergraduate medical training, and 10 h of specialist training. Better professional education ranked far above all other proposals for change (75% of countries that responded), and lack of education was seen as the key issue impeding good management of headache [12].

5.3.4 National Professional Organizations

A national professional organization for headache disorders (or headache chapter in another organization) existed in two-thirds of countries that responded, with a very marked difference between high- and upper-middle-income, on the one hand (71–76%), and low-income countries, on the other (16%) [12]. The true numbers might be much lower, since respondents were much more readily identified in countries where such organizations existed.

A minority (20%) of professional headache organizations participated in the construction of postgraduate training curricula on headache, and only 10% engaged in the development of undergraduate curricula [12]. Rather more (over one third) arranged conferences, raised awareness of headache-related issues or were involved in setting guidelines for diagnosis and treatment of headache (a low-cost opportunity for substantial service improvement).

5.3.5 A Template for Action

The *Atlas* went beyond descriptions of this dismal *status quo*, and the issuing of political messages to the world's national governments. It set out an account of the way forward, in a template for action. More is said of this in Chap. 14.

5.4 Concluding Remarks

What were the findings of this first global enquiry into these matters? They were that headache disorders were ubiquitous, prevalent, disabling and largely treatable (therefore meeting all criteria for priority), but under-recognized, underdiagnosed and undertreated. Very large numbers of people disabled by headache did not receive effective healthcare. Illness that could be relieved was not, and burdens, both individual and societal, persisted. The barriers responsible for this might vary throughout the world, but poor awareness of headache in a context of limited resources generally—and in healthcare in particular—was constantly among them [12]. In summary, the *Atlas* described "worldwide neglect of major causes of public ill-health, and the inadequacies of responses to them in countries throughout the world" [12]. Yet the financial costs to society through lost productivity were far greater than the healthcare expenditure on headache in any country.

These were messages from WHO directly to the governments of the world.

Raising awareness is the purpose of this monograph, and all of the topics introduced in this section are subjects of its later chapters.

References

1. World Health Organization. World health report 2001. Geneva: WHO; 2001.
2. Vos T, Abajobir AA, Abate KH, Abbafati C, Abbas KM, Abd-Allah F, Abdulkader RS, Abdulle AM, Abebo TA, Abera SF, Aboyans V, Abu-Raddad LJ, Ackerman IN, Adamu AA, Adetokunboh O, Afarideh M, Afshin A, Agarwal SK, Aggarwal R, Agrawal A, Agrawal S, Ahmadieh H, Ahmed MB, Aichour MTE, Aichour AN, Aichour I, Aiyar S, Akinyemi RO, Akseer N, Al Lami FH, Alahdab F, Al-Aly Z, Alam K, Alam N, Alam T, et al. Global, regional, and national incidence, prevalence, and years lived with disability for 328 diseases and injuries for 195 countries, 1990–2016: a systematic analysis for the global burden of disease study 2016. Lancet. 2017;390:1211–59.
3. GBD 2017 Disease and Injury Incidence and Prevalence Collaborators. Global, regional, and national incidence, prevalence, and years lived with disability for 354 diseases and injuries for 195 countries and territories, 1990–2017: a systematic analysis for the Global Burden of Disease Study 2017. Lancet. 2018;392:1789–858.
4. World Health Organization. Headache disorders and public health. Education and management implications. Geneva: WHO (WHO/MSD/MBD/00.9); 2000.
5. Steiner TJ. *Lifting The Burden*: the global campaign against headache. Lancet Neurol. 2004;3:204–5.

6. Steiner TJ. *Lifting The Burden*: the global campaign to reduce the burden of headache worldwide. J Headache Pain. 2005;6:373–7.
7. Steiner TJ, Birbeck GL, Jensen R, Katsarava Z, Martelletti P, Stovner LJ. *Lifting The Burden*: the first 7 years. J Headache Pain. 2010;11:451–5.
8. Steiner TJ, Birbeck GL, Jensen R, Katsarava Z, Martelletti P, Stovner LJ. The Global Campaign, World Health Organization and *Lifting The Burden*: collaboration in action. J Headache Pain. 2011;12:273–4.
9. Steiner TJ, Stovner LJ, Dua T, Birbeck GL, Jensen R, Katsarava Z, Martelletti P, Saxena S. Time to act on headache disorders. J Headache Pain. 2011;12:501–3.
10. *Lifting The Burden*. The Global Campaign against Headache. http://www.l-t-b.org.
11. Stovner LJ, Hagen K, Jensen R, Katsarava Z, Lipton R, Scher A, Steiner TJ, Zwart JA. The global burden of headache: a documentation of headache prevalence and disability worldwide. Cephalalgia. 2007;27:193–210.
12. World Health Organization, *Lifting The Burden*. Atlas of headache disorders and resources in the world 2011. Geneva: WHO; 2011.
13. Steiner TJ, Scher AI, Stewart WF, Kolodner K, Liberman J, Lipton RB. The prevalence and disability burden of adult migraine in England and their relationships to age, gender and ethnicity. Cephalalgia. 2003;23:519–27.
14. Castillo J, Munoz P, Guitera V, Pascual J. Epidemiology of chronic daily headache in the general population. Headache. 1999;39:190–6.
15. Schwartz BS, Stewart WF, Lipton RB. Lost workdays and decreased work effectiveness associated with headache in the workplace. J Occup Environ Med. 1997;39:320–7.
16. Steiner TJ, Antonaci F, Jensen R, Lainez JMA, Lantéri-Minet M, Valade D on behalf of the European Headache Federation and *Lifting The Burden*: the Global Campaign against Headache. Recommendations for headache service organisation and delivery in Europe. J Headache Pain. 2001;12:419–26.
17. International Headache Society Classification Subcommittee. The international classification of headache disorders, 2nd edition. Cephalalgia. 2004;24(suppl 1):1–160.

Part II
Quantifying Headache

Chapter 6
Epidemiological Methods for Headache Studies

Lars Jacob Stovner and Timothy J. Steiner

6.1 Introduction

The importance of epidemiological studies for headache science is now widely recognized. When headache was ranked the second most disabling disorder worldwide in the Global Burden of Disease 2016 study ([1]; also, Chaps. 5, 9 and 14), this was in large part the result of decades of headache epidemiological studies in many countries [2].

While much money and time had been committed to these studies, their methods and quality were variable [2–7]. A review of all previous studies found they had been performed, and reported, in quite different ways [2, 7]. This made it very difficult to interpret and summarize their results and, particularly, to compare the findings of studies performed in different settings and countries or at different times. Further, while quality varied, there were some studies that appeared well-enough performed, but reported in too little detail to make comparisons possible.

Headache epidemiological studies inform needs assessment, underpin service policy and gain acceptance of headache disorders as a public-health priority [6]. In addition, they can increase our understanding of causes and risk factors, thereby

L. J. Stovner (✉)
Department of Neuromedicine and Movement Science, NTNU Norwegian University of Science and Technology, Trondheim, Norway

Norwegian Advisory Unit on Headaches, Department of Neurology and Clinical Neurophysiology, St Olavs University Hospital, Trondheim, Norway
e-mail: lars.stovner@ntnu.no

T. J. Steiner
Department of Neuromedicine and Movement Science, NTNU Norwegian University of Science and Technology, Trondheim, Norway

Division of Brain Sciences, Imperial College London, London, UK
e-mail: t.steiner@imperial.ac.uk

T. J. Steiner, L. J. Stovner (eds.), *Societal Impact of Headache*, Headache,
https://doi.org/10.1007/978-3-030-24728-7_6

improving opportunities for treatment and prevention (see Chap. 10). Quality therefore matters in these studies. The need for better and standardized methodology, supported by guidelines for the design and performance of these studies, had been evident for some years [3, 4] when, in 2014, such guidelines were published [5]. The initiative came from *Lifting The Burden* (LTB), a UK-registered charitable non-governmental organization, which directs the Global Campaign against Headache in official relations with the World Health Organization (WHO). It was supported financially by LTB, the International Headache Society (IHS), the World Headache Alliance and the Norwegian University of Science and Technology in Trondheim, Norway.

Quality improvement was the main aim, not only to improve reliability of headache epidemiological studies but also so that resources directed towards them would be better spent [5]. Further, while the guidelines would primarily be useful in the planning and performance of new studies, they could also, it was believed, be applied to evaluation of the quality of studies previously published [5]. This chapter is based on the parts of these guidelines that deal with how to measure prevalence. The parts on how to measure burden and cost are the basis of Chap. 7.

An expert consensus group was convened, with two considerations in mind: inclusion of experience and competence in headache epidemiology and epidemiology in general, and international and cross-cultural relevance. To the latter end, members were drawn from all six WHO world regions. After a first draft had been circulated, and feedback received from all members, the group convened in Trondheim in September 2011 for a 3-day meeting. A preliminary manuscript then posted on the IHS website invited worldwide open consultation, which, along with feedback from staff at WHO, informed the final, published version [5].

The recommendations here are drawn from these guidelines. They relate specifically to studies of headache, or address issues of particular relevance to headache, with more general supporting discussion when needed. It is strongly advised that headache epidemiological studies be planned and performed in collaboration with a local epidemiologist, familiar with the population of interest and culture(s). While the focus of the recommendations is on adult studies, many apply equally to studies of children and/or adolescents and others can be applied with adaptation. There are some considerations specific to studies of the elderly, and attention is drawn to these. With regard specifically to the *reporting* of studies, the STROBE statements (http://www.strobe-statement.org/) [8, 9] should be consulted.

The recommendations apply most readily to primary headache disorders, principally migraine and tension-type headache (TTH) (see Chap. 2). They are not intended to be exclusive to these: the principles are relevant also to epidemiological studies of secondary headaches, provided that adequate definitions can be applied in questionnaires or other survey instruments. However, burdens arising from secondary headaches are, in general, more correctly attributed to the underlying disorders. Medication-overuse headache (MOH), a secondary headache by definition, is something of an exception. The recommendations expressly encompass MOH firstly because it arises only from a pre-existing, usually primary headache disorder and, secondly, because it unquestionably contributes to public ill health. They also embrace the broader group of headaches occurring on 15 or more days per month, again because these unquestionably contribute to public ill health. It is acknowledged later that these may be poorly characterized and, within a survey conducted by enquiries at single points in time, impossible to diagnose more specifically than as frequent headache.

6.2 Headache Epidemiology

Epidemiology is aptly described as "the study of distribution and determinants of disease frequency in human populations" [10]. Epidemiological studies are often classified as *descriptive* (setting out the distribution of disease among different groups) or *analytical* (elucidating determinants: i.e., risk factors or causes).

The usual focus of descriptive epidemiology in headache is *prevalence*, an estimate of how common a disease is, and expressed as a proportion (number of cases in a population divided by the number of individuals in that population). Also important is *incidence*, a measure of the risk of developing a condition within a specified period of time, expressed as a rate. *Remission* is the probability of a case becoming a non-case, through natural history or intervention, again within a specified period of time, and expressed as a rate. *Duration* of disease is the period between onset and remission. *Mortality* is important in epidemiology in general, but it has little relevance to primary headache disorders.

Incidence, duration, remission and prevalence are related not only conceptually but also mathematically, the last being the steady-state consequence of the first two, often summarized by the formula $P = ID$, where P = (point) prevalence, I = incidence per year and D = duration in years.

Headache terminology is unfortunately inconsistent, owing to the fact that headache is a chronic disorder with episodic manifestations. An "active headache disorder" is essentially characterized by the occurrence, at least once, of symptoms within the previous year [11]. Prevalence studies that adopt this definition of a case (i.e., a person who reports at least one headache episode during this time) necessarily use a timeframe of 1 year and usually report the findings as 1-year prevalence. Strictly speaking, however, such estimates describe the number of *current* cases (i.e., point prevalence). A different enquiry, defining a case only when symptoms are actually present ("headache now"), also estimates point prevalence, but of headache attacks, or headache as a symptom, not of a headache disorder. The terms "incidence" and "remission" can, similarly, be applied either to headache attacks or to headache disorders, although in practice they have generally referred to the latter, with specified time periods (e.g., incidence rate = number with first onset of headache per 100 person-years; remission rate = % of cases of headache disorder who then have no further attacks during 1 year of follow-up). These terms must be used carefully to avoid confusion.

These recommendations are of equal relevance to descriptive and analytical studies. But which of these is the *purpose* of the study must always be clear at the outset: it affects, fundamentally, the design of the study, the choice of study population, the size of the study sample and the information to be collected.

6.2.1 Ethical Issues

Ethical issues in epidemiological studies arise in their planning, conduct and reporting. Many are general. Ethical principles firmly and universally established in medical practice also apply to research in the form of headache epidemiological studies. These principles include respect for autonomy, non-maleficence, beneficence and justice [12], the last with particular reference to resource allocation in a context of limited resources (distributive justice, or equity). The ethics of the medical profession include veracity (truth-telling), fidelity (the keeping of promises) and confidentiality, and are based on the needs of patients (including potential and future patients), the responsibilities of doctors, the good of society as a whole and deserts. These have been discussed in detail elsewhere [13, 14].

Before they commence, epidemiological studies require approval by an appropriate ethics review board (ERB), usually local but, where one does not exist, from another legitimate, authoritative and competent source, such as WHO's Research Ethics Review Committee. Data protection also requires due consideration [14], and may, according to the laws of the country in which the study is conducted, require additional approvals.

Consent by participants in surveys is often implicit, and ongoing: respondents renew consent each time they provide an answer to an enquiry. Formal written consent at the start of the enquiry provides only evidence of consent at that moment, and may serve little purpose for that reason (although an ERB may require it). Consent must be informed, which requires that the purpose and nature of the survey are explained to each participant's satisfaction. Consent must also be voluntary, and participants allowed to withdraw from the study whenever they may wish.

Inducements to take part in a study that carries no risk of harm to the participant do not directly raise concerns. Both parties benefit: the researcher from the subject's participation and the subject from the inducement. However, they may raise concerns indirectly, since inducements are not of equal value to all potential subjects. Monetary inducements are more attractive to poorer people, and this does not respect the principle of equity. For the same reason, monetary inducements (and probably inducements of any sort) are likely to increase participation bias (an important quality issue discussed later).

When the inducement is the offer of needed healthcare, either free or to which the research subject would not otherwise have ready access, he or she may have little choice but to participate. Still the participant benefits. In the absence of risk of harm, even this may be considered acceptable, although a counterargument is that collecting data from needy people while offering them nothing in return is objectionable. Justification is forthcoming when the purpose of the survey is needs assessment—to inform the development of health services, which, later, will be provided for the benefit of the population being surveyed. But there is another important question, which goes beyond the ethics of reward: to what extent is there a duty of care upon researchers when untreated and possibly serious illness is discovered by a survey? This question is sometimes raised—especially in low-income countries. These recommendations cannot give a general answer: this must be a matter for local ERBs. Two points can be noted: first, surveys are commonly made by lay interviewers, who do not themselves diagnose and have no skills to recognize illness, let alone do anything to alleviate it; second, research that may benefit a society cannot be made too onerous, or it will never be done.

Data protection, and consent relating to the use of personal data, generally requires that participants are explicitly informed of each of the following:

- Where, in what form, how and by whom data relating to them will be held
- Who will have access to them
- The purpose(s) for which they will be used, with guarantees that they will be used for no other purpose (this implies that, if data are to be stored long-term for other purposes not yet foreseen, at least a general explanation of this intention should be given)
- How they will be destroyed once the purposes are achieved.

To reduce the possibility of misuse of personal data, the duration of their storage should be as short as possible. On the other hand, it is desirable, and regulators often require it, that original research data are stored for several years, for documentation and to enable detection of fraud in science. Clearly, personal data should be handled and stored safely, respecting the privacy of participants and in accordance with the laws and regulations for data storage in the country.

Resources are limited. Studies that waste them (whether financial resources or the willingness of subjects to take part) are unethical because of the opportunity cost: other studies will not be possible as a result. Under-resourced studies that cannot achieve their purpose are likely to be unethical because the resources are probably wasted. Unscientific studies certainly waste resources, and are unethical for this reason alone. Worse, they may generate misleading results.

Adherence to these recommendations should ensure appropriate allocation of resources, and their effective use, in headache epidemiological research. However, the need for *efficiency* calls for careful deliberation of whether a particular new headache epidemiological study is required at all, and of the need for high diagnostic precision, with large sample size and resource-demanding methods of data collection. In some circumstances, a new stand-alone study can be adequately replaced, with conservation of resources, by joining a larger health survey (see later).

6.2.2 Methodological Issues

The methodological issues arising with regard to the design of a headache epidemiological study are largely general, and are dealt with in general textbooks on epidemiology. Here, as noted earlier, we discuss those relating specifically or addressing issues of particular relevance to studies of headache. More general supporting discussion is added only when needed.

6.2.2.1 The Study Design

This should match the purpose of the study and take due account of available resources and the general conditions in the area(s) where the study will be performed. It must be described in sufficient detail that the study can be replicated.

Most studies on headache epidemiology are descriptive, with a cross-sectional design in which prevalence and burden are assessed at the same point in time. Studies with more analytical aims, to define causes of or risk factors for headache, usually have case–control or cohort designs. Case–control studies typically compare cases (who have the disease) with controls (who are similar persons without the disease) for prior exposure to one or more putative risk factors. In cohort studies, a group (cohort) of disease-free individuals are followed and assessed periodically to determine whether they have developed the disease of interest. Within the cohort, participants are categorized as exposed or not to a suspected causal factor; incidence rates are compared after a specified time in the exposed and unexposed categories.

Methodologies differ mostly in how study samples are selected; the principles for collecting data, engaging with participants and diagnosing headaches are similar. Therefore, while these recommendations mostly concern cross-sectional studies, they will be useful in all study designs.

6.2.2.2 The Population of Interest

This is sometimes referred to as the *sampling frame*, and is the population that it is wished to study. It includes every person so defined, and is always defined geographically as well, often, as by one or more additional characteristics. It should match the purpose of the study, and the selection should be explicitly justified. It must also be described in sufficient detail that the study can be compared with others.

In headache research, the population of interest is usually, but not always, the population of a whole country, or of a region larger or smaller than a country. However, depending on the aim of the study, the population of interest may be restricted to a specific age group (e.g., adults of working age, adolescents, school or pre-school children), to members of groups defined by ethnicity, culture or language, to workers in certain trades or professions or university students, to people with another particular disease, etc. These recommendations remain relevant to studies of these more selected groups.

Headache *patient* populations are rarely legitimate populations of interest, not just because they are highly selected but also because the criteria by which they are selected (often self-selected) are generally indeterminable. A study of such populations tells little about, and cannot be extrapolated to, either the general population or any more broadly defined population. An arguable exception occurs in the case of severe headache disorders (discussed later, under *Special issues*).

It is an advantage when the characteristics of the population of interest are known (distributions of age, gender, educational levels and socio-economic status, proportions living in rural and urban areas, etc.), since this allows evaluation of representativeness of the participating sample, and statistical adjustments with regard to these features when necessary.

6.2.2.3 Bias

Bias refers to errors that are systematic rather than random. In epidemiological studies, biases are of two main types: selection (or participation) bias and information (or measurement) bias.

Selection bias is commonly the consequence of an imperfect sampling procedure and/or a low participation proportion, resulting in a sample unrepresentative of the population of interest. With regard to gender and age composition, statistical adjustments for imbalance can be made if these properties are known for the population of interest. *Participation bias* ("interest bias") can result from the higher tendency of people with headache to participate in headache studies, because they have more personal interest in them.

Information bias, or a systematic error in measuring disease or exposure, may occur when the manner in which information is gathered varies systematically. For example, two interviewers, one in a city and the other in a rural area, may conduct the interview differently, with differences in findings that are erroneously attributed to area of habitation. Similarly, one interviewer who completes all interviews in one location first, then all those in another, may introduce systematic differences over time in the manner of interviewing (due to a learning curve, for example), again with spuriously different results from the two locations.

Biases are almost inevitable, but should be minimized. The likely causes of bias should be identified at outset, and due steps taken to manage them. Bias may not necessarily be of much consequence, depending on its magnitude and on whether it is differential (affecting some participants more than others) or non-differential (affecting all participants equally). The potential for bias, and the need to avoid or at least minimize it, drive many aspects of the planning, execution and analysis of a study.

6.2.2.4 Sample Selection

To include every member of the population of interest in an epidemiological survey is feasible only in a minority of studies. Instead, it is necessary to choose a smaller group of people (*the sample*) to whom access is possible. It is essential that this sample is *representative* of the population of interest, in order to be able to generalize the results from the sample to the whole population of interest. "Representative" means similar to the population of interest in all properties of relevance to (i.e., likely to influence) the objects of measurement (here, headache prevalence and/or burden). There is an assumption here that knowledge exists of what these properties are, which may not be entirely true. In the context of headache, representativeness clearly encompasses age and gender, which are known to affect headache prevalence. Also of relevance, probably, are socio-economic status, employment, area of habitation (rural or urban) and ethnicity, and possibly, in some settings, native language and/or tribal group. Methods that ensure or at least optimize representativeness with regard to a range of identified variables such as these are more likely to achieve the same with other, unrecognized variables.

Sampling introduces multiple opportunities for selection bias, which should be recognized and controlled. Sampling aims, first and foremost, to produce a group within the population of interest who are both accessible for survey and representative of it. Sampling *identifies* individuals to be surveyed, but usually does not, of itself, provide a *means of access* to these individuals, while the means of access is an important consideration when determining the sampling method.

Sampling uses either *probability* or *non-probability* methods. With the former, each member of the population of interest has an initial probability (which is larger than zero) of being selected, and this probability can be accurately determined; this is not the case with the latter. Non-probability methods include convenience sampling (selecting those who are at hand), judgemental sampling (selecting those judged to be best suited for the purpose), quota sampling (selecting quotas fulfilling particular traits) and snowball sampling (letting participants recruit future participants). With these methods, the degree to which the sample differs from the population of interest is uncontrolled, and selection bias is impossible to assess.

Probability sampling methods are therefore much to be preferred. With simple random sampling, all individuals within the population of interest have equal probability of being selected. Nonetheless, the method is vulnerable to sampling error: *by chance*, important characteristics of the sample such as gender or age distributions may not well reflect those of the whole population. Stratified sampling reduces this chance by dividing the population into sub-populations (strata), different with regard, for example, to age, gender and/or habitation, and randomly drawing the sample from within each of these strata, in parts in proportion to their size.

Both random sampling and stratified sampling are relatively easy when an overview of the population of interest exists—usually in the form of a register of all members of it. Selection can then be made directly from the register (usually by computer). A map showing all households in an area to be sampled can also serve the purpose of a register. Sampling by telephone is an established method [15]. Where telephones (landline or mobile) are widespread, but no population overview exists in the form of a complete telephone directory, random digit-dialling (area codes, followed randomly by as many digits as are typical for phone numbers in the areas) is an effective method of obtaining a random sample [15], but it risks bias because telephones are not evenly distributed among different age, gender and socio-economic groups.

Cluster sampling is an alternative in areas with no pre-existing overview of the population, but often preferable anyway because it is logistically efficient, reducing travel costs and time. Usually it involves selecting participants only from a limited number of defined geographical areas (e.g., blocks, streets or parts of villages, or perhaps schools) that are themselves chosen randomly. Areas can also be stratified according to socio-economic status, urban/rural location, etc. In *multistage cluster sampling*, smaller areas are selected randomly within larger areas, and this is repeated in many stages until the requisite number of small, surveyable areas are identified, spread around the region or country. In these ultimate units, all individuals, or a random selection of individuals or households, are contacted.

In many studies, rather than contacting individuals, it will be easier to contact *households* (people living together and sharing the same kitchen). Generally, in headache studies, only one of a household should be selected, because members of families are similar genetically, share their environment and have common lifestyles, effectively reducing variance when two or more are included. In order to avoid bias with regard to who will be home and answer the door, the interviewer should list all members of the household, then select the participant randomly from all those who are eligible, returning by appointment for the interview when that person is not present.

The study protocol should set out the method for *replacement*, when it is impossible to contact a selected person: for example, by pre-selecting more individuals than needed, or by extending the sampling process by visiting more randomly selected households than initially specified.

The *sample size* must be sufficient to achieve the study purpose(s), but not so large as to waste resources. In determining sample size, expected prevalence and desired precision of the estimates are the only factors to consider (not, as often believed, the size of the population of interest). Desired precision is not free from issues of resources and ethics: a larger sample than needed is wasteful, whereas a study with too small a sample for its purpose is futile, and also wasteful. Several statistical programs include sample-size calculations, and there is also a simple table in the published guidelines [5].

If the requirement is to estimate, with acceptable precision, the prevalence of different headache disorders, or of subtypes of a disorder (migraine in general and migraine with aura, for example), sample size is calculated with regard to the disorder or subtype assumed to be least prevalent. The same is true when estimates within subgroups or comparisons between them (e.g., males versus females, rural versus urban) are part of the purpose: the sample size must be calculated to include sufficient of the population in the smallest subgroup. To avoid inflating the overall sample unnecessarily, it is possible to "oversample" people in that particular subgroup (i.e., select more than the proportion in the population). Such people then have a higher (but known) chance of being selected than those in other subgroups, and correction is necessary when calculating overall prevalence.

A larger sample may also be needed to estimate burden than to estimate prevalence, because burden is not distributed equally among cases: most of it is accounted for by a minority of those with the disorder. For example, 3–4% of the population have most of the burden of migraine [16]; among all people with migraine, TTH or MOH, the relatively few with MOH have the highest individual burden [17].

Cluster sampling is assumed to reduce natural variance, and therefore requires larger sample sizes to obtain the same precision of estimates [18].

The sampling method should be explicitly justified, and it should be described in sufficient detail that the study can be replicated. Biases that might have arisen from the sampling procedure should be identified and discussed.

6.2.2.5 Accessing and Engaging Participants

The ways in which members of the sample are contacted (*access*), and their willing commitment to the enquiry procured (*engagement*), are important determinants of how carefully and completely they will respond and, therefore, of data quality.

Means of access clearly depends on what means of communication exist (telephone registries, email or home address lists, up-to-date maps of residential areas) and on infrastructure (e.g., means and ease of travel). Access methods compatible with *probability sampling* include visiting households and calling by telephone (landline or mobile), usually without prior warning (cold-calling) in either case, and letters mailed or emailed to participants selected from registers that provide addresses. In some settings, participants may be invited to come to the interviewer's office.

Cold-calling at households tends to yield a higher participation proportion (among people who are at home) than telephone interviews, which are easier for the interviewee to terminate. Both methods may give rise to selection bias, because certain types of person are more likely to stay at home, open the door or answer the phone. To increase participation proportion, it is often necessary to make more than one attempt to contact a person who does not answer first time. The study protocol should define how many attempts are made (commonly three), and when, before a person or a household is deemed impossible to contact. Certain types of household are more likely to be empty, or their phones unanswered, at particular times of the day: for example, working households will be selectively uncontactable during normal working hours, while older people may not open doors to strangers in the evening. The protocol should take these factors into consideration when stipulating schedules for repeated contacts.

Accessing participants by mail is cheap, and by email even cheaper, but these methods have two major disadvantages. They presume the use of self-administered questionnaires, which can give rise to misunderstandings and therefore data of low quality. They inevitably lead to selection bias because certain types of person are less inclined to reply.

Inviting prospective participants to the office of the interviewer allows face-to-face interview, and examination if necessary, but it is time-consuming for participants, likely therefore to discourage participation and promote selection bias with regard to who has the time to attend.

Methods involving *non-probability sampling* include stopping prospective participants in the street and using lists of telephone numbers or email addresses that happen to be available rather than complete registries. These are convenience samples, biased by whatever factors cause people to be on the street, or in a selective list, and rarely useful in headache epidemiology.

Engagement, the procurement of prospective participants' willing cooperation in a study, directly affects participation proportion and, therefore, participation bias. How it is done depends upon the means of access, and also is determined by certain characteristics of the prospective participants, such as literacy, language, cognitive ability and culture.

Face-to-face interviews are the most direct method of engagement, and the only method useful in populations with poor literacy. Their disadvantage is that they are time-consuming and therefore expensive. *Telephone interviews* are almost as direct but, unlike face-to-face interviews, do not allow physical examination.

Both face-to-face and telephone interviews allow clarification of questions. While generally thought to lead to more accurate answers, clarification may instead give rise to information bias, not only because the information given to those who ask is different from that given to those who do not, but also because different interviewers may give different clarifications. Therefore, if clarification is permitted, there should be clear, pre-specified limits to the extent of it, aiming to ensure that all interviewers do it in the same way. In a computer-assisted telephone interview (CATI), interviewers follow a script driven by a computer program. Face-to-face interviews can be computer-assisted in the same way. These methods permit only pre-scripted clarifications.

Self-administered questionnaires are a relatively cheap method, but require a high degree of literacy and some familiarity with answering questionnaires. The method provides no encouragement to respond and no opportunity for clarifications, generally resulting in low participation proportions and incomplete questionnaires.

Engagement in groups (e.g., by a teacher posing questions collectively to the pupils in the classroom) can be a cost-effective way of performing a study. Engagement through a third person may be the only way to gain contact with or information from some participants, for example small children through their parents. In some cultures, people can be engaged only through village elders or heads of households. With these methods, the risk of misunderstandings must be carefully evaluated. Additionally, lower sensitivity and specificity for detecting headache must be expected from such remote engagements.

Careful selection and adequate training of interviewers are of paramount importance, whether interviews are conducted face-to-face or by telephone. As to their selection, interviewing is a skill in itself: it should not be assumed that health personnel such as nurses, medical students or, especially, doctors are the best qualified to do it. Unless the interviewer is a headache specialist (see below), diagnoses should not be made during the interview but later, by applying an algorithm to the questionnaire responses [19]. It is therefore doubtful, in most surveys, whether clinical skills are important: it may be better to engage professionally trained interviewers who understand interview methodology and who follow the questionnaire and operations manual.

Adequate training of interviewers embraces a clear understanding of the nature and purpose of the survey, and a recognition of which questions are of particular importance or may need clarification. When there are multiple interviewers, training should be identical for each of them to ensure that data are collected in the same way by all, without introduction of information bias. While multiple interviewers almost inevitably introduce some degree of variability, more interviewers reduce the duration of the study, which, if long, can also be a source of variation.

When the interviewer is a headache specialist (a physician skilled in headache diagnosis and familiar with the culture and language of the respondent), not only can the diagnosis be made during the interview but, further, multiple diagnoses, where appropriate, can be made in the same participant. If examination and supplementary investigations are made, secondary headaches can be diagnosed. No validation of the diagnostic method is needed, since it can be assumed that optimal diagnostic methods are employed. Headache specialists, of course, may not explicitly use ICHD diagnostic criteria [11]: they have at their disposal and are likely to apply, as in the clinic, a broader, experienced-based and more inclusive set of criteria for diagnosis, which ICHD-based questionnaires can never match. High sensitivity can be expected for detecting relatively minor headache complaints and rare headaches.

In low-income countries, headache specialists are simply not available.

6.2.2.6 Participation and Non-participation

The *participation proportion* is an important result of a study; in particular it is important for evaluating bias. But it has no universal definition [9]. It is generally understood as the proportion of those *selected, contacted and eligible* who actually participate in the study meaningfully (i.e., provide answers to most questions). Calculation of participation proportion therefore excludes those in the preselected sample who a) were not contactable (because they had died, or moved away since the study was planned, or because no-one answered the phone or opened the door), or b) were contacted but found to be ineligible (because it was not possible to seek their consent, for whatever reason, or they did not fulfil the eligibility criteria [wrong age or gender, for example]).

In almost all cases, *non-participation* (among those contacted and eligible) results either from outright refusal to participate or, among those consenting to take part, from inability to cooperate usefully, perhaps answering only a few questions or providing conflicting responses.

Only a very high participation proportion, rarely achieved, guarantees *representativeness* (assuming correct sampling). Participation proportions >80% are considered excellent, and ≥70% acceptable, but even these do not secure representativeness. On the other hand, a low participation proportion does not necessarily mean the included sample is unrepresentative: this depends on the factors responsible for non-participation [9]. But usually, because probability of participation tends to vary between different subgroups of a sample (e.g., it may be particularly low among young males), a low participation proportion influences the overall results (i.e., it is a source of bias). In other words, both how many and who actually participate in the study are crucial to representativeness.

Since non-participation cannot be altogether avoided, all reasons for it (declined to participate, too sick to be interviewed, did not return the questionnaire, completed the questionnaire inadequately or inappropriately, etc.) should be listed, and, if possible, coupled with at least a demographic description of each non-participant. They can then be taken into account in evaluations of sample representativeness, and the likelihood, magnitude and influence of participation bias.

When participation proportion is low, representativeness may be estimated through a study of non-participants, although this is possible only when the initial sampling was from a register including contact details. Enquiry is usually by telephone, calling a random sample of non-participants, and it must be limited to a few key questions (e.g., age, gender, the screening question(s) for headache, perhaps one on headache frequency and a very few on diagnosis). This minimal dataset, at least showing whether non-participants are similar to or very different from participants in the main study, is highly valuable in assessing various types of selection bias. An additional question, asking why they did not participate initially, will inform discussion of selection bias. It may also help in the better design of future studies.

6.2.2.7 Method of Enquiry: The Study Instrument

A *structured questionnaire* (prescribed questions, with predefined response options) is usual both to identify (and diagnose) headache caseness and for enquiry into headache burden. Some questions may call for open answers (e.g., number of days with headache, names of medicines) but, generally, open answers are difficult to interpret and categorize; for diagnosis, they do not permit algorithmic determination (see below).

Structured questionnaires should, depending on the study purpose(s), include identifier(s), demographics (age, gender, education, employment, personal and/or household income, habitation [urban, rural], ethnicity [when relevant], etc.), screening and sieve questions, diagnostic questions, enquiry into symptom burden (headache frequency, duration, intensity, etc.) and one or more other elements of burden (disability, time loss, family burden, cost, etc.) ([19]; also, Chaps. 4 and 7).

Quality of the questionnaire is fundamental to the quality of the entire study: nothing can compensate for failures in data collection. Time and resources are well spent in developing a good questionnaire, and much attention should be paid to layout (clarity and ease of use reduce error rates), intelligibility, acceptability and content (how many diagnoses are necessary, and what aspects of burden are to be measured?).

Questionnaires should be *parsimonious*, and not include any questions that do not contribute to the study's purpose(s): irrelevant questions not only irritate participants but also create unnecessary workload. Further, questionnaires should avoid enquiries that are irrelevant to particular participants, by directing them past sections that are not applicable. Ideally, of course, all questions pertinent to the survey are answered clearly by every participant, but certain questions (screening question, diagnostic questions and, perhaps, key questions on burden) *must* be answered if the respondent is not to be classified as a non-participant.

A *pre-pilot study* in a small convenience sample drawn from patients in the clinic may be most useful to test whether questions are culturally inoffensive and that questionnaire length (time to complete) is acceptable.

Meticulous translation is then essential, following a rigorous translation protocol [20]. A larger *pilot study* in a convenience sample drawn from the population of interest should be conducted after translation to ensure that questions are understood correctly and discover those that may cause problems and require clarification. The pilot studies may uncover need for amendment(s) to the questionnaires or retranslation (and, potentially, retesting).

If the questionnaire is newly developed, validation in the language and specific setting of the study is highly desirable, at least of the diagnostic part (see below).

6.2.2.8 Case Definition and Diagnosis

In all headache epidemiological studies, it is of fundamental importance to define who is a case and who is not. How caseness is defined can greatly influence the results, and this concerns the definition of headache, and of its types or subtypes. "Migraine" may include all its types and subtypes (ICHD-3 codes 1.1–1.6) [11] in some studies, but only migraine with or without aura (ICHD-3 codes 1.1 and 1.2) [11] in others. "Migraine with aura" may or may not include the subtypes aura without headache and aura with non-migrainous headache. "Migraine" and "tension-type headache" may include both episodic and chronic types or be restricted to the former, with chronic types subsumed within the general category of headache occurring on 15 or more days per month.

In all studies, the timeframe should be defined. Caseness in headache epidemiological studies usually implies an active headache disorder, defined in ICHD-II as headache during the last year [21]; hence *1-year prevalence* is most used, and it allows the most comparisons with previous studies. Shorter timeframes (6-month and 3-month) are also quite common, but adopt different definitions of caseness.

Recall errors probably generate some information bias, not least because they are greater in the elderly. Obviously, these are greater over longer periods: very short and recent timeframes, such as *1-day prevalence* (headache today, or yesterday) avoid recall problems almost completely. Estimates of 1-day prevalence do not describe the proportion of the population with an active headache disorder, but they yield very accurate information on burden in the population ([22]; also, Chap. 7).

Headache yesterday is probably most correctly estimated when respondents are contacted directly by face-to-face interview or telephone, and not given the opportunity to choose when to answer. If the question is posed by letter, for example, it is conceivable (indeed, not unlikely) that people with headache on the day of receiving it will postpone answering until the first headache-free day, resulting in a spuriously high reported prevalence of headache yesterday.

Life-time prevalence ("Have you ever had headache?") has mostly been used for the rarer headache disorders such as cluster headache because it increases the likelihood of finding cases. It is also relevant in genetic epidemiological studies, which must eliminate those who have ever had the disorder from control groups. Here, recall error may be problematic, especially in the elderly; young people may have better recall, but there is no "long ago".

Lifetime, 1-year and 1-day prevalences can be ascertained in a single study with appropriate design and enquiry.

To detect cases, most studies use a two-stage procedure. First, a *screening question* asks participants whether they have headache or not (within the designated timeframe); second, those answering affirmatively are posed the diagnostic questions. In some studies, screening employs a relatively simple self-administered questionnaire, whereas, in the second stage, screen-positive participants are subjected to more thorough face-to-face or telephone interviews. Two-stage procedures are time-saving and avoid irrelevant enquiry, but are at risk from false-negative screening. Hence, sensitivity may be lower, particularly for minor headache complaints, than is achieved by subjecting all participants to full personal interview.

The screening question(s) that define headache caseness are of crucial importance, since the study results depend to a large degree on their exact phrasing. A neutral question (such as "Have you had headache during the last year?") will include almost all cases, even those for whom headache is only a minor nuisance, yielding higher prevalence estimates than a non-neutral question specifying degree, frequency, intensity or circumstances of its occurrence [23] ("Have you *suffered from* headache?", "Have you had *frequent* headache?", "Have you had *bad* headache?", "Have you had headache *not due to* hangover, head injury, flu or common cold?"). Screening questions should always be reported *verbatim*.

After a neutral question, additional questions can then *sieve* participants: identify, and perhaps exclude, those with very low frequency (e.g., <1/month), intensity or functional impairment, who are of less interest from medical or public-health perspectives.

Most headache epidemiological studies wish to distinguish between different *headache types*. For this purpose, diagnostic questions built into the structured questionnaire should, ideally, apply ICHD-3 criteria [11]. However, these criteria were primarily designed for clinical use and not for epidemiological enquiry, for which they are not particularly well-suited: their strict application requires that all participants are personally interviewed by a competent clinician and, in many cases, examined, which is rarely feasible. Additionally, they are expressed in technical language, which is particularly relevant in distinguishing between migraine and TTH, the two most common disorders. Questions about headache duration [2] require patients to consider untreated attacks, which they may never have, or last had long ago. There are no easy lay explanations of photo- and phonophobia. In epidemiological studies, there must be modifications of these criteria, which, therefore, should be tested in a validation study (see below). All modifications should be reported (not engulfed in the unhelpful expression, "modified ICHD criteria").

Migraine aura is very difficult to diagnose by questionnaire. For this reason, it should not dictate the broader diagnosis of migraine.

The group of disorders characterized by headache on 15 or more days per month present a particular problem, since precise diagnosis, from enquiry at a single point in time, is generally difficult and often impossible (or, at least, highly unreliable). The important subgroup with medication overuse can be identified, but labelled only as "probable MOH", since causation cannot be established.

Diagnoses are best made by *algorithm*, applied after interview to the recorded responses [19]. This separates the (non-expert) interviewer from the diagnostic process, and, when there are multiple interviewers, ensures uniformity in the process. The algorithmic flow is important: probable MOH should be diagnosed before the primary headaches, and migraine before TTH. Probable migraine and probable TTH follow (see below).

An alternative approach to diagnosing headache types is a *recognition-based method*, presenting descriptions (case vignettes) or pictorial representations of different headaches to participants [24]. Recognition-based diagnosis is appropriate and convenient—and may give the most accurate results—in certain settings and populations (especially young children).

6.2.2.9 "Definite" and "Probable" Diagnoses

ICHD-3 allows the diagnosis of *probable* headaches types when all but one of the diagnostic criteria for a disorder are met, provided that not all are met for another disorder [11]. For example, a headache cannot be diagnosed as probable migraine if it meets the criteria for TTH. In epidemiological studies, common experience is that about half of diagnoses are probable according to these rules [25, 26], while validation studies in subgroups of the same populations find, according to expert diagnoses, that fewer than 10% are probable. This may be a consequence of applying modified ICHD-3 criteria in the main study, but not in the validation; however, empirically, duration of (supposedly untreated) attacks appears to be unreliably reported.

"Probable migraine" and "probable TTH" are not separate diagnostic entities, and it is unhelpful to report them as though they were. Cases of "probable migraine", not meeting the criteria for TTH, are more probably migraine than anything else, and vice versa. The guidelines recommend that "definite migraine" and "probable migraine" be reported separately, then combined ("all migraine") for further analysis; and, similarly, "definite TTH" and "probable TTH" ("all TTH") [5]. When a diagnostic algorithm is applied, diagnoses must be made in the order dictated by ICHD-3 [11]: migraine, TTH, probable migraine, probable TTH.

6.2.2.10 How Many Diagnoses in Each Individual?

Participants in epidemiological surveys may have more than one headache type. This poses problems, since it may be difficult for them to remember which features belong to which headache type, and attribute them accordingly; only a headache specialist as interviewer can sort this out correctly. A solution, valid for public-health purposes, is to ask the participant to identify the *most bothersome headache* (the one, in his or her mind, that interferes most with life), and focus solely on this when responding. This approach, adopted in the Headache-Attributed Restriction, Disability, Social Handicap and Impaired Participation (HARDSHIP) questionnaire ([19]; also, Chap. 7), will tend to underestimate less troubling headache types, therefore systematically neglecting TTH among participants with both TTH and migraine. Arguably, the observed prevalence of TTH in studies where this is done should be inflated by the same proportion of those with migraine. This is rarely done: conservatism is preferred.

Multiple diagnoses require more questions, discouraging participation and leading to a lower participation proportion; studies should carefully assess their value. When the purpose is to assess population headache burden, it is neither realistic nor necessary to assess the burden attributable to each headache type in each person. For public-health purposes, it is more important to avoid double counting, which this might encourage.

6.2.2.11 Validation of the Questionnaire

Diagnostic accuracy is usually important. *Diagnostic validation* is performed preferably in a randomly selected sub-sample of participants in the main study; stratified sampling, according to caseness and diagnosis (no headache, migraine, TTH or probable MOH), can then ensure adequate numbers of each. Otherwise, a separate sample is drawn from the population of interest, but stratification is then not possible. Headache patients are *not* an acceptable substitute: their headache disorders are not representative of those of the population of interest, and, often with more knowledge of headache and experience of anamnesis, their performance is conditioned when answering questionnaires.

Validation requires that participants are re-interviewed by a headache expert (a physician skilled in headache diagnosis and familiar with the culture and language of the respondent), applying clinical skills to diagnose (the "gold standard") while being ignorant of the questionnaire diagnoses. To minimize discrepancies due to change in the headache itself, expert interviews should follow soon after the original diagnoses (no more than 1 month). They are preferably conducted face-to-face, but telephone interviews are an acceptable resource-conserving alternative when respondents are widely spread geographically.

Questionnaire-derived and expert diagnoses are then compared, which allows calculation of the instrument's sensitivity, specificity, positive and negative predictive values and kappa value for each diagnosis [27]. The precision (confidence interval) of the estimate for each diagnosis is dependent on the number with that diagnosis in the validation sample. Validations performed in the last decade have typically included 180–500 participants overall, drawn randomly as a sub-sample from the main study, giving relatively narrow confidence intervals for migraine and TTH [25–29] but not always for probable MOH [27]. Validation of the screening question ("Have you had headache ...?") is achieved in those who answered "No".

The validation study can inform and optimize the diagnostic algorithm: small amendments can be made (e.g., excluding from the diagnostic criteria for migraine the minimum duration of 4 h, which has been found empirically to cause problems), and the comparisons remade between questionnaire-derived and expert diagnoses, which may or may not lead to improvement. There is usually a trade-off between sensitivity and specificity: one increases at the expense of the other. Genetic studies require caseness certainty, and therefore high specificity; for most other studies, the algorithm that gives the highest overall diagnostic accuracy (sum of sensitivity and specificity) is preferable.

Validation is clearly not possible in countries with no headache experts (no gold standard available); yet, in such countries, studies of headache burden may be of particular importance. In these circumstances, it is advisable to employ a diagnostic questionnaire used and validated already, in multiple languages and cultures.

6.2.2.12 Data-Entry

Data should be recorded in the most practical way, which is usually on paper, but sometimes directly into computer. Highly portable tablet computers promise direct computer-entry as the way of the future, with the very great advantage of obviating data transcription.

When data must be transferred from source documents to computer, rigorous quality controls are essential, ideally employing full double data-entry (two people independently transcribe all data) to produce two full datasets. These are electronically compared to detect errors (inconsistencies), which are resolved by reference to the source documents. At minimum, the proportion of errors should be estimated in a subset of the data (e.g., 10% of items), entered twice. If this proportion (including its confidence interval) is judged likely to have more than negligible influence on the results to be reported, full double data-entry is required.

6.2.3 Special Issues

6.2.3.1 Studies of Particular Age Groups

In countries with obligatory schooling, representative samples of *children and adolescents* of school age can be obtained by selecting all, or a random sample, of the pupils of a representative sample of schools. This is a cluster-sampling method, and selected schools should reflect the diversities of the country or region with regard to socio-economic status and area of habitation (rural or urban). Interviews may be undertaken by specially trained interviewers, or by a teacher or school nurse. For small children, some information may have to be given by parents or teachers.

Somewhat different diagnostic criteria apply in these age groups, although still essentially based on ICHD-3 ([30]; also, Chap. 3). Diagnostic instruments require modification accordingly, and, of course, these and other measuring instruments must reflect the language and comprehension skills of the age range. Validation of the diagnostic method is as important as in studies on adults.

Studies in *elderly populations* (usually defined as >65 years of age) can expect lower prevalences of primary headache disorders and higher prevalences of secondary headaches, more comorbidities, reduced mental and physical capacities (which may affect engagement and ease of data collection), and lower workforce participation (which affects the impact of headache and the way burden is estimated). For these reasons, larger samples may be needed, and there may be more focus on diagnosis of secondary headaches—at least to avoid their misdiagnosis as primary headache disorders when these are the object of interest. Comorbidities, as potential confounders in estimations of burden, may also require greater consideration, and more importance attached to adjustments for comorbidities in analysis.

6.2.3.2 Studies of Rare Headaches

Prevalence of rare headaches is difficult to assess. Very large samples are needed and, because they are not easily identified through self-administered questionnaires, headache experts must usually make the diagnoses.

However, only rare headaches that are severe, for example, cluster headache and trigeminal neuralgia, are of any public-health interest. Conditions such as these demand medical attention, which, in societies with good access to medical care and well-kept electronic (i.e., searchable) records, makes it possible to detect potential cases by screening large clinic populations such as general practitioners' lists. Diagnoses, in far smaller numbers of candidates, can then be ascertained by expert interview [31].

Most published prevalence estimates of rare headaches are of lifetime prevalence, because cases are more numerous; but current prevalence (1-year or 1-day) is likely to be of greater interest.

6.2.3.3 Stand-Alone Studies Versus Large Health Surveys

A relatively long questionnaire, such as HARDSHIP ([19]; also, Chap. 7), is most suited to a study wholly dedicated to headache (*stand-alone study*).

The large burden arising from headache disorders should equally motivate analytical epidemiological studies to determine risk factors and causes of headache (see Chap. 10), some of which may be preventable. These purposes may not be achievable within the same studies that measure prevalence and burden: they require, in addition, collection and registration of relevant exposure data, and follow-up studies, possible only in *large health surveys* that register multiple disorders and potential risk factors.

However, large health surveys cannot feasibly include a full headache questionnaire; instead, the necessary minimum is a valid screening question for active headache disorder, some questions allowing determination of severity (frequency, intensity and duration), and ideally a question set for the diagnosis of migraine and TTH (as mutually exclusive diagnoses). Validation of these questions remains as important as in stand-alone studies.

6.3 Concluding Remarks

This chapter recounts, and slightly updates, consensus methodological guidelines for headache epidemiological studies first published in 2014 [5]. It makes recommendations covering ethical aspects, key epidemiological concepts and the methodological issues around study design, sample selection, accessing and engaging participants, study instruments, diagnosis of headache types and sources of error.

Its purpose is not to inform those who are planning studies (who should refer to the original) so much as to assist critical evaluation of published reports of headache prevalence and burden, given that these are of very variable quality.

References

1. Vos T, Abajobir AA, Abate KH, Abbafati C, Abbas KM, Abd-Allah F, Abdulkader RS, Abdulle AM, Abebo TA, Abera SF, Aboyans V, Abu-Raddad LJ, Ackerman IN, Adamu AA, Adetokunboh O, Afarideh M, Afshin A, Agarwal SK, Aggarwal R, Agrawal A, Agrawal S, Ahmadieh H, Ahmed MB, Aichour MTE, Aichour AN, Aichour I, Aiyar S, Akinyemi RO, Akseer N, Al Lami FH, Alahdab F, Al-Aly Z, Alam K, Alam N, Alam T, et al. Global, regional, and national incidence, prevalence, and years lived with disability for 328 diseases and injuries for 195 countries, 1990–2016: a systematic analysis for the Global Burden of Disease Study 2016. Lancet. 2017;390:1211–59.
2. Stovner LJ, Hagen K, Jensen R, Katsarava Z, Lipton R, Scher A, Steiner TJ, Zwart JA. The global burden of headache: a documentation of headache prevalence and disability worldwide. Cephalalgia. 2007;27:193–210.
3. Stovner LJ, Scher AI. Epidemiology of headache. In: Olesen J, Goadsby PJ, Ramadan NM, Tfelt-Hansen P, Welch KMA, editors. The headaches. 3rd ed. Philadelphia: Lippincott Williams & Wilkins; 2005. p. 17–26.
4. Steiner TJ, Stovner LJ, Al Jumah M, Birbeck GL, Gururaj G, Jensen R, Katsarava Z, Queiroz LP, Scher AI, Tekle-Haimanot R, Wang S-J, Martelletti P, Dua T, Chatterji S. Improving quality in population surveys of headache prevalence, burden and cost: key methodological considerations. J Headache Pain. 2013;14:87.
5. Stovner LJ, Al Jumah M, Birbeck GL, Gururaj G, Jensen R, Katsarava Z, Queiroz LP, Scher AI, Tekle-Haimanot R, Wang SJ, Steiner TJ. The methodology of population surveys of headache prevalence, burden and cost: principles and recommendations from the Global Campaign against Headache. J Headache Pain. 2014;15:5.
6. Vos T, Flaxman AD, Naghavi M, Lozano R, Michaud C, Ezzati M, Shibuya K, Salomon JA, Abdalla S, Aboyans V, Abraham J, Ackerman I, Aggarwal R, Ahn SY, Ali MK, Alvarado M, Anderson HR, Anderson LM, Andrews KG, Atkinson C, Baddour LM, Bahalim AN, Barker-Collo S, Barrero LH, Bartels DH, Basáñez MG, Baxter A, Bell ML, Benjamin EJ, Bennett D, Bernabé E, Bhalla K, Bhandari B, Bikbov B, Bin Abdulhak A, et al. Years lived with disability

(YLD) for 1160 sequelae of 289 diseases and injuries 1990–2010: a systematic analysis for the Global Burden of Disease Study 2010. Lancet. 2012;380:2163–96.

7. Stovner LJ, Andrée C. Prevalence of headache in Europe: a review for the Eurolight project. J Headache Pain. 2010;11:289–99.
8. Gallo V, Egger M, McCormack V, Farmer PB, Ioannidis JPA, Kirsch-Volders M, Matullo G, Phillips DH, Schoket B, Stromberg U, Vermeulen R, Wild C, Porta M, Vineis P. STrengthening the Reporting of OBservational studies in Epidemiology—Molecular Epidemiology (STROBE-ME): an extension of the STROBE statement. PLoS Med. 2011;8:e1001117.
9. Vandenbroucke JP, von Elm E, Altman DG, Gotzsche PC, Mulrow CD, Pocock SJ, Poole C, Schlesselman JJ, Egger M. Strengthening the Reporting of Observational Studies in Epidemiology (STROBE): explanation and elaboration. Epidemiology. 2007;18:805–35.
10. Hennekens CH, Buring JE. Epidemiology in medicine. Philadelphia: Lippincott, Williams & Wilkins; 1987.
11. Headache Classification Committee of the International Headache Society. The international classification of headache disorders. 3rd edition. Cephalalgia. 2018;38:1–211.
12. Beauchamp TL, Childress JF. Principles of biomedical ethics. 6th ed. New York: Oxford University Press; 2008.
13. Steiner TJ. Ethical issues in headache research and management. Report and recommendations. Cephalalgia. 1998;18:505–29.
14. Steiner TJ. Ethical issues arising from commercial sponsorship and from relationships with the pharmaceutical industry—report and recommendations of the Ethics Subcommittee of the International Headache Society. Cephalalgia. 2008;28(Suppl 3):1–25.
15. Olson SH, Kelsey JL, Pearson TA, Levin B. Evaluation of random digit dialing as a method of control selection in case-control studies. Am J Epidemiol. 1992;135:210–22.
16. Linde M, Dahlöf C. Attitudes and burden of disease among self-considered migraineurs—a nation-wide population-based survey in Sweden. Cephalalgia. 2004;24:455–65.
17. Linde M, Gustavsson A, Stovner LJ, Steiner TJ, Barré J, Katsarava Z, Lainez JM, Lampl C, Lantéri-Minet M, Rastenyte D, Ruiz de la Torre E, Tassorelli C, Andrée C. The cost of headache disorders in Europe: the Eurolight project. Eur J Neurol. 2012;19:703–11.
18. Schaeffer RL, Ott RL, Mendenhall W, Gerow KG. Elementary survey sampling. 7th ed. Belmont, CA: Duxbury Press; 2011.
19. Steiner TJ, Gururaj G, Andrée C, Katsarava Z, Ayzenberg I, Yu SY, Al Jumah M, Tekle-Haimanot R, Birbeck GL, Herekar A, Linde M, Mbewe E, Manandhar K, Risal A, Jensen R, Queiroz LP, Scher AI, Wang SJ, Stovner LJ. Diagnosis, prevalence estimation and burden measurement in population surveys of headache: presenting the HARDSHIP questionnaire. J Headache Pain. 2014;15:3.
20. Peters M, Bertelote JM, Houchin C, Kandoura T, Steiner TJ. Translation protocols. J Headache Pain. 2007;8(suppl 1):S40–7.
21. Classification Subcommittee of the International Headache Society. The international classification of headache disorders. 2nd edition. Cephalalgia. 2004;24(Suppl 1):1–160.
22. Yu S, He M, Liu R, Feng J, Qiao X, Yang X, Cao X, Zhao G, Fang Y, Steiner TJ. Headache yesterday in China: a new approach to estimating the burden of headache, applied in a general-population survey in China. Cephalalgia. 2013;33:1211–7.
23. Stovner LJ, Zwart JA, Hagen K, Terwindt G, Pascual J. Epidemiology of headache in Europe. Eur J Neurol. 2006;13:333–45.
24. Zwart JA, Dyb G, Stovner LJ, Sand T, Holmen TL. The validity of 'recognition-based' headache diagnoses in adolescents. Data from the Nord-Trondelag health study 1995–97, head-HUNT-youth. Cephalalgia. 2003;23:223–9.
25. Yu S-Y, Cao X-T, Zhao G, Yang X-S, Qiao X-Y, Fang Y-N, Feng J-C, Liu R-Z, Steiner TJ. The burden of headache in China: validation of diagnostic questionnaire for a population-based survey. J Headache Pain. 2011;12:141–6.
26. Ayzenberg I, Katsarava Z, Mathalikov R, Chernysh M, Osipova V, Tabeeva G, Steiner TJ. The burden of headache in Russia: validation of the diagnostic questionnaire in a population-based sample. Eur J Neurol. 2011;18:454–9.

27. Hagen K, Zwart JA, Aamodt AH, Nilsen KB, Brathen G, Helde G, Stjern M, Tronvik EA, Stovner LJ. The validity of questionnaire-based diagnoses: the third Nord-Trondelag health study 2006–2008. J Headache Pain. 2010;11:67–73.
28. Lipton RB, Dodick D, Sadovsky R, Kolodner K, Endicott J, Hettiarachchi J, Harrison W. A self-administered screener for migraine in primary care: the ID migraine validation study. Neurology. 2003;61:375–82.
29. Kukava M, Dzagnidze A, Mirvelashvili E, Djibuti M, Fritsche G, Jensen R, Stovner LJ, Steiner TJ, Katsarava Z. Validation of a Georgian language headache questionnaire in a population-based sample. J Headache Pain. 2007;8:321–4.
30. Wöber C, Wöber-Bingöl C, Uluduz D, Aslan TS, Uygunoglu U, Tüfekçi A, Alp SI, Duman T, Sürgün F, Emir GK, Demir CF, Balgetir F, Özdemir YB, Auer T, Siva A, Steiner TJ. Undifferentiated headache: broadening the approach to headache in children and adolescents, with supporting evidence from a nationwide school-based cross-sectional survey in Turkey. J Headache Pain. 2018;19:18.
31. Torelli P, Beghi E, Manzoni GC. Cluster headache prevalence in the Italian general population. Neurology. 2005;64:469–74.

Chapter 7
Methodology of Headache Measurement

Timothy J. Steiner and Lars Jacob Stovner

7.1 Introduction

This chapter discusses headache *measurement* in populations: prevalence estimation and quantification of headache-attributed burden. While there is academic interest in this, particularly for comparisons, its primary purpose is to inform health policy.

The focus is on the individual enquiry, addressed to a respondent within a sample who has been identified and engaged. The prior processes of selection and engagement are crucial: respondents not representative of the group for whom they speak will provide information that is at best meaningless and at worst misleading. These processes, *inter alia*, are discussed in Chap. 6.

The ideas and recommendations presented here come from a broad expert base and are supported by worldwide experience. Reduction of the burden of headache worldwide is the central purpose of the Global Campaign against Headache ([1–5]; also Chaps. 5 and 14). The Campaign's objectives require action supported by awareness, the latter underpinned by knowledge of the levels, nationally and worldwide, of headache-related ill health and healthcare need. Knowledge shows what

T. J. Steiner (✉)
Department of Neuromedicine and Movement Science, NTNU Norwegian University of Science and Technology, Trondheim, Norway

Division of Brain Sciences, Imperial College London, London, UK
e-mail: t.steiner@imperial.ac.uk

L. J. Stovner
Department of Neuromedicine and Movement Science, NTNU Norwegian University of Science and Technology, Trondheim, Norway

Norwegian Advisory Unit on Headaches, Department of Neurology and Clinical Neurophysiology, St Olavs University Hospital, Trondheim, Norway
e-mail: lars.stovner@ntnu.no

T. J. Steiner, L. J. Stovner (eds.), *Societal Impact of Headache*, Headache,
https://doi.org/10.1007/978-3-030-24728-7_7

manner of change—and how much—is required. It supports the humanitarian, economic and political arguments for change, and it signals the priority that should be accorded to action for change. The knowledge base is the foundation on which everything must be built.

The knowledge base, however, is incomplete. The Global Campaign began to address this 15 years ago, planning and implementing population-based studies in Georgia [6], India [7], China [8], Russia [9], Pakistan [10], Ethiopia [11], Zambia [12], Nepal [13], Mongolia, Saudi Arabia, Morocco, Benin, Cameroon and Peru [not yet published], and providing intellectual support for the 10-country Eurolight project [14]. Required for these were both a standardized protocol [15] and a survey instrument, the Headache-Attributed Restriction, Disability, Social Handicap and Impaired Participation (HARDSHIP) questionnaire [16].

The questionnaire is the basis of this chapter. There is, inevitably, some overlap with and repetition of the content of Chap. 6.

7.2 The HARDSHIP Questionnaire

Many people, not only the group providing expert opinion from a variety of backgrounds but also local investigators from over 20 countries, were involved in the design of HARDSHIP. The diagnostic questions have been the subject of several validation studies, in India (translated into Kannada) [7], China (translated into Mandarin Chinese) [8], Russia (translated into Russian) [9] and Pakistan (translated into Urdu) [10]. HARDSHIP has undergone testing in many cultures and settings: so far in 20 countries and 19 languages.

HARDSHIP is a structured questionnaire which may be administered by medical or (more usually) trained lay interviewers (see Chap. 6). It has a modular design [16]: separate question sets cover demographic characteristics (Table 7.1), screen for caseness (headache disorder present or not) (Table 7.2), diagnose headache type (Tables 7.3, 7.4, and 7.5) and address each of the several quantifiable components of burden (see Chap. 4) (Tables 7.6, 7.7, 7.8, 7.9, 7.10, 7.11, and 7.12). The modular design renders it highly amenable to adaptation. Separate modules, each of which may be included or not according to study purpose, time constraints, resources available and cultural sensitivities, cover the quantifiable range of components of headache-attributed burden (Table 7.6).

7.2.1 Demographic Enquiry

This preliminary enquiry (Table 7.1) is essential. It characterizes the sample, and allows comparison between those who have been selected and the population of interest from whom they are drawn, and of whom they are intended to be representative (see Chap. 6).

Ideally the enquiry will reflect all factors that may influence prevalence and/or burden of headache, but in practice this objective is limited by the availability of data characterizing the entire population. National census statistics are commonly available for gender and age distributions. Even when they are not, these are of such prime importance in headache epidemiology that they must be known in the sample. Social situation (especially wealth), habitation (urban or rural) and ethnicity and/or culture may be important influencers of prevalence or burden, and are therefore of some interest.

Table 7.1 Demographic module in HARDSHIP

Question	Response options
Demographic enquiry	
What is your age?	Number of years
What is your gender?	Male/female
Habitation	Urban/semi-urban/rural [alternatively: urban/rural]
Social situation enquiry	
What is your marital status?	Single/married/widowed/separated or divorced
Are you living with a household partner? (husband or wife, or an unmarried partner of either gender in a stable relationship)	No/yes
Which of these is closest to your personal situation?	Employed or self-employed/homemaker or housewife/student/unemployed/retired
Which of these best describes your work?	Professional/semi-professional/skilled worker/semi-skilled worker/unskilled worker [these categories are suggestions; they should be adapted and/or supplemented as appropriate for the country]
What is your total net household income per year? [alternatively: What is your total net personal income?]	Five bands corresponding to the national household income quintiles, so that one-fifth of the population falls into each income category; [in the alternative, five bands corresponding to national per capita income quintiles]
How many years did you complete in full-time education?	Number of years at school or places of higher education
What is your native language (the language you first learned to speak)?	Name of language
What language do you usually speak in your own home? [this question may, if appropriate, be replaced or supplemented by questions on ethnicity]	Name of language

Table 7.2 Screen module in HARDSHIP

Question	Response options
Have you ever had a headache in your lifetime?	No/yes
Have you had a headache during the last 12 months?	No/yes
During the last 30 days, on how many of these days did you have a headache?	Number of days

Table 7.3 Frequent headache module (15 or more days/month) in HARDSHIP

Question	Response options
How long do these headaches usually last?	Number of minutes/number of hours/never goes away
Do you take any medication to *treat* these headaches?	No/yes
What medication do you use most to treat these headaches? And what other medications do you also take for this purpose?	None/name(s) of the most-used and other medications
Altogether, on how many days in the last 30 days did you take these medications?	Number of days

Table 7.4 Diagnostic module in HARDSHIP

Question (addressed to the headache type described as most bothersome when more than one type is reported)	Response options
How often do you have this type of headache?	Every day/number of days per month/number of days per year
How long does this type of headache usually last?	Number of minutes/number of hours/never goes away
Is your last answer with or without medication? And, if appropriate: How long would it last if you did not take medication?	With/without Number of minutes/number of hours/number of days
How bad is this type of headache usually?	Not bad/quite bad/very bad
There are many ways of describing a headache, but most are either throbbing or pressing. Thinking still of this type of headache, which best describes the pain?	Throbbing or pulsating/pressing, squeezing or tightening
Is the pain of this type of headache usually on only one side of the head?	No/yes
Does exercise (like walking or climbing stairs) tend to make it worse?	No/yes
Thinking still of this type of headache, how does it affect your ability to do day-to-day activities?	Can do everything as normal/cannot do some things/can do nothing
With this type of headache, do you usually feel nauseated (as though you may vomit or throw up)?	No/yes
With this type of headache, do you usually actually vomit (throw up)?	No/yes
When you have this type of headache, does daylight or other lighting bother you? In other words, do you prefer to be in the dark?	No/not sure/yes
When you have this type of headache, does noise bother you? In other words, do you prefer to be in the quiet?	No/not sure/yes

Table 7.5 Sensitivities and specificities of the HARDSHIP diagnostic question set, for migraine and tension-type headache, in published studies

	Migraine		Tension-type headache	
Study	Sensitivity	Specificity	Sensitivity	Specificity
India [7][a]	0.63	0.85	0.57	0.81
China [8][b]	0.83	0.99	0.51	0.99
Russia [9][c]	0.77	0.82	0.64	0.91
Pakistan [10][d]	0.74	0.87	0.60	0.92

[a]Translated into Kannada
[b]Translated into Mandarin Chinese
[c]Translated into Russian
[d]Translated into Urdu

Table 7.6 The components of headache-attributed burden covered by modules within the HARDSHIP questionnaire (with references to other tables)

1. Symptom burden (Table 7.4)
2. Treatments, and health-resource utilization (Table 7.7)
3. Disability and productive time losses (Tables 7.8 and 7.9)
4. Interictal burden (Table 7.10)
5. Quality of life and subjective well-being (Tables 7.11 and 7.12)
6. Perception of control (Table 7.13)
7. Overall individual burden (willingness to pay for treatment as a summary measure) (Table 7.14)
8. Cumulative burden (impact on education, career and earnings) (Table 7.15)
9. Effects on relationships, love life and family dynamics (Table 7.16)
10. Burden on others, including household partner and children (Table 7.17)
11. Financial cost (Tables 7.7, 7.8, and 7.9)

Table 7.7 Health-resource utilization module in HARDSHIP

Question	Response options
Many different medications may be used successfully to treat headache. Some are prescription-only, while others can be bought over the counter. Please look at this list. Which of these have you used in the last month?	Nothing at all/number of days for each of a country-specific list of medications
Are there any other medications you have used to treat your headache in the last month?	Name(s) of medication(s) and number of days for each
Medications to prevent headaches are usually taken daily. Are you taking any of these now? If so, how long for?	None/number of weeks or months for each of a country-specific list of medications
Many people with headache treat themselves, but others need professional advice. Have you had professional advice about your headaches in the last year? Who from, and how many times?	No-one/number of times for each of a country-specific list of healthcare providers
Most people with headache do not require any investigations, but occasionally these tests are done. Because of your headaches, have you had any of these tests in the last year?	None/MRI brain scan/CT brain scan/X-rays of the neck/eye tests (for glasses)/blood tests [the list may be adapted or supplemented as appropriate for the country]
Have you, in the last year, been admitted to hospital because of your headaches?	No/yes, and total number of days in hospital

Table 7.8 Disability (lost productivity) module in HARDSHIP

Question	Response
On how many days in the last 3 months could you not go to work or school because of your headaches?	Number of days
On how many days in the last 3 months could you do less than half your usual amount in your job or schoolwork because of your headaches?	Number of days
On how many days in the last 3 months could you not do any household work because of your headaches?	Number of days
On how many days in the last 3 months could you do less than half your usual amount of household work because of your headaches?	Number of days
On how many days in the last 3 months did you miss family, social or leisure activities because of your headaches?	Number of days

Table 7.9 HARDSHIP module on headache yesterday

Question	Response options
Did you have a headache yesterday?	No/yes
If yes, was this the type of headache you have just been describing? [i.e., the headache type that has been diagnosed]	No/yes
Please think about the headache you had yesterday. How long did it last?	All day/number of hours
How bad was this headache yesterday?	Not bad/quite bad/very bad
Please think about everything you wanted to do yesterday if you had not had a headache. How much of this did you actually do?	Nothing/less than half/more than half/everything
Was yesterday a workday (either at your job or at school)?	No/yes
If yes, because of your headache, did you miss work or school yesterday?	No/arrived late, took time out during the day or left early (plus total number of hours lost)/missed the whole day
If you were at work or school with your headache yesterday, how much of your work did you get done?	Nothing/less than half/more than half/everything
Will you able to make up for this today or later?	No/partly/completely/not applicable
Please think about household work or general chores that you wanted to do yesterday if you had not had headache. How much of this did you actually do?	Nothing/less than half/more than half/everything
Please think about leisure and social activities that you wanted to do yesterday if you had not had headache. How much of this did you actually do? (please tick one box)	Nothing/less than half/more than half/everything
What treatment did you take for the headache you had yesterday?	Nothing at all/names of all medications and the number of times each was taken

Table 7.10 HARDSHIP module on interictal burden

Question	Response options
When (how long ago) was the last day when you did not have a headache?	Number of days (if no headache yesterday, enter 1 day)/number of weeks/cannot remember
On that day, were you anxious or worried about your next headache episode?	No/yes
On that day, was there anything you could not do or did not do because you wanted to avoid getting a headache?	No/yes
On that day, did you feel completely free from all headache-related symptoms?	No/yes

Table 7.11 HARDSHIP module on quality of life (adapted from [26])

Question	Response options
These questions should be answered by all respondents, including those without headache.	
How would you rate your quality of life?	Very poor/poor/neither poor nor good/good/very good
How satisfied are you with your health?	Very dissatisfied/dissatisfied/neither satisfied nor dissatisfied/satisfied/very satisfied
How satisfied are you with your ability to perform your daily living activities?	Very dissatisfied/dissatisfied/neither satisfied nor dissatisfied/satisfied/very satisfied
How satisfied are you with yourself?	Very dissatisfied/dissatisfied/neither satisfied nor dissatisfied/satisfied/very satisfied
How satisfied are you with your personal relationships?	Very dissatisfied/dissatisfied/neither satisfied nor dissatisfied/satisfied/very satisfied
How satisfied are you with the conditions of your living place?	Very dissatisfied/dissatisfied/neither satisfied nor dissatisfied/satisfied/very satisfied
Do you have enough energy for everyday life?	Not at all/a little/moderately/mostly/completely
Have you enough money to meet your needs?	Not at all/a little/moderately/mostly/completely

Table 7.12 HARDSHIP module on subjective well-being (adapted from [27])

Question	Response options
These questions should be answered by all respondents, including those without headache.	
Overall, how satisfied are you with your life nowadays?	0–10 (where 0 is not at all satisfied and 10 is completely satisfied)
Overall, to what extent do you feel that the things you do in your life are worthwhile?	0–10 (where 0 is not at all worthwhile and 10 is completely worthwhile)
Overall, how happy did you feel yesterday?	0–10 (where 0 is not at all happy and 10 is completely happy)
Overall, how anxious did you feel yesterday?	0–10 (where 0 is not at all anxious and 10 is completely anxious)

7.2.2 Screen Questions

These are crucial. They define caseness and avoid superfluous enquiry among those without headache. At the same time, if formulated inappropriately they jeopardize the enquiry by excluding cases. Neutral questions are recommended ([15]; also, Chap. 6), since qualifiers (as in "Have you *suffered* from headache?", "Have you had *frequent* headache?" or "Have you had headache *not due to hangover, trauma, flu or common cold*?") introduce subjective interpretations into the definition of caseness.

The third question in Table 7.2 leads to additional enquiry (especially into medication use) in those who report 15 or more days (Table 7.3).

7.2.3 Diagnostic Enquiry

Diagnosis in epidemiological enquiry must follow ICHD criteria [17], because these are the common language of definition and description of headache disorders [15]. However, ICHD criteria were not designed for this purpose, and are not particularly well suited to it ([15]; also, Chap. 6). Diagnoses are *not* made by the interviewer(s): responses to the diagnostic questions (Table 7.4) are transformed into diagnoses algorithmically [16]. The ICHD criteria must therefore be built into a structured questionnaire, although this is not how diagnoses are usually made in clinical settings. Open questions are difficult to interpret and categorize, and do not permit algorithmic determination.

The likelihood of multiple headache types occurring in a single respondent is recognized, and the potential confusion arising therefrom is minimized by asking the respondent to identify, and focus upon, the one that is subjectively the most bothersome (see Chap. 6). Diagnostic questions, and subsequent enquiries into burden, are directed expressly at this headache type. Headache occurring on 15 or more days/month is separated from episodic headache and categorized as with or without medication overuse (Table 7.3); it cannot be diagnosed algorithmically beyond this. MOH is diagnosable in cross-sectional studies only as an association of medication overuse with frequent headache (there is no evidence available of causation) [15]. Therefore, all such cases are *probable* MOH, and it is important to recognize this limitation during analyses and interpretation.

Certain criteria distinguishing between migraine and TTH pose particular problems in population surveys [15]. First, empirically it has been found difficult to gather correct responses on headache duration [18], requiring patients to consider *untreated* attacks, which they may never have or last had long ago. This results in a high proportion of probable diagnoses because duration criteria appear unfulfilled [17]. Second, there are no easy lay explanations of photo- and phonophobia, which are technical concepts, and even more difficult is to specify what degrees of photo- and phonophobia fulfil migraine criteria in ICHD [17]. False-positive responses, more likely when answers are forced (because the response option of “don’t know” is diagnostically unhelpful), push diagnoses towards migraine. HARDSHIP includes a “not sure” option (Table 7.4), and applies a rule that “not sure” implies absence of the symptom. The reasoning is that presence of a symptom creates a definite awareness of it, and only its absence allows uncertainty.

Diagnostic validation studies have been conducted in a number of countries, with results so far published from India [7], China [8], Russia [9] and Pakistan [10] (Table 7.5). Specificities for migraine and TTH were high (range 0.82–0.99) but, in all studies, sensitivity was better for migraine (range 0.63–0.83) than for TTH (0.51–0.64), and relative insensitivity to TTH has been confirmed in all languages and cultures in which HARDSHIP has been used. The problem is attributable partly to the diagnostic questions being necessarily tied to ICHD, which makes it difficult to resolve because there is very limited scope for change. More particularly, though, it is due to the nature of TTH itself. Being usually a mild-to-moderate headache, TTH is more likely than migraine to go unreported. Beyond this, because it lacks specific features, it is diagnosed through absence of the features characteristic of migraine, and, therefore, effectively by default.

7.2.4 *Burden Enquiry*

Multiple modules within HARDSHIP address the recognizable components of headache-attributed burden (Table 7.6).

The common symptoms of pain, nausea, vomiting, photophobia and phonophobia are addressed in HARDSHIP in the diagnostic module (Table 7.4). The enquiry into burden requires quantity estimation, rather than merely establishing whether or not a symptom is present, as in diagnosis. Pain can be quantified at individual level in terms of frequency, subjectively in terms of intensity and somewhat unreliably, it has been noted empirically [18], in terms of duration. Nausea, photophobia and phonophobia are almost impossible to quantify, but their occurrence can be recorded and frequencies expressed as group statistics.

Disability attributed to headache is also difficult to quantify completely. Common proxies are lost time and reduced productivity, for which well-validated instruments exist [19, 20]. HARDSHIP imports the Headache-Attributed Lost Time (HALT-90) index [20] (Table 7.8). Reliability of recall is an issue here. Burden questions have commonly been limited to a 3-month timeframe [19, 20] as a compromise between the limits of recall and the purpose of enquiry. When the latter is the assessment of an individual patient for therapeutic reasons, the period must be long enough to be representative of that individual. In large-group studies, this is quite unnecessary: different considerations apply, because population- rather than individual-representativeness is sought [20]. Variations of HALT that record over shorter timeframes of 1 month (HALT-30) and 1 week (HALT-7) [20] have been tested empirically [21] and can be used instead.

Enquiry into headache yesterday (effectively HALT-1) (Table 7.9) avoids recall problems almost altogether [20, 22–25]. It cannot describe the proportion of the population with an active headache disorder, but it yields very reliable information on burden in each individual and, potentially, a rather precise estimate of population burden on a particular day and therefore on any day (assuming no major seasonal variation). A large sample is necessary, because 1-day prevalence of episodic headache disorders is obviously much lower than 1-year prevalence. This module probably should not be used except in an unscheduled interview (face-to-face or telephone [15]): when the questionnaire is delivered to a person who happens to have headache on that day, he or she may well postpone answering it until their next headache-free day. The result would be a spuriously high count of headache yesterday.

Interictal burden arises because headache attacks are unpleasant, and those who experience them frequently are likely to worry about when the next may occur, and/or attempt to eliminate possible triggers through lifestyle compromise (see Chap. 4). Enquiry into these is possible, at least in terms of prevalence (Table 7.10). Interictal burden, which is continuous, is likely to affect subjective well-being and may be sufficient to impair quality of life. It is perhaps adequately, if not specifically, captured by measures of these. HARDSHIP imports, as modules, WHOQoL-8 [26] (Table 7.11) and the four questions on subjective well-being taken from the UK-ONS 2012 survey [27] (Table 7.12). Interictal burden is also a major factor in perception of control (Table 7.13).

Willingness-to-pay (WTP), established by the "bidding game" method (Table 7.14), is used as an overall summary measure of individual burden, unlikely to be comprehensive but attractive for its simplicity [15]. Its reliability as a burden measure remains unclear: its hypothetical nature allows a potential disconnection between what respondents *say* they will pay and what they actually *will* pay when confronted by the reality. And WTP of course is very much constrained by ability to pay. Nevertheless, this form of enquiry has been used to assess sustainability of healthcare initiatives in resource-poor countries [28].

Table 7.13 HARDSHIP module on perception of control

Question	Response options
Do you feel that your employer and work colleagues understand and accept your headaches?	No/partly/yes, fully
Do you feel that your family and friends understand and accept your headaches?	No/partly/yes, fully
Do you avoid telling people that you have headaches?	No/yes
Taking into account everything you do to treat your headaches, how well do you think you control them?	Not at all/a little/quite well/completely

Table 7.14 HARDSHIP module on overall burden (willingness-to-pay)

Question	Response options
Imagine that there is a treatment you can buy. If you take it, your headaches will no longer bother you. How much would you be willing to pay every month for this treatment? [In the questions below, 5× (in national currency units) should be set at a level at which 50% of respondents are expected to say "yes"]	
1. Would you pay 5× a month?	No/yes [if no, go to question 2; if yes, go to question 5]
2. Would you pay 2× a month?	No/yes, and agreed amount [if no, go to question 3; if yes, agree an amount between 2× and 5× to end this enquiry]
3. Would you pay 1× a month?	No/yes, and agreed amount [if no, go to question 4; if yes, agree an amount between 1× and 2× to end this enquiry]
4. Would you pay anything?	No/yes, and agreed amount [if no, end this enquiry; if yes, agree an amount between 0 and 1× and end this enquiry]
5. Would you pay 10× a month?	No, and agreed amount/yes [if no, agree an amount between 5× and 10× to end this enquiry; if yes, go to question 6]
6. Would you pay 20× a month?	No, and agreed amount/yes [if no, agree an amount between 10× and 20× to end this enquiry; if yes, go to question 7]
7. Would you pay 50× a month?	No, and agreed amount/yes [if no, agree an amount between 20× and 50× to end this enquiry; if yes, go to question 8]
8. Would you pay 100× a month?	No, and agreed amount/yes, and agreed amount [if no, agree an amount between 50× and 100× to end this enquiry; if yes, agree an amount of 100× or more and end this enquiry]

Financial costs are direct (healthcare and treatment costs) and indirect (lost-productivity costs from absenteeism and reduced effectiveness at work). Chapter 12 explores these in detail.

Cumulative burden, accruing over a lifetime (see Chap. 4), cannot be fully assessed until late in lifetime. Furthermore, attribution may be uncertain. Nevertheless, a consequence of recurring inability to work may be decreased probability of promotion, and a consequence of lost school-time may be reduced career opportunities. These are potentially heavy burdens, and should be captured as best they can (Table 7.15). Also at least potentially cumulative are the effects on relationships, love life and family dynamics (Table 7.16).

Burden on others, unaffected by headache themselves, is also addressed by HARDSHIP (Table 7.17). Subjective interpretations are unavoidable. A full account necessitates enquiries among the others, which in practical terms may be possible only among close family members.

Healthcare resource consumption (Table 7.7) is relatively easy to enquire into, albeit subject to recall error. It should also be easy to establish who pays for it (the patient, employer, insurer or society via the State). It is less easy to attach accurate

Table 7.15 HARDSHIP module on cumulative burden (impact on education, career and earnings)

Question	Response options
Have your headaches interfered with your education?	No/yes, I did less well/yes, I did not attempt something/yes, I gave up early
Do you believe your headaches have made you less successful in your career?	No/yes, I have done less well/yes, I have attempted less/yes, I have taken an easier job/yes, I have taken long-term sick leave/yes, I have retired early/yes, I am on a disability pension
Have your headaches reduced your earnings?	No/yes

Table 7.16 HARDSHIP module on relationships, love life and family dynamics

Question	Response options
These questions to be asked only when appropriate	
In the last 3 months, have your headaches caused difficulties in your love life?	No/yes
Have your headaches ever caused a long-term relationship or partnership to break down?	No/yes, temporarily/yes, permanently
Have your headaches affected your choices with regard to family planning?	No/yes, I have had fewer children/yes, I have avoided having children/yes, they have made it harder to conceive/yes, I have avoided oral contraception

Table 7.17 HARDSHIP module on burden on others (household partner and children)

Question	Response options
All these questions to be asked only when appropriate	
During the last 3 months, have your headaches caused one or more of your children to miss school?	No/yes, and total number of days
During the last 3 months, have your headaches prevented you from taking an interest in your children?	No, or less than once a month/yes, once or more a month/yes, once or more a week/yes, every day
During the last 3 months, have your headaches caused your partner to lose time from work?	No/yes, and total number of days
During the last 3 months, have your headaches caused your partner to miss social activities?	No/yes, and total number of occasions

costs to individual items of healthcare, perhaps necessitating separate research into healthcare costs in the country or region in question, but it has been done [29]. Indirect costs of lost productivity (included in Tables 7.8 and 7.9) are by far the greater part of the overall financial cost of headache [29, 30]. They may be borne by individuals, but commonly fall upon employers and/or insurers, and are a drain on national economies.

7.3 Concluding Remarks

A very broad base of expert opinion contributed to the evolution of HARDSHIP and question choice. It has undergone testing in many cultures and settings, 20 countries and 19 languages. Its modular design has facilitated this, rendering it highly amenable to adaptation to suit purpose, resource availability (especially time) and cultural sensitivities.

Demographic enquiry and sample characterization, at the very least encompassing age and gender, are a mandatory preliminary to burden enquiry. Diagnostic enquiry is constrained by ICHD-3, while ICHD-3 is not well suited to epidemiological use. The question set adopted should be locally validated; when this is not possible, reliance is placed on the validations of HARDSHIP in multiple other settings.

Enquiry into burden permits considerable scope for a variety of approaches, and adaptation according to purpose. While not all components of burden need be addressed, symptom burden and lost productivity should always be among those that are.

References

1. Steiner TJ. *Lifting The Burden*: the global campaign against headache. Lancet Neurol. 2004;3:204–5.
2. Steiner TJ. *Lifting The Burden*: the global campaign to reduce the burden of headache worldwide. J Headache Pain. 2005;6:373–7.
3. Steiner TJ, Birbeck GL, Jensen R, Katsarava Z, Martelletti P, Stovner LJ. *Lifting The Burden*: the first 7 years. J Headache Pain. 2010;11:451–5.
4. Steiner TJ, Birbeck GL, Jensen R, Katsarava Z, Martelletti P, Stovner LJ. The global campaign, World Health Organization and *Lifting The Burden*: collaboration in action. J Headache Pain. 2011;12:273–4.
5. *Lifting The Burden*. The Global Campaign against Headache. http://www.l-t-b.org.
6. Katsarava Z, Kukava M, Mirvelashvili E, Tavadze A, Dzagnidze A, Djibuti M, Steiner TJ. A pilot methodological validation study for a population-based survey of the prevalences of migraine, tension-type headache and chronic daily headache in the country of Georgia. J Headache Pain. 2007;8:77–82.
7. Rao GN, Kulkarni GB, Gururaj G, Rajesh K, Subbakrishna DK, Steiner TJ, Stovner LJ. The burden of headache disorders in India: methodology and questionnaire validation for a community-based survey in Karnataka state. J Headache Pain. 2012;13:543–50.
8. Yu S-Y, Cao X-T, Zhao G, Yang X-S, Qiao X-Y, Fang Y-N, Feng J-C, Liu R-Z, Steiner TJ. The burden of headache in China: validation of diagnostic questionnaire for a population-based survey. J Headache Pain. 2011;12:141–6.
9. Ayzenberg I, Katsarava Z, Mathalikov R, Chernysh M, Osipova V, Tabeeva G, Steiner TJ. The burden of headache in Russia: validation of the diagnostic questionnaire in a population-based sample. Eur J Neurol. 2011;18:454–9.
10. Herekar AD, Herekar AA, Ahmad A, Uqaili UL, Ahmed B, Effendi J, Alvi SZ, Steiner TJ. The burden of headache disorders in Pakistan: methodology of a population-based nationwide study, and questionnaire validation. J Headache Pain. 2013;14:73.
11. Zebenigus M, Tekle-Haimanot R, Worku DK, Thomas H, Steiner TJ. The prevalence of primary headache disorders in Ethiopia. J Headache Pain. 2016;17:110.

12. Mbewe E, Zairemthiama P, Yeh H-H, Paul R, Birbeck GL, Steiner TJ. The epidemiology of primary headache disorders in Zambia: a population-based door-to-door survey. J Headache Pain. 2015;16:30.
13. Manandhar K, Risal A, Steiner TJ, Holen A, Koju R, Linde M. Estimating the prevalence and burden of major disorders of the brain in Nepal: methodology of a nationwide population-based study. J Headache Pain. 2014;15:52.
14. Andrée C, Stovner LJ, Steiner TJ, Barré J, Katsarava Z, Lainez JM, Lanteri-Minet M, Mick G, Rastenyte D, Ruiz de la Torre E, Tassorelli C, Vriezen P, Lampl C. The Eurolight project: the impact of primary headache disorders in Europe. Description of methods. J Headache Pain. 2011;12:541–9.
15. Stovner LJ, Al Jumah M, Birbeck GL, Gururaj G, Jensen R, Katsarava Z, Queiroz LP, Scher AI, Tekle-Haimanot R, Wang SJ, Steiner TJ. The methodology of population surveys of headache prevalence, burden and cost: principles and recommendations from the global campaign against headache. J Headache Pain. 2014;15:5.
16. Steiner TJ, Gururaj G, Andrée C, Katsarava Z, Ayzenberg I, Yu SY, Al Jumah M, Tekle-Haimanot R, Birbeck GL, Herekar A, Linde M, Mbewe E, Manandhar K, Risal A, Jensen R, Queiroz LP, Scher AI, Wang SJ, Stovner LJ. Diagnosis, prevalence estimation and burden measurement in population surveys of headache: presenting the HARDSHIP questionnaire. J Headache Pain. 2014;15:3.
17. Classification Committee of the International Headache Society. The international classification of headache disorders, 3rd edition. Cephalalgia. 2018;38:1–211.
18. Stovner LJ, Hagen K, Jensen R, Katsarava Z, Lipton R, Scher A, Steiner TJ, Zwart JA. The global burden of headache: a documentation of headache prevalence and disability worldwide. Cephalalgia. 2007;27:193–210.
19. Lipton RB, Stewart WF, Sawyer J, Edmeads JG. Clinical utility of an instrument assessing migraine disability: the Migraine Disability Assessment (MIDAS) questionnaire. Headache. 2001;41:854–61.
20. Steiner TJ, Lipton RB on behalf of *Lifting The Burden*: The Global Campaign against Headache. The Headache-Attributed Lost Time (HALT) indices: measures of burden for clinical management and population-based research. J Headache Pain. 2018;19:12.
21. Selekler MH, Gökmen G, Steiner TJ. Productivity impact of headache on a heavy-manufacturing workforce in Turkey. J Headache Pain. 2013;14:88.
22. Yu S, He M, Liu R, Feng J, Qiao X, Yang X, Cao X, Zhao G, Fang Y, Steiner TJ. Headache yesterday in China: a new approach to estimating the burden of headache, applied in a general-population survey in China. Cephalalgia. 2013;33:1211–7.
23. Andrée C, Steiner TJ, Barré J, Katsarava Z, Lainez JM, Lampl C, Lantéri-Minet M, Rastenyte D, Ruiz de la Torre E, Tassorelli C, Stovner LJ. Headache yesterday in Europe. J Headache Pain. 2014;15:33.
24. Ayzenberg I, Katsarava Z, Sborowski A, Obermann M, Chernysh M, Osipova V, Tabeeva G, Steiner TJ. Headache yesterday in Russia: its prevalence and impact, and their application in estimating the national burden attributable to headache disorders. J Headache Pain. 2015;16:7.
25. Steiner TJ, Rao GN, Kulkarni GB, Gururaj G, Stovner LJ. Headache yesterday in Karnataka state, India: prevalence, impact and cost. J Headache Pain. 2016;17:74.
26. da Rocha NS, Power MJ, Bushnell DM, Fleck MP. The EUROHIS-QOL 8-item index: comparative psychometric properties to its parent WHOQOL-BREF. Value Health. 2012;15:449–57.
27. Office for National Statistics. First ONS annual experimental subjective well-being results. London: ONS; 2012. http://www.ons.gov.uk.
28. Lampl C, Steiner TJ, Mueller T, Mirvelashvili E, Djibuti M, Kukava M, Dzagnidze A, Jensen R, Stovner LJ, Katsarava Z. Will (or can) people pay for headache care in a poor country? J Headache Pain. 2012;13:67–74.
29. Linde M, Gustavsson A, Stovner LJ, Steiner TJ, Barré J, Katsarava Z, Lainez JM, Lampl C, Lantéri-Minet M, Rastenyte D, Ruiz de la Torre E, Tassorelli C, Andrée C. The cost of headache disorders in Europe: the Eurolight project. Eur J Neurol. 2012;19:703–11.
30. Hu XH, Markson LE, Lipton RB, Stewart WF, Berger ML. Burden of migraine in the United States. Disability and economic costs. Arch Intern Med. 1999;159:813–8.

Chapter 8
The Global Burden of Headache in Published Studies

Lars Jacob Stovner and Timothy J. Steiner

8.1 Introduction

Headache epidemiology is a relatively new discipline: the first studies appeared at the start of the 1970s [1]. From the outset, studies on prevalence of headache or migraine were performed, first and foremost, to document how common and widespread these disorders were and to evaluate their negative consequences (burden) at the societal level. This knowledge was needed, and to an extent still is, to support arguments for resource-allocation to healthcare for headache as well as to research. To some degree, these objectives have been attained, and headache disorders are now on the health agenda in many countries (see Chap. 5). However, this endeavour is far from finished, and there are still many areas of the world where the headache epidemiology is incompletely known, and important aspects of headache burden that have not been captured.

Another, also important potential of epidemiological studies is that they can detect causes and mechanisms of disease. These are *analytical* epidemiological studies (see Chap. 10), in contrast to the *descriptive* studies presented in this chapter.

L. J. Stovner
Department of Neuromedicine and Movement Science, NTNU Norwegian University of Science and Technology, Trondheim, Norway

Norwegian Advisory Unit on Headaches, Department of Neurology and Clinical Neurophysiology, St Olavs University Hospital, Trondheim, Norway
e-mail: lars.stovner@ntnu.no

T. J. Steiner (✉)
Department of Neuromedicine and Movement Science, NTNU Norwegian University of Science and Technology, Trondheim, Norway

Division of Brain Sciences, Imperial College London, London, UK
e-mail: t.steiner@imperial.ac.uk

T. J. Steiner, L. J. Stovner (eds.), *Societal Impact of Headache*, Headache,
https://doi.org/10.1007/978-3-030-24728-7_8

A very special methodology for assessing prevalence and burden has been developed in the Global Burden of Disease (GBD) study, the methods and results of which are described in Chap. 9. For headache *prevalence*, GBD bases its estimates almost exclusively on the individual studies dealt with in this chapter. For *burden*, however, GBD uses a method specifically developed for its purpose of making comparisons between widely different disorders. The individual studies, on the contrary, have historically assessed headache burden in many different ways, with little agreement in the literature on how to measure burden, and only a minority doing so in a meaningful way. Comparisons based on these, from country to country and even within countries, are very difficult.

If it was not already apparent, GBD's endeavour to measure and compare the burdens of all major disorders globally (see Chap. 9) has highlighted the need for more standardized methods. For headache, guidelines for measuring prevalence and burden were published in 2014 [2], and these are recounted in some detail in Chap. 6.

This chapter presents, from published studies, summary estimates of the prevalence of the principal headache disorders, discusses the potential effects of methodological differences and gives examples of how these studies measure the burden of headache.

8.2 Prevalence Studies

For estimates of headache prevalence (and burden), studies are useful only if they are reasonably representative of the population of a defined area. This excludes studies confined to patient populations, or to selected groups, although some that concern only a particular age range (children, adolescents, adults, the elderly) are of interest and usable. In the case of studies of specific headache types, only those appearing after the introduction of the first International Classification of Headache Disorders (ICHD-1) in 1988 are included here [3].

An overview of studies performed up to 2006 [4] showed global prevalences (with, generally, a time-frame of 1 year, which is the definition of an active headache disorder according to ICHD [3]) of 46% for *headache*, 11% for *migraine*, 42% for *tension-type headache* (TTH) and 3.4% for the group of disorders characterized by *headache on 15 or more days per month*. There were, then, few or no studies from large and populous countries or regions, such as Russia, India, China, Pakistan and large parts of Africa, in which lived half the population of the world [4].

This review is now being updated, with more than 100 new papers on prevalence. Importantly, there are now many more and good studies from the regions that were so incompletely covered previously. The revised global estimates, based on simple averaging of studies published both before and after 2006, indicate only slightly higher prevalences of all headache (48.0%) and of migraine (11.2%), and lower prevalence of TTH (23.4%), but markedly higher prevalence of headache on 15 or more days per month (5.0%) (Fig. 8.1). These estimates differ somewhat from those

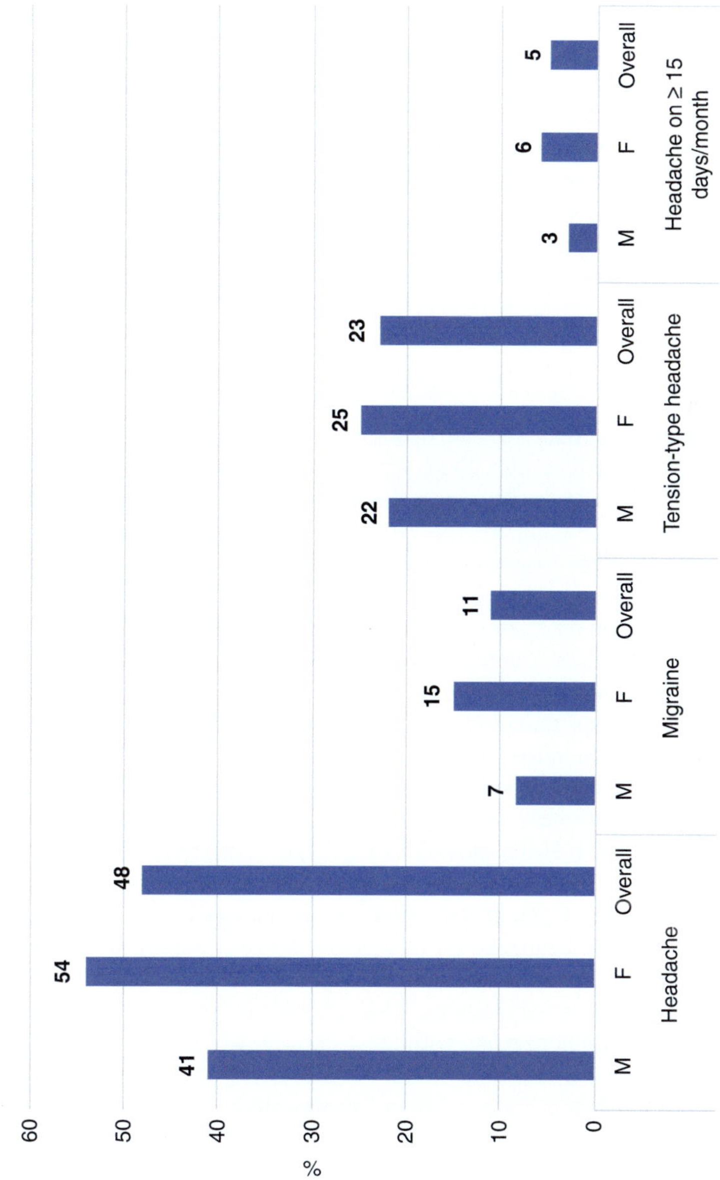

Fig. 8.1 Global headache prevalences by gender and overall, averaged from all published studies in the updated review (see Introduction)

of GBD2016 ([5]; also, Chap. 9) where, for example, the 1-year prevalences were 14.4% for migraine and 26.1% for TTH. The reasons are many. First and foremost, GBD estimates are based on rather intricate mathematical modelling, not only adjusting for age and gender composition of the populations but also taking account of the size of the population and the methodological quality of each study performed. GBD also imputes prevalences in countries where no data exist. In addition, there may be differences with regard to whether probable migraine and probable TTH were included in estimates.

There are large variations between studies. For migraine in both genders, prevalence estimates vary from 0.9% in a Chinese study among those over 60 years of age [6] to 43% among adults in a study from Italy [7]. Similarly, for TTH, prevalence estimates range from 0.7% in youths aged 12–14 in Thailand [8] to 49% in German adolescents [9]. For headache on 15 or more days per month, they range from 0.5% in a Turkish study of teenagers [10] to 19% among adults in Zambia [11]. These extreme variations may partly reflect real differences between countries and age groups, but, probably and to a large extent, also differences in methodology (discussed later).

Mean prevalence estimates for the different headache types in the world's continents, in studies before and after 2006, are shown in Fig. 8.2. They appear to show that, for all headache and for migraine, there are marked increases in Africa, Asia and Central/South America, stable prevalence in Europe, and a decrease in North America. For TTH, there are, apparently, marked increases in Africa and Asia, stable prevalences in Europe and Central/South America, and a decrease in North America. For headache on 15 or more days per month, estimates indicate a marked increase in Africa, moderate increases in Asia, North America and Europe, and stable prevalence in Central/South America. It is not possible to tell whether these changes are real, perhaps due to changes in causal factors, or in age and/or gender compositions of the populations, or whether they are due to methodological changes (for example, in diagnostic criteria).

Chronic migraine has been the subject of much interest (and some controversy) during the last decade. It is the most disabling type of migraine, for which it is of particular importance that new and more effective treatments are developed. Unrecognized in ICHD-1 [3], chronic migraine is defined in the latest version of ICHD (ICHD-3) [12] as headache on 15 or more days per month, with the features of migraine headache on at least eight of these, for at least 3 months. ICHD-3 expressly distinguishes chronic migraine from MOH [11]. Very few truly population-based studies have been performed with these criteria, while others have employed various modifications [13]. A review of all of these [14] found reported prevalences ranging between 0.5% and 5.4%, while a German study using the stricter criteria from ICHD-2 (15 or more days per month of headache with migraine features) [15] found a prevalence of only 0.3%, falling to 0.09% when those with medication overuse were excluded [16]. A more recent German study found only 0.02% with chronic migraine [17]. Among teenagers in Germany, 0.27% reportedly had chronic migraine, but only 0.07% complied with the strict criteria [18]. In an Italian study, only 0.2% had chronic migraine [19]. In Turkey, of 1.8% reportedly with chronic

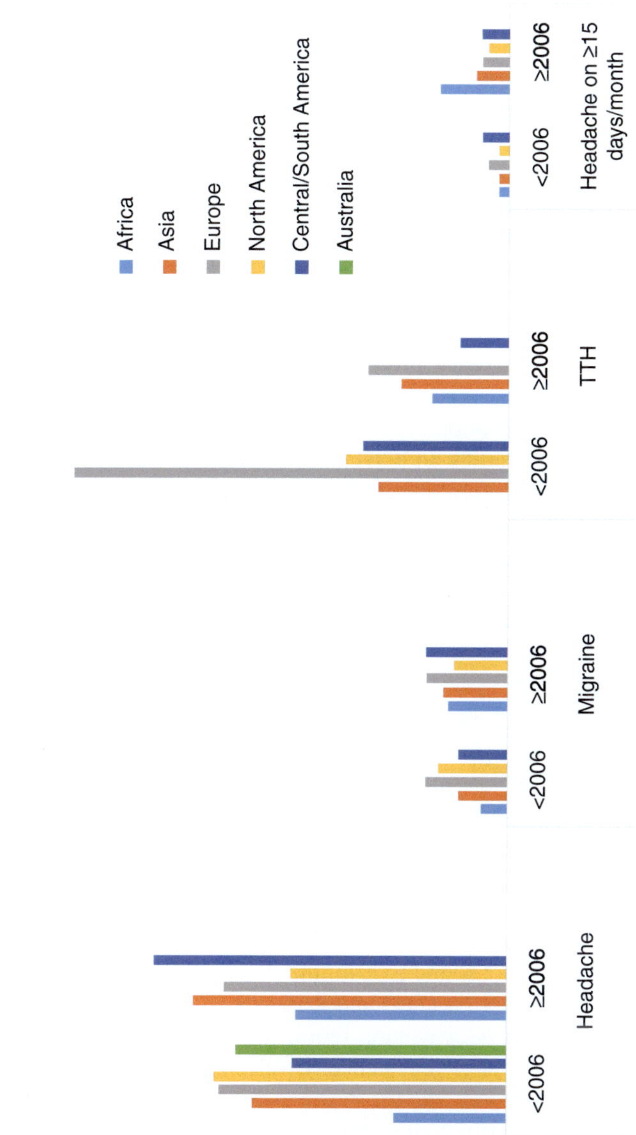

Fig. 8.2 Headache prevalences by continent in studies published before and after 2006

migraine, only 0.4% were without MOH [20]. In the same country, 1.5% of adolescents reportedly had chronic migraine [21]. In the USA, a large questionnaire survey (the CAMEO study) among more than 160,000 people above 12 years of age found a prevalence of 0.91% without medication overuse, but with a definition of chronic migraine that required only one of the 15 or more headache days per month to have migraine features [22]. In another US study among 12–17-year-olds, chronic migraine, without medication overuse, was found in 0.8% [23]. In Norway, among those aged 30–44 years, the prevalence of chronic migraine not including MOH was 0.01%, and of probable chronic migraine 0.1% [24]. In Egypt, 3.3% reportedly had chronic migraine, but only 1.4% without medication overuse [25]. In Georgia, the reported prevalence was 1.4%, not including those with MOH [26].

These variations particularly reflect differences in diagnostic criteria. Chronic migraine appears to be uncommon, but argument continues over its definition, and its true prevalence will remain very uncertain meanwhile [13].

Medication overuse headache (MOH) can be regarded as a complication of one of the primary headaches, usually migraine or TTH (see Chap. 2). ICHD-2 criteria required the diagnosis to be made only after successful treatment, by medication withdrawal, as proof of causation [15, 27]. This may be feasible in the clinic, but it is not in epidemiological studies. In ICHD-3, the diagnosis can be made on frequencies of headache and medication intake alone [28]. Herein lies much of the problem with chronic migraine since, among those with any highly frequent headache, medication overuse is common but its effect in causation is often unknown.

Probable MOH (pMOH: headache on 15 or more days per month *and* medication overuse) was found to affect 0.9% of adults in Georgia [26] and 1% in Spain [29, 30]. In the HUNT studies in Norway, from the 1990s, probable MOH was reported in 1% of adults [31] and 0.5% of adolescents [32], whereas a more recent study in the same country found 1.7% in young adults [33]. In Germany, a recent study found a prevalence of 2% among adults [34]. A large population-based study in Sweden, in which 44,300 people were interviewed by telephone, found MOH in 1.8%, markedly more among women (2.5%) than men (0.9%), and with a peak at around 50 years of age [35]. In Karnataka state, India, the prevalence was 1.2% [36]. The Eurolight study, which compiled data of varying population representativeness from nine European countries, found 3.1% with pMOH [37], almost the same as in the most population-based study among these, in Lithuania (3.2%) [38]. The lowest percentages were found in Ethiopia (0.7%) [39] and China (0.6%) [40], and the highest in Zambia (7.1%) [11] and Russia (5.3%) [41].

Cluster headache (CH) is quite rare, requiring studies in large populations for reasonably precise estimates of prevalence. Until now, mostly lifetime prevalence has been reported. Furthermore, the diagnosis is difficult to make by questionnaire, and requires interview, ideally face-to-face, by a headache specialist. In the Vågå study, where this was done in more than 1800 inhabitants of a Norwegian rural community, a lifetime prevalence of 0.33% was found [42]. A study in an Italian town among more than 10,000 patients registered in the lists of general practitioners (representative, in this country, of the general population), questionnaires or telephone interviews were used to screen the population, and suspected cases interviewed for confirmation by a headache specialist. By this method, the lifetime prevalence was found to be 0.28% [43]. These are not dissimilar to the 0.2% found in a Swedish twin registry study [44].

In Germany, however, where suspected CH cases in a population-based study were detected by questionnaire and interviewed by a neurologist, reported prevalence was only 0.12% [45]. In Georgia, a door-to-door survey using recognition-based diagnosis (see Chap. 6) found a single case among 1145 participants, corresponding to 0.09% [46], but with 95% confidence limits of 0.26%. A prevalence of 0.09% was also found in Teheran (Iran): three cases detected among more than 3500 participants in a door-to-door survey using trained interviewers with some medical education [47]. In Ethiopia, medical personnel interviewing screen-positive cases among 1105 textile mill workers found five with CH or other trigeminal autonomic cephalalgia (0.45%) [48].

8.2.1 Relations to Age and Gender

Most headache epidemiological studies demonstrate clear relations to these demographic factors. All headache types are more common in females than in males (Fig. 8.1). The difference between males and females is greatest for migraine and headache on 15 or more days per month (male/female ratio = 0.5 for both), less for all headache (0.76) and least for TTH (0.86).

There are also some relations to age. Figure 8.3 shows mean prevalences for the headache types in studies with mean age over 18 years compared to those with mean

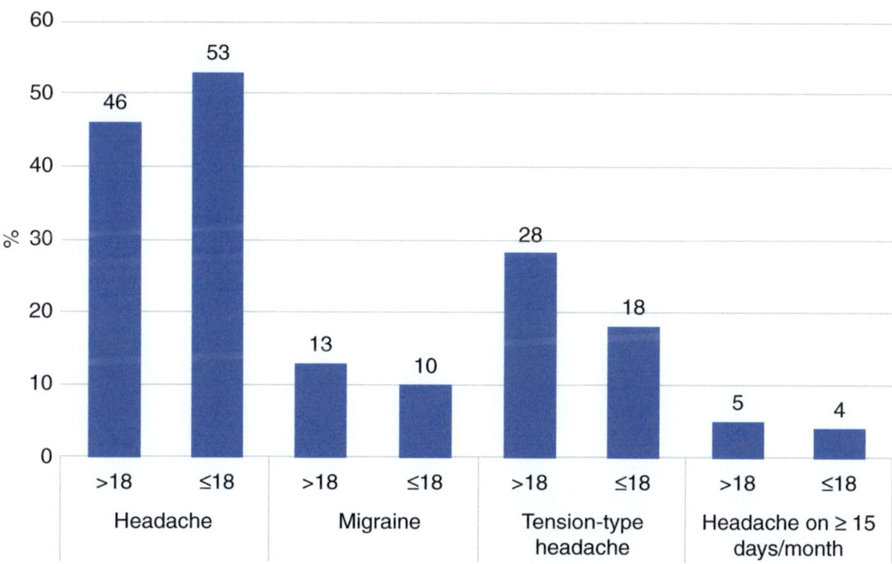

Fig. 8.3 Global headache prevalences by mean age of participants (>18 or ≤18 years), averaged from all published studies in the updated review (see Sect. 8.1)

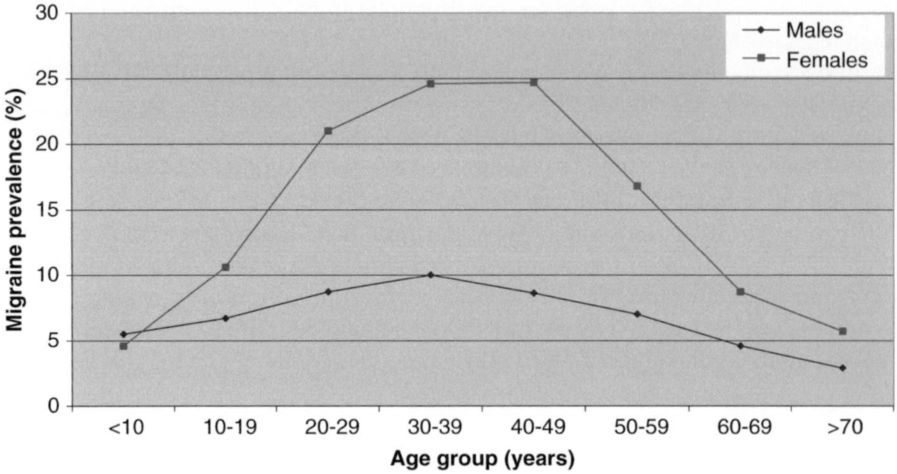

Fig. 8.4 Migraine prevalence by age and gender (reproduced from [49] by courtesy of *European Journal of Neurology*)

age of 18 years or less. All headache is more prevalent among the younger group (adult/young ratio = 0.87), contrary to the trend in all headache types, which are more common among adults (migraine: 1.3; TTH: 1.6; headache on 15 or more days per month: 1.2). This, of course, is paradoxical, but the explanation is found in Chap. 3. Many studies in children and adolescents report migraine and TTH while ignoring large proportions with headache meeting the criteria for neither (undifferentiated headache (see Chap. 3)).

Migraine is most clearly related to these demographic factors. Figure 8.4 shows its relations to both gender and age, using pooled data from several European studies [49]. In the age group below 10 years, migraine prevalence is almost equal among boys and girls (boys even slightly higher). After this age, prevalence is much higher among females, with a peak between 20 and 50 years during which prevalence is 2–3 times higher among females. After 50, there are marked declines in both genders, but particularly in females.

For all headache, age and gender distribution largely reflects that of TTH, with less marked increase during adolescence but similar decline with old age, and smaller differences between the genders (Fig. 8.5).

CH shows a marked male preponderance [50]. Previously, male:female ratios have been found of 4.8:1 for the episodic subtype and 6.3:1 for the chronic subtype, but these may have diminished during the last few decades, possibly reflecting changes in lifestyle among both genders (especially smoking habits) [50, 51].

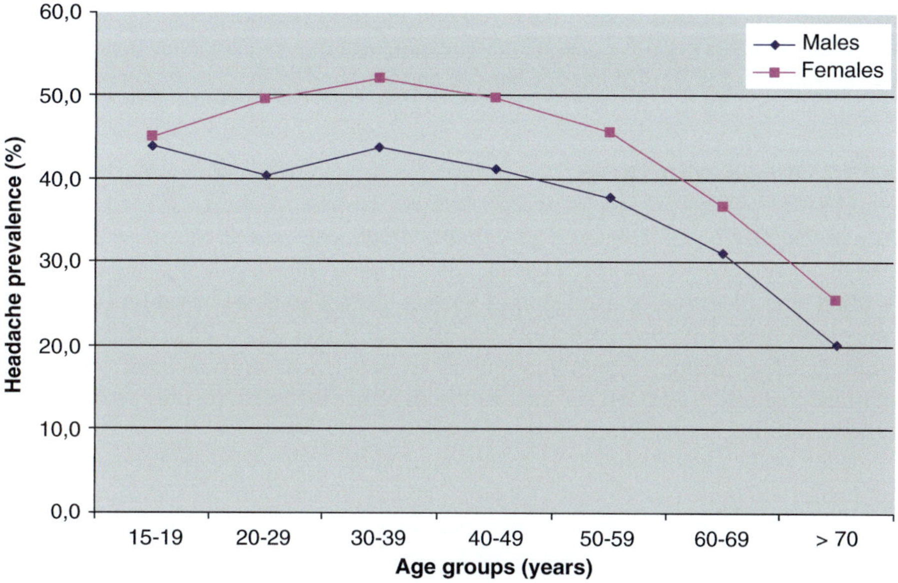

Fig. 8.5 All-headache prevalence by age and gender (reproduced from [49] by courtesy of *European Journal of Neurology*)

8.2.2 Methodological and Other Extraneous Sources of Variation

Headache prevalences are often found to vary considerably, within the same country and over relatively short periods. These differences must, clearly, have methodological causes. The methodological issues arising in population-based headache studies have been covered in detail in Chap. 6. The most important will be briefly mentioned here.

8.2.2.1 Screening Question

Many studies are performed in a two-stage manner, where there is first a screening question to establish whether a person has headache or not, and the screen-positives are then subjected to more thorough enquiry. It is empirically evident that the nature of the screening question has a great impact on how people answer, on how many proceed to the second stage, and hence on the estimate of prevalence. A neutral question ("have you had headache …?") tends to yield much higher prevalences than a question specifying some level of severity (e.g., "Have you *suffered from* headache …?") or frequency ("have you had *recurring* headaches …?"), or including other qualifiers ("Have you had a headache *not due to* hangover, head trauma, flu, common cold?") ([49]; also, Chaps. 6 and 7).

8.2.2.2 Diagnostic Criteria

The potentially potent influence of variable diagnostic criteria has been discussed earlier, in relation to chronic migraine. The criteria themselves, the way they are applied, and inclusion or exclusion of various headache types or subtypes all play large roles in determining prevalence estimates. It makes a very large difference, for example, if estimates of migraine and TTH prevalences only include those with definite diagnoses (all ICHD criteria fulfilled) rather than definite plus probable (all criteria fulfilled but one) (see Chaps. 6 and 7).

Many studies report only definite migraine and/or TTH, some report definite and probable, and quite a few do not specify, making comparisons very difficult (if not meaningless). When probable cases are included, prevalence estimates often increase dramatically. For example, in Russia, the reported prevalence of definite migraine is 10.8%, but of both definite and probable it is 20.3% [41]. Definite TTH affects 25.4%, both definite and probable affect 30.9%. Similar large proportions with probable migraine, doubling the overall estimate, have been found in USA (definite 14.7%, probable 14.6%) [52], France (11.2% and 10.1%) [53] and Nepal (17.5% and 17.2%) [54]. In a few studies where the diagnosis has been made face-to-face by headache experts, the proportions with probable diagnoses are smaller (Denmark: 16% definite, 1.8% probable [55]; Norway: 17.2% definite, 2.4% probable [56]). Future modelling of published prevalence data (in GBD, for example) must find a way to adjust according to whether or not probable diagnoses are included, or when this is unknown.

8.2.2.3 Multiple Diagnoses

Also with some influence is whether only one diagnosis is made, or more than one, when multiple types are present in a survey participant. Often, for good reasons, only one diagnosis is allowed, typically the most bothersome (see Chap. 6). Since migraine and TTH are often comorbid, this will usually lead to underestimates of TTH.

8.2.2.4 Participation Proportion

This may, through injection of bias, be a highly significant factor. For example, people affected by headache may be more interested in participation, which may spuriously inflate prevalence estimates. Participation bias of this and other sorts is more likely when participation proportion is low (see Chap. 6).

8.2.2.5 Other Sources of Variation

In addition to these methodological causes of largely spurious variations, other influences introduce variations that are real. For example, headache prevalence estimates are particularly dependent on the age and gender composition of the population of interest, because of the relationships described above (Figs. 8.2, 8.3, 8.4, and 8.5). Some differences can be expected in societies with very different proportions of young or older people.

Samples may not correctly reflect age and gender compositions of the population of interest from which they are drawn. This is a methodological issue (see Chap. 6). In all studies, it is advisable to adjust observed (sample) prevalences for age and gender distributions in the source population.

8.3 Burden Studies

The burden of a disease is the sum of all the negative effects a disease has on individuals, and on society. It has many dimensions [2], described in some detail in Chaps. 4 and 7. There are symptom burden (the direct burden of suffering from pain and associated symptoms), disability burden (impaired functional ability) and its consequential lost-productivity burden, interictal burden (restrictions between attacks) and cumulative burden (negative consequences that accrue over the years). In addition are financial burdens, including financial costs to both the individual and the society, dealt with in Chap. 12.

8.3.1 Symptom Burden

This direct burden is estimated as experienced during headache episodes (the *ictal state*). A measure can be the time spent with a certain level of pain, measured on a Likert scale 0–3 (0: no pain; 1: mild pain; 2: moderate [or "quite bad"] pain; 3: severe [or "very bad"] pain), calculated from the product of average duration of headache episodes and headache frequency (*time in ictal state*). In a previous study, such a measure was used to compare the impact of migraine with that of TTH [4]. In GBD2010, symptom burden was measured for these disorders using, instead of headache intensity, a disability weight (DW) for the ictal state established through a global consultation exercise from a brief description of the "average" condition (see Chap. 9). With this method, migraine was ranked as seventh most disabling disorder worldwide [57] (although the term "disabling" here refers more generally to lost health (see Chap. 4)). Later GBD studies have raised this ranking to 2nd [58, 59].

These methods depend on participants' recall, usually over 3 months, to establish averages for duration and frequency. In several studies, symptom burden has been measured in a more reliable way by asking participants to describe headache yesterday, almost completely eliminating recall errors (see Chap. 7). In China, for example, 3.8% of the population had quite bad or very bad headache yesterday (hence on any day) (see Chap 6). From duration of headache yesterday, it could be calculated that 1.4% had headache of this intensity at any moment [60]. Using the same methods of calculation, the proportion of people with bad or very bad headache at any time was 3.2% in Russia [61] and 2.4% in nine European countries [62].

8.3.2 Disability, Lost Time and Consequential Cost

Disability is the loss of function related to the disorder. We know this is large. For example, it has been estimated in USA that 300,000 people stay in bed each day (for 24 h) because of headache [63].

Disability often leads to lost time from important activities. In many studies conducted with the support of *Lifting The Burden* (LTB) [64], lost time has been measured by the Headache-Attributed Lost Time (HALT) questionnaire [65], a derivative of the Migraine Disability Assessment (MIDAS) instrument [66]. HALT measures time lost during the preceding 3 months not only from paid work but also from household chores and leisure activities, counting (for paid work and household chores) days of complete absence and days with productivity reduced by more than half. LTB studies use a very similar methodology in many other respects, making them highly comparable (Table 8.1).

Table 8.1 Days lost (mean and [SD]) from various activities due to migraine, tension-type headache (TTH) or probable medication-overuse headache (pMOH) during the preceding 3 months in studies supported by *Lifting The Burden*

	Days lost from paid work			Days lost from household work			Days lost from leisure		
	Migraine	TTH	pMOH	Migraine	TTH	pMOH	Migraine	TTH	pMOH
Ethiopia [67]	2.9 [5.9]	1.3 [3.0]	19 [31.9]	4.8 [8.3]	1.1 [3.4]	14.4 [23.6]	0.8 [1.7]	0.2 [0.5]	4.1 [9.1]
Eurolight [37][a]	3.2 [8.6]	1.0 [5.7]	14.2 [26.1]	4.6 [9.2]	1.3 [5.7]	21.4 [26.7]	2.1 [5.0]	0.6 [3.9]	9.0 [16.2]
India [68]	1.4 [4.1]	0.4 [1.9]	4.1 [11.8]	2.1 [4.0]	0.8 [2.3]	9.7 [11.0]			
Nepal [69]	1.9 [4.6]	0.9 [3.1]	8.0 [16.4]	3.5 [6.5]	1.3 [2.8]	8.9 [13.6]	0.8 [4.9]	0.2 [4.9]	1.2 [2.9]
Russia [70]	1.9 [2.8]	0.8 [1.8]	5.6 [8.7]				0.6 [1.4]	0.4 [1.0]	1.9 [5.1]
Zambia [71]	4.1 [6.6]	1.4 [2.8]	4.8 [8.2]	4.2 [7.4]	1.1 [3.0]	4.5 [7.3]	1.3 [2.8]	0.4 [1.2]	1.0 [1.8]
Mean	2.6	1.0	10.2	3.8	1.1	12.5	1.1	0.4	3.4

[a]Mean of studies in nine European countries (Austria, Germany, France, Italy, Lithuania, Luxembourg, Netherlands, Spain and the UK). These studies are probably oversampling headache patients

The table indicates considerable variations in findings between these studies, which may reflect work, life and/or other cultural differences, but lost time per person for pMOH is on average 3–4 times that of migraine and 10–11 times that of TTH. It can be calculated that migraine causes a mean of 0.9 lost days per month from paid work, 1.3 days from household work and 0.4 days from leisure activities. The corresponding figures for TTH are 0.3, 0.4 and 0.1, and for pMOH 3.4, 4.2 and 1.1 days per month.

Far fewer data exist for children and adolescents. PedMIDAS, a questionnaire developed for children, is quite similar to MIDAS but focuses more on school and homework than on work or household activities, in addition to leisure activities (play, sports) [72]. In a Turkish study of 7721 students aged 9–7 years, approximately 10% reported migraine (lifetime prevalence), with more than 10 days affected by it during the preceding 3 months [73]. Approximately 0.8 schooldays were completely lost and 0.5 days partially, while the students functioned at school with less than half their ability on approximately 2.5 days.

In some LTB studies, questions on headache yesterday were accompanied by questions on how much was done (all, more than half, less than half or nothing of that expected) when yesterday was a workday, enabling calculation of lost working capacity. In the Eurolight study, a mean of 27% of participants in the nine countries reported headache yesterday. This was certainly an overestimate, since not all samples in Eurolight were population-based, but in Lithuania, with sampling door-to-door and face-to-face interviews, headache yesterday was reported by 12% [38]. After adjustment for different sources of error, it was calculated that at least 0.7% (possibly 2–3 times more) of all working capacity in Europe was lost to headache [62]. In a nationally representative study in Russia, 14.5% had headache yesterday, with a calculated loss of 4% of workforce capacity [61]. In Karnataka state in India, 6% reported headache yesterday and a loss of 3% of all productive capacity [74]. The highest prevalence of headache yesterday was seen in Zambia (19%), with an estimated 11% productivity loss [71].

8.3.3 *Quality of Life*

Quality of life (QoL) is presumably affected by all aspects of headache-attributed burden. Measures of QoL in people with headache, while non-specific and not highly sensitive, perhaps provide an overall (summary) quantification. It is nonetheless a problematic measure, since it has no intuitive units.

The SF-36 is a widely used instrument to measure QoL, in eight dimensions. In a US study [75], where migraineurs were recruited from a medication trial, it was found that migraineurs had lower QoL than the general US population, most markedly for bodily pain, physical role limitations and social functioning. Since then, QoL has been measured also in population-based studies on headache epidemiology and burden (Table 8.2), by using SF-36 or other instruments. Generally, headache patients have reduced QoL compared to the general population, and on many dimensions.

Table 8.2 Quality-of-life (QoL) estimates in population-based headache epidemiological studies

Country [reference]	QoL instrument	Principal findings
France [76]	SF 36	People with migraine had significantly lower scores than headache free controls on all SF-36 dimensions, and lower scores on the pain dimension than people with other headaches.
Netherlands [77]	SF-36	People with migraine in a population-based study had lower scores on all dimensions compared with controls, the negative influence being greater than that of asthma, for example, and increasing with headache frequency.
Spain [78]	SF-36	Two population-based studies among people with headache on 15 or more days per month showed negative influences similar in those with migraine or TTH but especially marked in those with medication overuse, who had lower scores on all dimensions but particularly on role physical and bodily pain. Headache frequency was more important for QoL than headache intensity.
UK [79]	SF-36	In a population-based study, people with migraine with high or moderate disability had clear reductions in all dimensions.
US and UK [80]	SF-12	In both countries, people with migraine had lower scores than controls on both components (physical and mental) after adjusting for socioeconomic status and for comorbid depression. However, in those with both migraine and depression, QoL was further reduced.
France [81]	QvM	QoL was found to be lowest among those with headache on 15 or more days per month, intermediate among those with migraine and highest in people with other forms of episodic headache.
Nepal [69]	WHOQoL-8	Scores were lower in people with headache than in those without, correlated negatively with intensity and frequency of headache, and were lowest in people with pMOH.

QvM qualité de vie et migraine, *SF-36* short form survey, 36 items, *SF-12* short form survey, 12 items, *WHOQoL-8* World Health Organization Quality of Life instrument, 8 items, *pMOH* probable medication overuse headache

Comorbid conditions may add to the total burden of illness in people with headache. European population-based studies have demonstrated that depression and/or anxiety occur 2–3 times more often among those with migraine than in the general population [80, 82], while, as noted above, depression adds to QoL impairment in migraine [80]. This may be as important a factor for non-migrainous headache [83], but it is not known how this comorbidity influences QoL in other headache disorders. In addition, it has been found, both in Finnish children [84] and in Norwegian adults [85], that headache is also comorbid with other bodily pain.

8.3.4 Headache Impact on Family, Friends and Social Activities

Headache also affects the spouses, partners and children of people with it, and their ability to participate in household chores and social activities. A few population-based studies have measured these important aspects of headache burden,

Table 8.3 Impact on family, friends and social activities

Country or study [reference]	Headache type	Negative impact due to headache
US and UK [86]	Migraine	During last 3 months: • Reduced ability to do household chores: >60% marked impact • Missed family or social activities: 45% • Influence on relation with their children: >60% • Children missing school because of parents' migraine: 10% • Impaired ability to be a good partner: 46% • Partners had reduced ability to do household chores: 24% • Partners had missed family or social events: 20% Person affected had had fewer children because of migraine: 5% Person affected had avoided having children: 0.4%
Sweden [87]	Migraine	Negative influence on: • Attendance at work: 76% • Family situation: 67% • Leisure time: 59% • Social position: 37% • Sexual life: 43% • Love: 31% • Finding friends: 10%
Eurolight[a] [37]	Migraine	Children had missed school: 2% Prevented caring for the child: 18% Negatively affect love life: 18% Had fewer children or avoided having children: 5.5% Divorce or separation: 0.7%
	TTH	Children had missed school: 2% Prevented caring for the child: 8% Negatively affect love life: 6% Had fewer children or avoided having children: 1.1% Divorce or separation: 0.3%
	MOH	Children had missed school: 5% Prevented caring for the child: 50% Negatively affected love life: 49%% Had fewer children or avoided having children: 21.1% Divorce or separation: 7%

[a]Mean of studies in nine European countries (Austria, Germany, France, Italy, Lithuania, Luxembourg, Netherlands, Spain and the UK). These studies are probably oversampling people with headache

summarized in Table 8.3. It affects sexual life and, in a small minority of cases, can cause break-up of relations. It may also reduce ability and willingness to have children.

8.3.5 *Interictal Burden of Headache*

Headaches also affect the lives of people outside the attacks. This is a dimension rarely captured directly in studies, but is probably reflected in QoL impairments reported, especially, by people with migraine. In the Eurolight study, so-called

Table 8.4 Interictal burden of headache

Country [reference]	Impact	Migraine	TTH
Sweden [87]	Incomplete recovery between attacks	57% (9% more marked)	
Eurolight[a] [88]	Incomplete recovery between attacks	26%	19%
	Anxiety for next attack	11%	3%
	Lifestyle compromise to avoid attacks	15%	5%
	Rarely or never in control of headache	15%	9%
	Reluctant to tell others about headache	30%	27%
	Families and friends do not understand headache	10%	10%
	Employers and colleagues do not understand headache	12%	7%
	Time in interictal state	317 days/year	331 days/year

[a]Mean of studies in nine European countries (Austria, Germany, France, Italy, Lithuania, Luxembourg, Netherlands, Spain and the UK). These studies are probably oversampling people with headache

interictal burden (see Chap. 4) was measured through questions about recovery between attacks, anxiety for the next attack, lifestyle compromise to avoid attacks, the degree to which people felt in control of their headache, and how peoples' family, employer and colleagues accepted their disease [88] (Table 8.4).

8.3.6 Cumulative Burden

This is the sum of the enduring consequences of headache built over a lifetime, often rooted in childhood and adolescence (see Chaps. 3 and 4). Headache in young people during the formative years of education, and later when building careers and families, can and does adversely affect all three (see Chaps. 4 and 7). In the Eurolight study, 11.8% of participants believed they had done less well in education because of headache, 5.9% reported reduced earnings and 7.4% that their careers had suffered [89]. These may be relatively small proportions, but they are very heavy burdens.

Although clearly an extremely important aspect of headache burden cumulative burden is rarely assessed.

8.3.7 Burden of Cluster Headache

There are generally few good data on the burden of other headaches than migraine, TTH or MOH, and none based on population-based studies. Clinic-based samples are probably not representative of patients in the general populations, while the rarity of some of these other headaches makes population-based studies on the burden associated with them hard to conduct. This is true for CH, which, presumably, is a cause of very high burden on affected individuals.

CH-attributed burden has been evaluated in a Danish study in a neurological department [90]. Among 85 randomly selected CH patients, 78% reported restrictions in daily living during cluster periods and 13% also outside these periods. CH had caused lifestyle changes in 96%, mostly related to sleeping habits and avoidance of alcohol. Work was markedly affected, and, during the preceding year, those patients who were working had lost a mean of 9 workdays. When at work during a cluster period, 40% of patients reported only 60% working efficiency. One-third reported that CH had limited their careers, 16% had lost their jobs and 8% had taken early retirement because of CH.

A web-based study recruited 1134 people with CH from all over the USA [91]. This study found that 55% of participants had contemplated suicide and 2% had tried to commit suicide. Because of their headache, 17% had lost their jobs and 8% were out of work. Almost half had lost from 1–10 days of work during the preceding year, and 20% more than 11 days.

8.4 Concluding Remarks

Headache epidemiological studies have been crucial in the acknowledgement of headache as a major public-health problem. When the literature was reviewed in 2007 [4], there were large parts of the world where prevalence was unknown. Since then, new studies performed by LTB and others have filled many of the biggest gaps. A better view has emerged from published studies of the global burden of headache, but it is not yet a complete view. The challenge now is to improve methods generally, and standardize them across all studies ([2]; also, Chaps. 6 and 7), so that comparisons between countries and regions, and over time, can explain the differences that undoubtedly exist.

References

1. Waters WE. The epidemiological enigma of migraine. Int J Epidemiol. 1973;2:189–94.
2. Stovner LJ, Al Jumah M, Birbeck GL, Gururaj G, Jensen R, Katsarava Z, Queiroz LP, Scher AI, Tekle-Haimanot R, Wang SJ, Steiner TJ. The methodology of population surveys of headache prevalence, burden and cost: principles and recommendations from the global campaign against headache. J Headache Pain. 2014;15:5.
3. Headache Classification Committee of the International Headache Society. Classification and diagnostic criteria for headache disorders, cranial neuralgias and facial pain. Cephalalgia. 1988;8(Suppl 7):1–96.
4. Stovner LJ, Hagen K, Jensen R, Katsarava Z, Lipton R, Scher A, Steiner T, Zwart JA. The global burden of headache: a documentation of headache prevalence and disability worldwide. Cephalalgia. 2007;27:193–210.

5. Global Burden of Disease Headache Collaborators. Global, regional, and national burden of migraine and tension-type headache, 1990–2016: a systematic analysis for the Global Burden of Disease Study 2016. Lancet Neurol. 2018;17:954–76.
6. Zhang Y, Shi Z, Hock D, Yue W, Liu S, Zhang Y, Liu S, Zhao L, Lu H, Guan Y, Wang X, Wsiniewski T, Ji Y. Prevalence of primary headache disorders in a population aged 60 years and older in a rural area of northern China. J Headache Pain. 2016;17:83.
7. Allena M, Steiner TJ, Sances G, Carugno B, Balsamo F, Nappi G, Andrée C, Tassorelli C. Impact of headache disorders in Italy and the public-health and policy implications: a population-based study within the Eurolight project. J Headache Pain. 2015;16:100.
8. Visudtibhan A, Boonsopa C, Thampratankul L, Nuntnarumit P, Okaschareon C, Khongkhatithum C, Chiemchanya S, Visudhiphan P. Headache in junior high school students: types & characteristics in Thai children. J Med Assoc Thail. 2010;93:550–7.
9. Milde-Busch A, Blaschek A, Heinen F, Borggrafe I, Koerte I, Straube A, Schankin C, von Kries R. Associations between stress and migraine and tension-type headache: results from a school-based study in adolescents from grammar schools in Germany. Cephalalgia. 2011;31:774–85.
10. Unalp A, Dirik E, Kurul S. Prevalence and clinical findings of migraine and tension-type headache in adolescents. Pediatr Int. 2007;49:943–9.
11. Mbewe E, Zairemthiama P, Yeh HH, Paul R, Birbeck GL, Steiner TJ. The epidemiology of primary headache disorders in Zambia: a population-based door-to-door survey. J Headache Pain. 2015;16:515.
12. Headache Classification Committee of the International Headache Society (IHS). The international classification of headache disorders, 3rd edition. Cephalalgia. 2018;38:1–211.
13. Steiner T. Can we know the prevalence of MOH? Cephalalgia. 2014;34:403–4.
14. Natoli J, Manack A, Dean B, Butler Q, Turkel C, Stovner L, Lipton R. Global prevalence of chronic migraine: a systematic review. Cephalalgia. 2010;30:599–609.
15. Classification Subcommittee of the International Headache Society. The international classification of headache disorders. 2nd edition. Cephalalgia. 2004;24:1–160.
16. Straube A, Pfaffenrath V, Ladwig KH, Meisinger C, Hoffmann W, Fendrich K, Vennemann M, Berger K. Prevalence of chronic migraine and medication overuse headache in Germany-the German DMKG headache study. Cephalalgia. 2010;30:207–13.
17. Yoon MS, Manack A, Schramm S, Fritsche G, Obermann M, Diener HC, Moebus S, Katsarava Z. Chronic migraine and chronic tension-type headache are associated with concomitant low back pain: results of the German headache consortium study. Pain. 2013;154:484–92.
18. Fendrich K, Vennemann M, Pfaffenrath V, Evers S, May A, Berger K, Hoffmann W. Headache prevalence among adolescents—the German DMKG headache study. Cephalalgia. 2007;27:347–54.
19. Ferrante T, Castellini P, Abrignani G, Latte L, Russo M, Camarda C, Veronesi L, Pasquarella C, Manzoni GC, Torelli P. The PACE study: past-year prevalence of migraine in Parma's adult general population. Cephalalgia. 2012;32:358–65.
20. Ertas M, Baykan B, Orhan EK, Zarifoglu M, Karli N, Saip S, Onal AE, Siva A. One-year prevalence and the impact of migraine and tension-type headache in Turkey: a nationwide home-based study in adults. J Headache Pain. 2012;13:147–57.
21. Ozge A, Sasmaz T, Bugdayci R, Cakmak SE, Kurt AO, Kaleagasi SH, Siva A. The prevalence of chronic and episodic migraine in children and adolescents. Eur J Neurol. 2013;20:95–101.
22. Buse D, Manack A, Serrano D, Reed M, Varon S, Turkel C, Lipton R. Headache impact of chronic and episodic migraine: results from the American Migraine Prevalence and Prevention study. Headache. 2012;52:3–17.
23. Lipton RB, Manack A, Ricci JA, Chee E, Turkel CC, Winner P. Prevalence and burden of chronic migraine in adolescents: results of the chronic daily headache in adolescents study (C-dAS). Headache. 2011;51:693–706.
24. Grande RB, Aaseth K, Gulbrandsen P, Lundqvist C, Russell MB. Prevalence of primary chronic headache in a population-based sample of 30- to 44-year-old persons. The Akershus study of chronic headache. Neuroepidemiology. 2008;30:76–83.

25. Kandil MR, Hamed SA, Fadel KA, Khalifa HE, Ghanem MK, Mohamed KO. Migraine in Assiut Governorate, Egypt: epidemiology, risk factors, comorbid conditions and predictors of change from episodic to chronic migraine. Neurol Res. 2016;38:232–41.
26. Katsarava Z, Dzagnidze A, Kukava M, Mirvelashvili E, Djibuti M, Janelidze M, Jensen R, Stovner LJ, Steiner TJ. Primary headache disorders in the Republic of Georgia: prevalence and risk factors. Neurology. 2009;73:1796–803.
27. Olesen J, Bousser MG, Diener HC, Dodick D, First M, Goadsby PJ, Gobel H, Lainez MJ, Lance JW, Lipton RB, Nappi G, Sakai F, Schoenen J, Silberstein SD, Steiner TJ. New appendix criteria open for a broader concept of chronic migraine. Cephalalgia. 2006;26:742–6.
28. Headache Classification Committee of the International Headache Society. The international classification of headache disorders, 3rd edition (beta version). Cephalalgia. 2013;33:629–808.
29. Castillo J, Munoz P, Guitera V, Pascual J. Epidemiology of chronic daily headache in the general population. Headache. 1999;39:190–6.
30. Colas R, Munoz P, Temprano R, Gomez C, Pascual J. Chronic daily headache with analgesic overuse: epidemiology and impact on quality of life. Neurology. 2004;62:1338–42.
31. Zwart JA, Dyb G, Hagen K, Svebak S, Holmen J. Analgesic use: a predictor of chronic pain and medication overuse headache: the Head-HUNT study. Neurology. 2003;61:160–4.
32. Dyb G, Holmen TL, Zwart JA. Analgesic overuse among adolescents with headache: the Head-HUNT-Youth study. Neurology. 2006;66:198–201.
33. Aaseth K, Grande RB, Kvaerner KJ, Gulbrandsen P, Lundqvist C, Russell MB. Prevalence of secondary chronic headaches in a population-based sample of 30-44-year-old persons. The Akershus study of chronic headache. Cephalalgia. 2008;28:705–13.
34. Katsarava Z, Diener HC. Medication overuse headache in Germany. Cephalalgia. 2008;28:1221–2.
35. Jonsson P, Hedenrud T, Linde M. Epidemiology of medication overuse headache in the general Swedish population. Cephalalgia. 2011;31:1015–22.
36. Kulkarni GB, Rao GN, Gururaj G, Stovner LJ, Steiner TJ. Headache disorders and public ill-health in India: prevalence estimates in Karnataka state. J Headache Pain. 2015;16:67.
37. Steiner TJ, Stovner LJ, Katsarava Z, Lainez JM, Lampl C, Lanteri-Minet M, Rastenyte D, Ruiz de la Torre E, Tassorelli C, Barre J, Andrée C. The impact of headache in Europe: principal results of the Eurolight project. J Headache Pain. 2014;15:31.
38. Rastenyte D, Mickeviciene D, Stovner LJ, Thomas H, Andrée C, Steiner TJ. Prevalence and burden of headache disorders in Lithuania and their public-health and policy implications: a population-based study within the Eurolight project. J Headache Pain. 2017;18:53.
39. Zebenigus M, Tekle-Haimanot R, Worku DK, Thomas H, Steiner TJ. The prevalence of primary headache disorders in Ethiopia. J Headache Pain. 2016;17:110.
40. Yu S, Liu R, Zhao G, Yang X, Qiao X, Feng J, Fang Y, Cao X, He M, Steiner T. The prevalence and burden of primary headaches in China: a population-based door-to-door survey. Headache. 2012;52:582–91.
41. Ayzenberg I, Katsarava Z, Sborowski A, Chernysh M, Osipova V, Tabeeva G, Yakhno N, Steiner TJ. The prevalence of primary headache disorders in Russia: a countrywide survey. Cephalalgia. 2012;32:373–81.
42. Sjaastad O, Bakketeig LS. Cluster headache prevalence. Vågå study of headache epidemiology. Cephalalgia. 2003;23:528–33.
43. Torelli P, Beghi E, Manzoni GC. Cluster headache prevalence in the Italian general population. Neurology. 2005;64:469–74.
44. Ekbom K, Svensson DA, Pedersen NL, Waldenlind E. Lifetime prevalence and concordance risk of cluster headache in the Swedish twin population. Neurology. 2006;67:798–803.
45. Katsarava Z, Obermann M, Yoon MS, Dommes P, Kuznetsova J, Weimar C, Diener HC. Prevalence of cluster headache in a population-based sample in Germany. Cephalalgia. 2007;27:1014–9.
46. Katsarava Z, Dzagnidze A, Kukava M, Mirvelashvili E, Djibuti M, Janelidze M, Jensen R, Stovner LJ, Steiner TJ. Prevalence of cluster headache in the Republic of Georgia: results of a population-based study and methodological considerations. Cephalalgia. 2009;29:949–52.

47. Shahbeigi S, Fereshtehnejad SM, Mohammadi N, Golmakani MM, Tadayyon S, Jalilzadeh G, Pakdaman H. Epidemiology of headaches in Tehran urban area: a population-based cross-sectional study in district 8, year 2010. Neurol Sci. 2013;34:1157–66.
48. Takele GM, Tekle Haimanot R, Martelletti P. Prevalence and burden of primary headache in Akaki textile mill workers, Ethiopia. J Headache Pain. 2008;9:119–28.
49. Stovner LJ, Zwart JA, Hagen K, Terwindt G, Pascual J. Epidemiology of headache in Europe. Eur J Neurol. 2006;13:333–45.
50. Manzoni GC. Male preponderance of cluster headache is progressively decreasing over the years. Headache. 1997;37:588–9.
51. Ekbom K, Svensson DA, Traff H, Waldenlind E. Age at onset and sex ratio in cluster headache: observations over three decades. Cephalalgia. 2002;22:94–100.
52. Patel NV, Bigal ME, Kolodner KB, Leotta C, Lafata JE, Lipton RB. Prevalence and impact of migraine and probable migraine in a health plan. Neurology. 2004;63:1432–8.
53. Lanteri-Minet M, Valade D, Geraud G, Chautard MH, Lucas C. Migraine and probable migraine--results of FRAMIG 3, a French nationwide survey carried out according to the 2004 IHS classification. Cephalalgia. 2005;25:1146–58.
54. Manandhar K, Risal A, Steiner TJ, Holen A, Linde M. The prevalence of primary headache disorders in Nepal: a nationwide population-based study. J Headache Pain. 2015;16:95.
55. Rasmussen BK, Jensen R, Olesen J. A population-based analysis of the diagnostic criteria of the International Headache Society. Cephalalgia. 1991;11:129–34.
56. Hagen K, Zwart JA, Aamodt AH, Nilsen KB, Brathen G, Helde G, Stjern M, Tronvik EA, Stovner LJ. A face-to-face interview of participants in HUNT 3: the impact of the screening question on headache prevalence. J Headache Pain. 2008;9:289–94.
57. Steiner TJ, Stovner LJ, Birbeck GL. Migraine: the seventh disabler. J Headache Pain. 2013;14:1.
58. GBD 2016 Disease and Injury Incidence and Prevalence Collaborators. Global, regional, and national incidence, prevalence, and years lived with disability for 328 diseases and injuries for 195 countries, 1990–2016: a systematic analysis for the Global Burden of Disease Study 2016. Lancet. 2017;390:1211–59.
59. GBD 2017 Disease and Injury Incidence and Prevalence Collaborators. Global, regional, and national incidence, prevalence, and years lived with disability for 354 diseases and injuries for 195 countries and territories, 1990–2017: a systematic analysis for the Global Burden of Disease Study 2017. Lancet. 2018;392:1789–858.
60. Yu S, He M, Liu R, Feng J, Qiao X, Yang X, Cao X, Zhao G, Fang Y, Steiner TJ. Headache yesterday in China: a new approach to estimating the burden of headache, applied in a general-population survey in China. Cephalalgia. 2013;33:1211–7.
61. Ayzenberg I, Katsarava Z, Sborowski A, Obermann M, Chernysh M, Osipova V, Tabeeva G, Steiner TJ. Headache yesterday in Russia: its prevalence and impact, and their application in estimating the national burden attributable to headache disorders. J Headache Pain. 2014;15:7.
62. Andrée C, Steiner TJ, Barré J, Katsarava Z, Lainez JM, Lampl C, Lanteri-Minet M, Rastenyte D, Ruiz de la Torre E, Tassorelli C, Stovner LJ. Headache yesterday in Europe. J Headache Pain. 2014;15:33.
63. Hu XH, Markson LE, Lipton RB, Stewart WF, Berger ML. Burden of migraine in the United States: disability and economic costs. Arch Intern Med. 1999;159:813–8.
64. Steiner TJ. *Lifting The Burden*: the global campaign against headache. Lancet Neurol. 2004;3:204–5.
65. Steiner TJ, Lipton RB on behalf of *Lifting The Burden*: The Global Campaign against Headache. The Headache-Attributed Lost Time (HALT) Indices: measures of burden for clinical management and population-based research. J Headache Pain. 2018;19:12.
66. Lipton RB, Stewart WF, Sawyer J, Edmeads JG. Clinical utility of an instrument assessing migraine disability: the Migraine Disability Assessment (MIDAS) questionnaire. Headache. 2001;41:854–61.

67. Zebenigus M, Tekle-Haimanot R, Worku DK, Thomas H, Steiner TJ. The burden of headache disorders in Ethiopia: national estimates from a population-based door-to-door survey. J Headache Pain. 2017;18:58.
68. Rao GN, Kulkarni GB, Gururaj G, Rajesh K, Subbakrishna DK, Steiner TJ, Stovner LJ. The burden of headache disorders in India: methodology and questionnaire validation for a community-based survey in Karnataka state. J Headache Pain. 2012;13:543–50.
69. Manandhar K, Risal A, Linde M, Steiner TJ. The burden of headache disorders in Nepal: estimates from a population-based survey. J Headache Pain. 2015;17:3.
70. Ayzenberg I, Katsarava Z, Sborowski A, Chernysh M, Osipova V, Tabeeva G, Steiner TJ. Headache-attributed burden and its impact on productivity and quality of life in Russia: structured healthcare for headache is urgently needed. Eur J Neurol. 2014;21:758–65.
71. Mbewe E, Zairemthiama P, Paul R, Birbeck GL, Steiner TJ. The burden of primary headache disorders in Zambia: national estimates from a population-based door-to-door survey. J Headache Pain. 2015;16:513.
72. Hershey AD, Powers SW, Vockell AL, LeCates S, Kabbouche MA, Maynard MK. PedMIDAS: development of a questionnaire to assess disability of migraines in children. Neurology. 2001;57:2034–9.
73. Akyol A, Kiylioglu N, Aydin I, Erturk A, Kaya E, Telli E, Akyildiz U. Epidemiology and clinical characteristics of migraine among school children in the Menderes region. Cephalalgia. 2007;27:781–7.
74. Steiner TJ, Rao GN, Kulkarni GB, Gururaj G, Stovner LJ. Headache yesterday in Karnataka state, India: prevalence, impact and cost. J Headache Pain. 2016;17:74.
75. Osterhaus JT, Townsend RJ, Gandek B, Ware JE. Measuring the functional status and well-being of patients with migraine headache. Headache. 1994;34:337–43.
76. Michel P, Dartigues JF, Lindoulsi A, Henry P. Loss of productivity and quality of life in migraine sufferers among French workers: results from the GAZEL cohort. Headache. 1997;37:71–8.
77. Terwindt GM, Ferrari MD, Tijhuis M, Groenen SM, Picavet HS, Launer LJ. The impact of migraine on quality of life in the general population: the GEM study. Neurology. 2000;55:624–9.
78. Guitera V, Muñoz P, Castillo J, Pascual J. Quality of life in chronic daily headache: a study in a general population. Neurology. 2002;58:1062–5.
79. Lipton RB, Liberman JN, Kolodner KB, Bigal ME, Dowson A, Stewart WF. Migraine headache disability and health-related quality-of-life: a population-based case-control study from England. Cephalalgia. 2003;23:441–50.
80. Lipton RB, Hamelsky SW, Kolodner KB, Steiner TJ, Stewart WF. Migraine, quality of life, and depression: a population-based case-control study. Neurology. 2000;55:629–35.
81. Duru G, Auray JP, Gaudin AF, Dartigues JF, Henry P, Lantéri-Minet M, Lucas C, Pradalier A, Chazot G, Hasnaoui AE. Impact of headache on quality of life in a general population survey in France (GRIM2000 study). Headache. 2004;44:571–80.
82. Kececi H, Dener S, Analan E. Co-morbidity of migraine and major depression in the Turkish population. Cephalalgia. 2003;23:271–5.
83. Zwart JA, Dyb G, Hagen K, Odegard KJ, Dahl AA, Bovim G, Stovner LJ. Depression and anxiety disorders associated with headache frequency. The Nord-Trondelag health study. Eur J Neurol. 2003;20:147–52.
84. Anttila P, Metsahonkala L, Mikkelsson M, Helenius H, Sillanpaa M. Comorbidity of other pains in schoolchildren with migraine or nonmigrainous headache. J Pediatr. 2001; 138:176–80.
85. Hagen K, Einarsen C, Zwart JA, Svebak S, Bovim G. The co-occurrence of headache and musculoskeletal symptoms amongst 51,050 adults in Norway. Eur J Neurol. 2002;9:527–33.
86. Lipton RB, Bigal ME, Kolodner K, Stewart WF, Liberman JN, Steiner TJ. The family impact of migraine: population-based studies in the USA and UK. Cephalalgia. 2003;23:429–40.
87. Linde M, Dahlöf C. Attitudes and burden of disease among self-considered migraineurs--a nation-wide population-based survey in Sweden. Cephalalgia. 2004;24:455–65.

88. Lampl C, Thomas H, Stovner LJ, Tassorelli C, Katsarava Z, Lainez JM, Lanteri-Minet M, Rastenyte D, Ruiz de la Torre E, Andree C, Steiner TJ. Interictal burden attributable to episodic headache: findings from the Eurolight project. J Headache Pain. 2016;17:9.
89. Steiner TJ, Stovner LJ, Katsarava Z, Lainez JM, Lampl C, Lanteri-Minet M, Rastenyte D, Ruiz de la Torre E, Tassorelli C, Barré J, Andrée C. The impact of headache in Europe: principal results of the Eurolight project. J Headache Pain. 2014;15:31.
90. Jensen RM, Lyngberg A, Jensen RH. Burden of cluster headache. Cephalalgia. 2007;27:535–41.
91. Rozen TD, Fishman RS. Cluster headache in the United States of America: demographics, clinical characteristics, triggers, suicidality, and personal burden. Headache. 2012;52:99–113.

Chapter 9
Headache in the Global Burden of Disease (GBD) Studies

Lars Jacob Stovner, Emma Nichols, Timothy J. Steiner, and Theo Vos

9.1 Introduction

In some sense, it is true that migraine appeared on the global health map in 2001, when the World Health Organization (WHO) published its *World Health Report* of the Global Burden of Disease 2000 study (GBD2000) [1]. Before that, some doctors, in particular headache specialists, some people affected by headache and their organizations were aware of the impact of headache disorders on personal health and well-being. To some degree, they were aware also of their economic impact at individual and societal levels. However, perception of headache as a major public-health concern was mostly lacking, even in these circles. The influence of GBD, from GBD2000 and through its later iterations, has been far-reaching, and not least for the headaches. If the current neglect of headache disorders abates in years to come, the contributory importance of GBD must be recognized.

L. J. Stovner (✉)
Department of Neuromedicine and Movement Science, NTNU Norwegian University of Science and Technology, Trondheim, Norway

Norwegian Advisory Unit on Headaches, Department of Neurology and Clinical Neurophysiology, St Olavs University Hospital, Trondheim, Norway
e-mail: lars.stovner@ntnu.no

E. Nichols · T. Vos
Institute for Health Metrics and Evaluation (IHME), University of Washington, Seattle, WA, USA
e-mail: eln1@uw.edu; tvos@uw.edu

T. J. Steiner
Department of Neuromedicine and Movement Science, NTNU Norwegian University of Science and Technology, Trondheim, Norway

Division of Brain Sciences, Imperial College London, London, UK
e-mail: t.steiner@imperial.ac.uk

T. J. Steiner, L. J. Stovner (eds.), *Societal Impact of Headache*, Headache,
https://doi.org/10.1007/978-3-030-24728-7_9

The aim of this chapter is to provide an overview of the GBD project from its commencement, with a particular focus on headache. We explain the methodology relevant to headache used in GBD2016 and present the main results from this study (for which we have earlier published a thorough analysis [2]). We mention a few methodological changes that were made with regard to headache in GBD2017. Finally, we point to some challenges that should be addressed in future GBD iterations.

9.2 History of the GBD Studies with a Focus on Headache

9.2.1 GBD1990

This first GBD project, commissioned by the World Bank in 1991 and undertaken collaboratively by the Bank and WHO, was the background for the Bank's report, *Investment in Health* [3]. It was intended to be used by governments and non-governmental organizations (NGOs) to prioritize efforts in healthcare provision and research. Three goals, still highly relevant, were central to the project [4]:

1. To decouple epidemiological assessment of the magnitude of health problems from advocacy of particular health policies or interventions by interest groups
2. To include, in international health-policy debates, information on non-fatal health outcomes along with information on mortality
3. To undertake the quantification of health problems in time-based units that could also be used in economic appraisal

Goals 2 and 3 were fulfilled by establishing a new measure, disability-adjusted life years (DALYs), which are the sum of years of life lost (YLLs) through early mortality and years lived with disability (YLDs). YLL calculations for a disease are based on a set standard life expectancy at the age of each early death, itself derived from a life table combining the lowest observed age-specific mortality rates in any population greater than five million. YLDs are estimated as the number of years lived with a disorder (or with a health state attributable to it) multiplied by a disability weight (DW) for that disorder (or health state).

YLDs are highly relevant to headache disorders, whereas YLLs are not (headache disorders are not considered to be underlying causes of death), but neither migraine nor any other headache disorder were part of GBD1990.

9.2.2 GBD2000

This follow-up to GBD1990 was undertaken by WHO. It included data on a larger number of conditions, while providing burden estimates for all 21 WHO health regions.

Unlike its predecessor, GBD2000 recognized the importance of mental and neurological disorders and included migraine within these [1]. It used a rather intricate but relatively unsophisticated disease model to estimate overall disability attributable to migraine [5, 6]. Consultations with experts determined the distribution, in the population, of different attack severities (mild, moderate, severe) and their frequencies, and made assumptions about disease duration (between 15 and 45 years) and attack duration (24 h untreated and 6 h treated). A disability weight (DW) based on some previous estimates, on a scale from 0 to 1, was assigned to each attack severity (mild: 0.05; moderate: 0.16; severe: 0.7), and to the periods between attacks, for those with relatively frequent attacks (more than one per week), a DW of 0.03 was assigned. For the different world regions, GBD2000 assumed different proportions of treated and untreated attacks. Combining these DWs proportionately, an overall average DW of 0.03 was assigned to each person with untreated migraine and a DW of 0.007 to each person with treated migraine.

As in later iterations, prevalence estimates were based on population-based studies applying the then-current classification of the International Headache Society (IHS); for GBD2000, this was ICHD-I [7]. Studies included were mostly from Western Europe and North America, with a few from South America, East Asia and the Middle East and one from Africa [5]. Based on these epidemiological data, age-standardized prevalences (i.e. adjusted for age distributions in the different world regions) varied considerably: for women from 17% in parts of Europe to 3% in parts of Africa, and for men from 5.5% to 1%, with world prevalences of 7.9% for women and 2.8% for men [5]. In the whole world, men experienced 0.7 YLDs per 1000 person-years and women 1.8 YLDs per 1000 person-years. In the *World Health Report 2001* [1, 5], migraine accounted for 1.4% of all YLDs, which placed it among the top 20 (19th) disabling disorders worldwide. In women of all ages, it accounted for 2.0% of YLDs, putting it in 12th place. Even with no mortality (0 YLLs), migraine was the 19th highest cause of DALYs in young women (15–44 years).

GBD2000 was updated each year until 2004, when migraine fell out of the list of the 20 most disabling disorders, possibly owing to slight adjustments to some of the DWs.

All in all, the burden calculation for migraine in GBD2000 was complicated, not very transparent and based on several questionable assumptions. Nevertheless, the significance of GBD2000 for headache was considerable. It was later stated that

> "*With the publication of data on burden of migraine in WHR 2001, WHO recognises headache disorders as a high-priority public health problem and as such they deserve higher attention...*" [6].

9.2.3 GBD2010, GBD2013 and GBD2015

GBD2010 was a major revision, with regard not only to its breadth and scope (many more conditions and risk factors) but also to its innovative methods and use of a wide variety of data sources. The project was described as a "*systematic, scientific effort to quantify the magnitude of health loss due to diseases, injuries, and risk factors by age, sex, and geography for specific points in time*" [8].

GBD was now led by the newly established (2007) Institute for Health Metrics and Evaluation (IHME) at the University of Washington, Seattle, USA, with funding from the Bill and Melinda Gates Foundation. The study had become a truly global endeavour, representing the work of several high-ranking institutions (Harvard University, Imperial College London, Johns Hopkins University, University of Queensland, University of Tokyo and WHO), and altogether included 486 scientists from 302 institutions in 50 countries [9].

In GBD2010, the methodology was substantially revised. While earlier GBD iterations had been based on disease incidence, which is very relevant for prevention but for which there are limited data for many disorders, GBD2000 estimates were instead based on prevalence measures. For these, there were far more data, particularly for the chronic and episodic disorders. Extensive mathematical disease models were introduced to enable use of all available data (rather than selecting a single "most appropriate" source for a particular geographical location) and to provide estimates for all countries and all age and gender groups at different time points. Instead of expert opinions as the basis for determining DWs, these were now to be derived from "lay descriptions" of all health states in a so-called *pairwise comparisons* method, with, eventually, over 60,000 people participating in nine country surveys and an open internet survey. Descriptions of two hypothetical persons with different, randomly selected health states were presented to respondents, who were asked to indicate which person in their view was the healthier of the two. The rationale behind the method was the intuition that conditions perceived as relatively similar in their effect on health would create more disagreement (i.e. closer to 50/50 responses), while conditions very different in their effect would create less (e.g. 90/10 responses). By comparing all responses, conditions could be ranked from most to least effect on health. Still no exact DW could be assigned: this was achieved by another set of pairwise comparisons, this time of population health programmes. Respondents were asked to compare the health benefits of 30 different life-saving or disease-prevention programmes: for example, one that prevented 1000 rapid deaths and another that prevented a number of cases, varying between 2000 and 10,000, of a non-fatal disease. In this way, health conditions were placed on a 0–1 scale, where 0 was perfect health and 1 was disability deemed equivalent to death.

For headache disorders, now including both migraine and TTH, the method of YLD estimation had in some ways become much less intricate. In contrast to GBD2000, where three levels of migraine attack severity were described and each assigned a DW, in GBD2010 and subsequently, only one (ictal) health state was defined for migraine and one for TTH. This was sensible, because there were limited data on the population distributions of different attack severities. To achieve this, the lay descriptions of the health states attempted to capture, for each disorder, the "mean" headache attack. Thus, in GBD2010, the DW for migraine (ictal state) was 0.434 [10]: during an attack, health loss was equated to 43.4% of death. The corresponding DW for TTH was 0.040 [10].

Data sources for headache from GBD2010 onwards were, mostly, published population-based studies of prevalence identified by regular PubMed searches (using the terms *headache epidemiology*, *headache prevalence*, *migraine epidemiology* and *migraine prevalence*) and through scrutiny of reference lists in published papers. Some data were also solicited from the GBD network of collaborators, allowing, for example, the inclusion of data from not-yet-published LTB studies. Studies subsequent to the publication of ICHD-I in 1988 [7] were considered, with some earlier studies after appropriate adjustments of the data.

A weakness of GBD2000 was that the large majority of headache studies were from Western Europe and North America; at that time, there were few data from large and populous areas of the world (South East Asia, Eastern Europe, large parts of Africa and mainland China). Some of the few studies existing from outside Europe and North America encompassed many different disorders and gave unrealistically low prevalence estimates (e.g. a study from Saudi Arabia reported a lifetime prevalence of headache overall of only 8% [11]). Prevalence data for GBD2010 were taken from a 2007 review of all published prevalence and burden studies [12], which used explicit quality criteria for acceptance of studies [13]. The result was inclusion of many more studies than those available for GBD2000, but still evidence was lacking from important countries and several regions. Therefore, *Lifting The Burden* (LTB) [14] supplied supplementary data from new population-based studies performed in Russia [15], China [16, 17] and India [18].

GBD2010 was thus able to report on TTH as well as migraine, while GBD2013 and GBD2015, each including further headache epidemiological studies, added estimates for MOH.

9.3 GBD2016 and GBD2017

9.3.1 Methods

A full description and analysis of the methods and results of GBD2016 in relation to headache have been published [2]; the following relates mostly to GBD2016, with GBD2017 mentioned only where the methods differ.

In GBD2016, the number of collaborators increased to more than 2500, from 133 countries [19]. GBD2016 used a hierarchical list of 328 diseases and injuries with four levels of increasing diagnostic detail ("granularity"), in which migraine and TTH were on level 3, under neurological disorders (level 2) and non-communicable diseases (level 1). GBD2017 introduced a new category of "headache disorders" at level 3, displacing migraine and TTH to level 4. At level 5 of the hierarchy, GBD2016 listed 2989 *sequelae*: the direct consequences of disease or injuries, each mapped to a parsimonious set of 235 health states. GBD2016 considered MOH a *sequela* of either migraine or TTH rather than a separate entity, and the burden attributed to

MOH was added to the burden estimates for each of these disorders according to the proportions believed to arise from them (migraine: 73%; TTH: 27%) [20, 21].

YLDs in GBD reflect the number of years lived with a disorder, adjusted for the attributable health loss expressed in the DW assigned to it. For most diseases, YLDs for a certain year are calculated as prevalence times DW. For episodic disorders such as headaches, the DW pertains only to the symptomatic (ictal) state, and YLD calculations are based on estimates of time in this state.

GBD2016 (and GBD2017) used variations of the DWs, which were first introduced in GBD2013 as participation expanded in the surveys whereby they were quantified (see above). Thus, the DW for migraine (symptomatic state) was increased very slightly to 0.441, and the DW for TTH was diminished very slightly to 0.037. The DW for MOH, included for the first time in GBD2013, was 0.223 [22]. Table 9.1 shows these and the DWs of some other disorders for comparison.

GBD2016 analyzed data from 195 countries and territories grouped into 21 geographical regions and seven super-regions based on geographical proximity and epidemiological similarity of countries [19]. Countries were also scored according to a sociodemographic index (SDI), a composite measure of income, education and fertility meant to capture, roughly, their level of "development" over time [19].

Table 9.1 Disability weights (DWs) for headache disorders, and selected other conditions for comparison (headache disorders in bold typeface; from [22], the last update of DWs, used in GBD 2013 and later iterations)

Condition	Disease weight	95% CI
Schizophrenia, acute stage	0.778	0.606–0.900
Major depressive disorder, severe episode	0.658	0.477–0.807
Epilepsy, severe, ≥1/month	0.552	0.375–0.710
AIDS, no retroviral treatment	0.547	0.382–0.715
Stroke, long-term consequences, severe	0.552	0.377–0.707
Metastatic cancer	0.451	0.307–0.600
Migraine	**0.441**	**0.294–0.588**
Moderate depressive episode	0.396	0.267–0.531
Acute myocardial infarction, days 1–2	0.432	0.288–0.579
Low back pain, most severe, with leg pain	0.384	0.256–0.518
Neck pain, most severe	0.304	0.202–0.415
Diarrhoea, severe	0.247	0.164–0.348
Epilepsy, less severe, ≤1/month	0.263	0.173–0.367
Crohn's disease or ulcerative colitis	0.231	0.156–0.320
Medication overuse headache	**0.223**	**0.146–0.313**
Heart failure, severe	0.179	0.122–0.251
Severe anaemia	0.149	0.101–0.209
Major depressive disorder, mild episode	0.145	0.099–0.209
Asthma, uncontrolled	0.133	0.086–0.0192
Tension-type headache	**0.037**	**0.022–0.057**
Mild angina pectoris	0.033	0.020–0.052
Stroke, long-term consequences, mild	0.019	0.010–0.032
Infertility, primary	0.011	0.005–0.021

Data sources in GBD2016 included United States (US) medical claims data, for the years 2000, 2010 and 2012. GBD2017 omitted these because of the large adjustments needed to make them comparable with data from population-based studies.

Migraine data were extracted from 135 studies in GBD2016, covering 16 of the 21 GBD world regions; TTH data came from 76 studies in 16 regions; MOH data came from 37 studies in seven regions [19]. For migraine, 13 studies provided data on frequency and duration of attacks, collectively indicating that people with migraine spend, on average, 8.5% of their time in the symptomatic state. For TTH, seven studies indicated 4.7% of time in this state. Frequency and duration were generally categorized, and it was presumed that the mean of the upper and lower limits fairly represented each category. For MOH, only one study provided data [15], indicating that people with MOH have headache on a mean of 23.1 days per month.

9.3.1.1 Comprehensiveness

GBD studies employ extensive mathematical modelling in order to make them comprehensive: that is, to provide estimates of incidence, prevalence, mortality and remission rate for all included disease states in all countries, in all age groups and both genders, and at different time points. The so-called *compartmental disease model* provides the relationships between these variables, and can be used to estimate those missing (e.g. there are very few data on incidence for headache disorders). For all headaches, mortality is set at zero, as is occurrence below 5 years of age.

For most disorders, including the headaches, data are scarce or lacking for many countries, regions and age groups, the methods used to estimate prevalence (and incidence) have been heterogenous, and available data are of varying quality (because, for example, of varying case definitions, age categories and representativeness of population samples (see Chaps. 6 and 7)). To enable comprehensiveness in spite of these problems, GBD has developed a so-called *Bayesian meta-regression method* called DisMod-MR. This mathematically models disease variables such as prevalence and incidence by combining the methods of meta-analysis (using weighted averages of many data points) with estimates of associations ("regressions") between, for example, prevalence of a disorder and covariates. For headache, these covariates are the fixed effects of gender and of methodological characteristics of studies ("study level covariates" (see below)) and the random effects of geography (region, country). *Bayesian* means that the method uses *priors* (initial estimates), derived from other countries, to make final estimates for a certain gender-age group for a country where data are missing.

9.3.1.2 Adjustment

As to *study level covariates*, these are taken from the published guidelines on performance and quality evaluation of studies on headache prevalence, burden and cost [13]. From GBD2015 onwards, all headache epidemiological studies have been scored according to a modified version (dichotomized variables) of these criteria, considering representativeness of the population, quality of sampling, headache recall period, participation proportion, survey method, validation of diagnostic instrument and the way in which ICHD criteria were applied. In Dismod-MR, these variables are evaluated as potential covariates for adjustment of data.

In the migraine epidemiological studies in GBD2016, only two of these factors appeared to play a role: low participation proportion and poor survey method. The US claims data apparently underestimated prevalence grossly, by almost 90%, yet their age pattern was consistent with that of US surveys and they were used after adjustment because they provided detailed estimates by state in the USA. For TTH, adjustments were required for survey method, low participation proportion, poor sampling method, poor application of ICHD criteria and lack of validation of the diagnostic instrument. Claims data underestimated TTH prevalence by approximately 85%. For MOH, adjustments were required for poor application of ICHD criteria and low participation proportion.

9.3.1.3 Borrowing Strength Over Space and Time

By these means, a best guess can be made even where no data exist. Where there are no data for an age group, gender or a time point, estimates are made from those adjacent. For countries with data, final estimates are still, to some degree, informed by those from the whole world, super-region and region, making them less vulnerable to bias and random effects. In GBD terminology, estimates "borrow strength over space and time".

Each new GBD cycle will include not only new data from the preceding year(s) but also newly available old data concerning past years. Since DisMod is continuously upgraded and refined, new covariates, and values for them, are introduced, and diagnostic entities may be changed. Hence, new estimations affect the whole time series, implying that, for example, migraine estimates for 1990 may not be the same in GBD2010 as in GBD2016 or GBD2017.

9.3.1.4 Comorbidity Correction

Since many people suffer from the consequences of two or more conditions, especially with aging, simply adding DWs can result in a combined DW greater than 1, which does not have meaning. To avoid overestimation of the burden, both on the individual and at societal level, comorbidity correction for YLDs is the final step.

Comorbidities are considered to be independent of each other: that is, they co-occur by chance, according to their respective prevalences. (Dependent comorbidity is recognized when two disorders tend to co-occur more often than would be expected by chance. Dependent comorbidities are incompletely known, computationally very challenging and probably do not make a large difference to estimates when corrections are made for age.)

In GBD, comorbidity corrections are performed for each gender, age, time and location group. The following example concerns only two comorbid conditions, but the model can include more. In a person with two disorders A and B, with different DWs (DW_A and DW_B), the total ("cumulative") DW is calculated by the formula $DW_{A+B} = [1 - (1 - DW_A)*(1 - DW_B)]$. This can intuitively be understood as follows: when a person already with disorder A develops disorder B, the DW of the second disorder is calculated on the basis not of full health but of the health remaining after DW_A has been deducted. So, in the example, if $DW_A = 0.5$ and $DW_B = 0.4$, the cumulative $DW_{A+B} = 0.7$.

The cumulative DW combines the DWs of two (or more) disorders, but, often, interest is only in the resultant DW of one disorder after comorbidities have been taken into account. This is determined by first calculating the attributable DWs with respect to the disorder of interest, and then taking the population averages of attributable DWs in all individuals in the population. This yields comorbidity-corrected YLDs for the disorder in the population. To continue the example, consider a population of 1000 in which disorder A (the disorder of interest) has a prevalence of 10% (100 people affected) and disorder B 5% (50 people affected); furthermore, comorbidity here is solely due to chance. Among the 100 with disorder A, five will also have disorder B. To the 95 without, $DW_A = 0.5$ is applied. Among the five, the disability attributable to A is 0.3, represented by $DW_{attrib} = 0.5*0.6$, where 0.6 is the health remaining after deduction of DW_B. In the population of 1000, the comorbidity-corrected DW among the 100 people with A is only 0.49, calculated as [(95*0.5) + (5*0.3)]/100.

9.3.2 *Headache Estimates in GBD2016*

Results have been extracted from relevant parts of the GBD2016 capstone paper on prevalences and YLDs for all diseases [19] and from the publication of headache results [2].

GDB2016 reported almost three billion people affected by headache disorders: 1.90 billion (95% uncertainty interval (UI): 1.71–2.10 bn) had TTH and 1.04 billion (1.00–1.09 bn) had migraine. Globally, TTH was the third most prevalent disorder (after dental caries and latent tuberculosis infection) and migraine eighth [19]. Global age-standardized prevalences were 26.1% (95% UI: 23.6–29.0) for TTH (30.8% [28.0–34.0] in women and 21.4% [19.2–23.9] in men) and 14.4% (13.8–15.0) for migraine (18.9% [18.1–19.7] in women and 9.8% [9.4–10.2] in men). Age-standardized prevalences of both TTH and migraine varied considerably through the different GBD regions and were almost twice as high in Western Europe and Australasia as in Eastern sub-Saharan Africa (Fig. 9.1). The numbers in the different regions (Fig. 9.2) demonstrate that approximately 40% of all people with migraine (430 million) or TTH (770 million) in the world were living in South Asia or East Asia.

Migraine was responsible for 45.1 (29.0–62.8) million YLDs globally in 2016, and TTH for 7.2 (4.6–10.5) million. Global age-standardized YLD rates (YLDs/100,000 population) were, for migraine, 599.0 (386.0–833.3) (777.6 [500.4–1083.6] in women, 422.3 [274.3–586.7] in men) and, for TTH, 95.9 (61.5–140.0) (114.6 [73.6–162.4] in women, 77.4 [49.6–113.2] in men). Figure 9.3 shows the

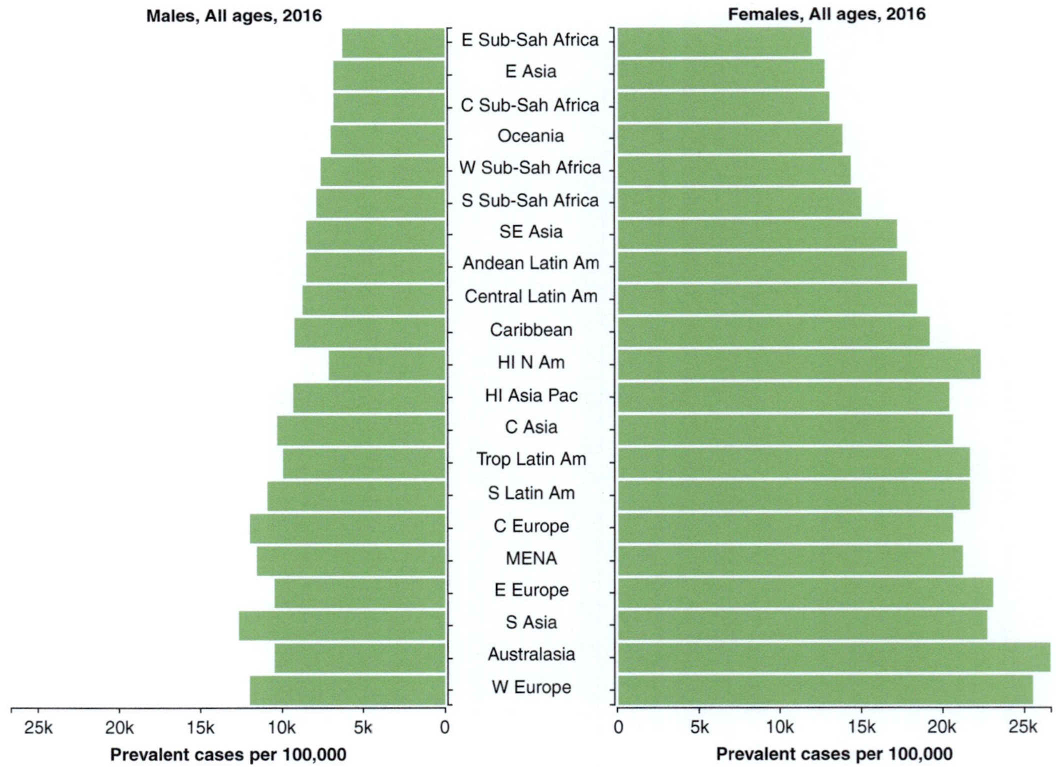

Fig. 9.1 Age-standardized prevalences (per 100,000 population) in males (left) and females (right), ranked by total, in the different GBD regions (in alphabetical order: Andean Latin America, Australasia, Caribbean, Central Asia, Central Europe, Central Latin America, Central sub-Saharan Africa, East Asia, Eastern Europe, Eastern sub-Saharan Africa, High Income Asia Pacific, High Income North America, Middle East and North Africa, Oceania, South Asia, Southeast Asia, Southern Latin America, Southern sub-Saharan Africa, Tropical Latin America, Western Europe, Western sub-Saharan Africa) (from [19])

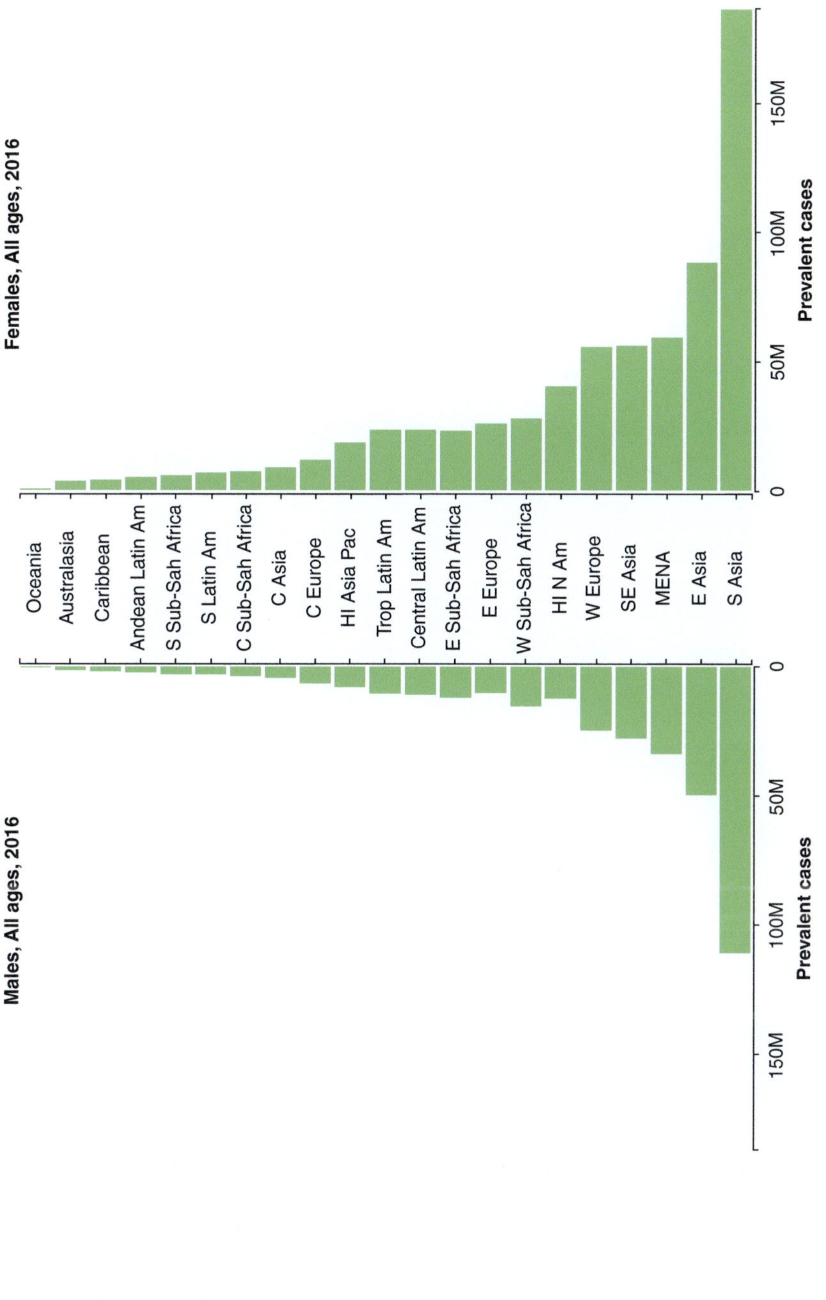

Fig. 9.2 Age-standardized numbers of cases in males (left) and females (right) in the different GBD regions (for explanation of regions, see legend to Fig. 9.1) (from [19])

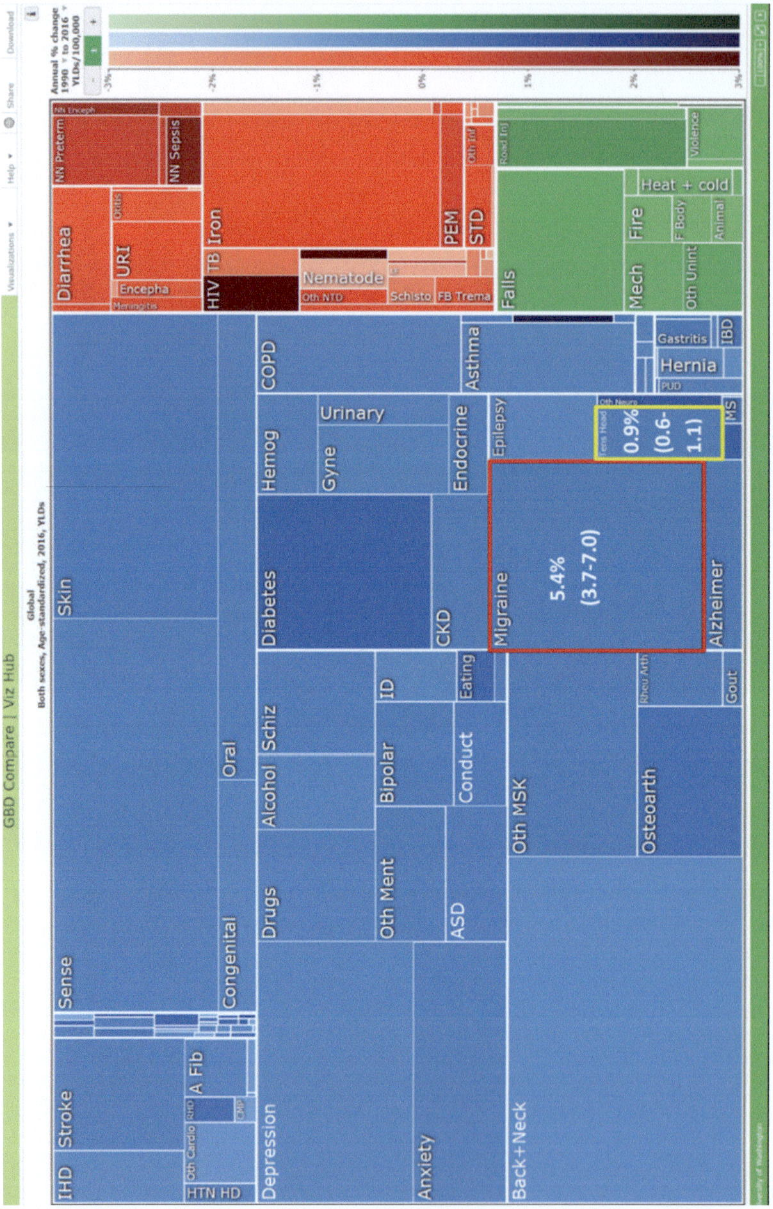

Fig. 9.3 Headache on the global disease map. Graphical presentation of the relative proportions (age-standardized) of YLDs for all disorders (level 3) in 2016, in both genders and all world regions (blue area: non-communicable diseases; green area: injuries; red area: nutritional, mother-child and communicable diseases (from IHME interactive website: https://vizhub.healthdata.org/gbd-compare/). We have emphasized migraine (red outline) and tension-type headache (yellow outline), and indicated percentage YLDs of the global total

percentages of all YLDs caused by each disorder analyzed at cause-level 3, highlighting migraine (5.4% of all YLDs) and TTH (0.9%). At level 4, the most specific (granular) cause level, migraine was the second cause of disability (after back pain) in 1990, 2006 and 2016 [19] and, in GBD2016, the first cause of disability in people under 50 years [23]. In terms of percentage of all YLDs, migraine was first in two regions, second in nine, third in five, fourth in two, fifth in two and sixth in one. Globally, TTH was 28th in 1990, 2006 and 2016 [19]. Absolute number of YLDs for migraine increased by 32.3% between 1990 and 2006 and by 14.3% between 2006 and 2016, but the mean changes in age-standardized YLD rates were small (−0.4% and +1.1%, respectively). For TTH, there were also marked increases in absolute rates over the two periods (32.7% and 15.4%, respectively), but not in age-standardized rates (−0.7% and +0.4%). Migraine, along with low back pain, ranked among the top 10 causes of YLDs (age-standardized) in all 195 countries [19].

Figure 9.4 relates YLD rates to age for migraine and TTH. Both disorders were most burdensome at ages 35–45 years, whereafter the burdens of both, but particularly of migraine, tapered to less than a third of the peak value by age 85. However, the figure shows that headache, and in particular migraine, represented a substantial burden in young and elderly people.

Figure 9.5 shows there was no obvious relation between the burdens (DALY rates) of migraine and TTH and SDI in the different groups of countries.

With regard to DALYs, these are the same as YLDs for migraine and TTH, since no mortality is attributed to headache. Globally, in both genders and all ages, migraine caused 1.9% (1.3–2.5) of all DALYs, 2.7% (1.8–3.6) of those in women and 1.2% (0.8–1.7) of those in men. The corresponding numbers for TTH were 0.3% (0.2–0.4) for both genders, 0.4% (0.3–0.5) in women and 0.2% (0.2–0.3) in men. Table 9.2 shows the proportion of all YLDs and DALYs for the neurological conditions, stroke and some pain conditions. This shows that migraine is second after low back pain with regard to YLDs and third after low back pain and stroke with regard to DALYs. Among the purely neurological disorders, it is by far the most burdensome.

9.4 Comments

The GBD studies have recently been described as "a systematic scientific effort to quantify the comparative magnitude of health loss from diseases, injuries and risks by age sex, and population over time" [24]. GBD makes use of a wide variety of data sources on diseases and risk factors, thereby enhancing the value of all the single studies, enabling corrections for comorbidities, associations and known sources of error. There are several limitations to the estimates on headaches that must be taken into consideration and amended, but they nevertheless give a clear message to the world about the importance of headache for global public health.

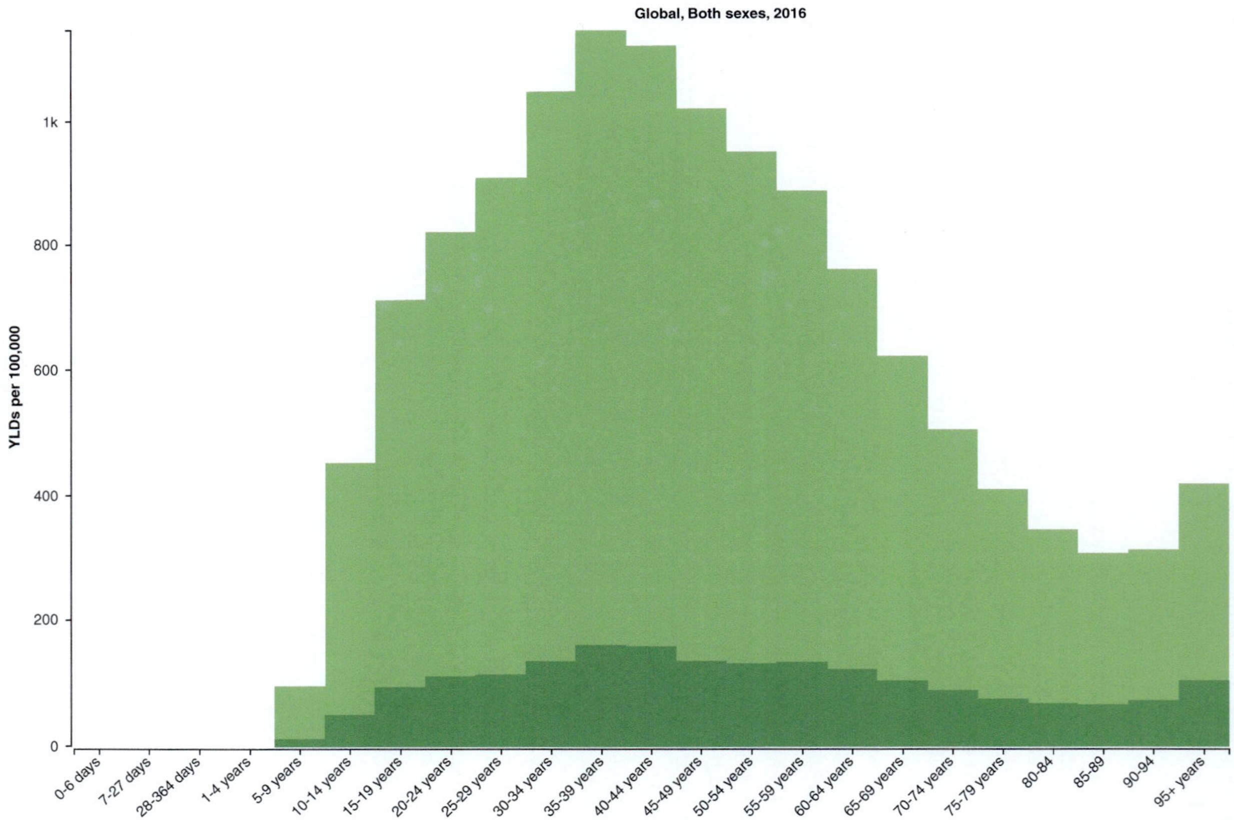

Fig. 9.4 Global YLD rates (YLDs per 100,000 population) for migraine (light green) and tension-type headache (dark green) for both genders by age (from IHME interactive website (https://vizhub.healthdata.org/gbd-compare/))

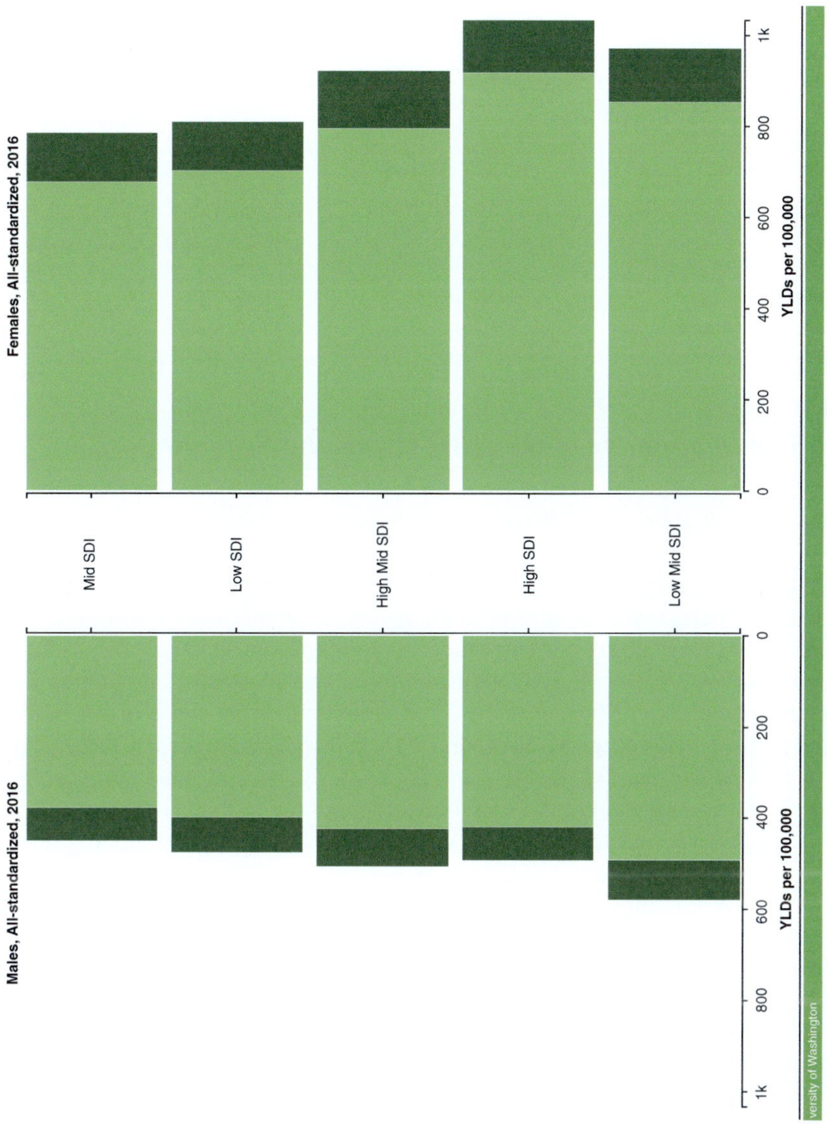

Fig. 9.5 YLD rates (YLDs per 100,000 population) in the five regions defined by sociodemographic index (SDI) for migraine (light green) and TTH (dark green) in men (left) and women (right) (from IHME interactive website (https://vizhub.healthdata.org/gbd-compare/))

Table 9.2 DALYs and YLDs as percentages of all DALYs and YLDs, globally for both genders and all ages, for migraine and TTH compared with other important neurological disorders, stroke and pain conditions (from IHME interactive website (http://viz.healthmetricsandevaluation.org/gbd-compare/))

Condition	DALYs [95% UI]	YLDs [95% UI]
Low back pain	2.4 [1.9–3.0]	7.2 [6.0–8.3]
Stroke	4.9 [4.5–5.3]	1.8 [1.4–2.2]
Neck pain	1.2 [0.9–1.6]	3.6 [3.0–4.3]
Other musculoskeletal disorders	1.3 [0.9–1.7]	3.6 [2.8–4.7]
Neurological disorders		
Alzheimer's disease	1.2 [1.0–1.4]	0.8 [0.6–1.0]
Migraine	**1.9 [1.3–2.5]**	**5.6 [4.0–7.2]**
Epilepsy	0.6 [0.5–0.7]	0.9 [0.7–1.2]
Parkinson's disease	0.1 [0.1–0.2]	0.1 [0.1–0.1]
Multiple sclerosis	0.0 [0.0–0.1]	0.1 [0.1–0.1]
Tension-type headache	**0.3 [0.2–0.4]**	**0.9 [0.7–1.1]**
Other neurological disorders	0.2 [0.1–0.2]	0.2 [0.2–0.3]

9.4.1 The Importance of the GBD Headache Estimates

GBD has shown that headache disorders, and in particular migraine, are among the principal causes of disability all over the world, particularly in women. In 2016, migraine and TTH affected nearly three billion people globally, causing 7% of all YLDs and 2% of all DALYs in spite of no mortality. Migraine was the second cause of disability, and particularly burdensome during the most productive years of life, while its impact was not negligible among children and adolescents, or among the middle-aged and elderly. Migraine is by far the most important cause of morbidity among the purely neurological disorders (except for stroke when measured in DALYs). Among the painful disorders, migraine is the second most burdensome globally, after low back pain (a mixture of disorders).

The increases in headache YLDs over the years are most probably due to growth and aging of the world's population, since YLD rates (per 100,000) have remained stable. On DALY rankings, the headaches are higher in 2016 than in 1990 because of a decrease in the relative importance of fatal disorders during these years.

GBD also documents that headache is not a western disorder, confined to the rich part of the world. In contrast, some of the highest prevalences are found in some low- and middle-income countries. It has previously been shown that many countries are undergoing a double set of transitions: a demographic transition from high to low mortality and fertility, accompanied by an epidemiological transition from high to low rates of communicable diseases, maternal diseases and childhood mortality, with an increase in relative importance of non-communicable diseases. Both transitions are strongly linked to changes in the SDI. However, headaches seem little affected by these transitions, as there is no obvious relation between SDI level and headache YLD rates. Therefore, it can be predicted that the relative importance of headache for public health will increase as the importance of fatal diseases decrease. Of course, in many poor countries, people suffer the double burden of both communicable and non-communicable diseases: one does not lessen the other.

Finally, GBD shows that the large majority of people with migraine in the world live in countries where medications of proven efficacy are either unavailable or unaffordable for the majority, and where there is little medical attention given to headache. This gives a strong call for improving health care for headache, and embedding it within existing healthcare systems (see Chaps. 13, 14, and 15). The call sounds everywhere: not only in the richest countries. Studies in several developing countries have demonstrated large national productivity losses due to headache: 1.3% in China [17], 1.6% in Ethiopia [25], 1.9% in Zambia [26], 3% in India [27] and 5.6% in Nepal [28]. If only part of this lost productivity can be recovered through better treatment, investments in improved health services will be highly cost-effective (see Chap. 15).

9.4.2 Limitations in GBD Methods and Headache Burden Estimates

Lack of data is still a limitation. Although a number of headache epidemiological studies in the last decade have included large and populous regions of the world, such as Russia, China, India and parts of Africa, where no data existed before, it remains the case that the majority of studies are from a few high-income regions, and there are still five regions wholly undocumented for migraine. No data exist for the large populations of Indonesia, Vietnam, Bangladesh, Egypt, South Africa and the Democratic Republic of Congo. In sub-Saharan Africa, only five countries have any data on headache. For TTH and MOH, the data are even more scarce. In addition, there are very few population-based studies that provide good estimates of average headache duration and frequency, which are necessary for calculation of time spent in the symptomatic state. Further, there is a need to update results in many places, to gather more reliable data and, perhaps, to monitor secular trends in headache epidemiology.

In GBD, DisMod-MR makes it possible to adjust results of studies according to methodological norms for how to perform and evaluate studies. An important aspect not taken into account in this model is the distinction between definite and probable diagnoses of migraine and TTH. Definite diagnoses fulfil all main diagnostic ICHD criteria, whereas probable diagnoses fail to fulfil one of these. The latter, as noted, are relatively common in epidemiological studies because data gathering is unavoidably less searching and thorough than in clinical settings. Studies that have reported both definite and probable migraine have found similar prevalences of each (see Chap. 7).

Importantly, probable diagnoses do not represent separate nosological entities (see Chap. 6). In clinical settings, they are useful for patients in whom there is diagnostic uncertainty pending confirmation (or refutation) later. This is not the case in epidemiological studies, and, unless probable diagnoses are included within either migraine or TTH, large numbers of people with headache—perhaps half—will not be counted. However, until now, the vast majority of studies of migraine have reported only definite migraine or are silent on the issue.

Studies investigating who received probable migraine diagnoses in epidemiological studies have found the great majority failed on attack duration, reporting attacks of less than 4 h (e.g. [29–31]). Otherwise, the characteristics of definite and probable migraine are similar, and the latter is associated with considerable disability and suffering. GBD needs to develop methods to include probable migraine, addressing its omission from most historical data; otherwise, much disability will be unaccounted for. While GBD2017 began the process, the methods need further refinement. Similar arguments can be made for probable TTH, although the missed YLDs are far fewer because of the much lower DW of TTH.

Another problem is the handling of the chronic headache disorders: those characterized by headache on 15 or more days per month for more than 3 months. Many of these will fall into the categories of chronic migraine, chronic TTH or MOH, but these diagnoses generally cannot be made with any certainty in epidemiological studies, which are mostly based on structured questionnaires administered by lay interviewers or self-administered (see Chaps. 6 and 7). Probable MOH may be identified where headache on 15 or more days per month is associated with medication overuse (see Chap. 7), but otherwise these undoubtedly disabling headaches are not captured by the diagnoses used in GBD. It is not clear how this problem might be solved: future epidemiological studies cannot easily improve the recognition of chronic migraine and chronic TTH.

Despite efforts to adjust for methodological differences between studies, some of the variation between countries may be due to measurement error. Efforts to standardize the methods for studies on prevalence and burden of headache, and adherence to the published guidelines ([13]; also, Chaps. 6 and 7), will, hopefully, make future comparisons more reliable of headache-attributed burden across geographical borders and over time periods.

The fact that SDI, when applied across countries and cultures, is not reflected in differences in headache prevalence does not eliminate the possibility that socioeconomic factors are important within a country or region. A socioeconomic gradient, to the effect that low socioeconomic status is linked to higher headache prevalence, has been shown in high-, middle- and low-income countries [15, 32–34].

In conclusion, there are still major limitations in GBD headache burden estimations, but they are, by far, the most precise and comprehensive that we have.

9.4.3 The Challenge for Future GBD Headache Studies

GBD estimates will now be updated annually. They will include more data from countries where none existed, and reflect a continuing development of the methods of imputation of data for countries with little direct evidence.

This requires continued work also in headache. For the headache research community, it must be a priority regularly to feed data of high quality to the project. Whatever is the motivation to do headache epidemiological studies in the future, these studies should be conducted so as to be relevant and informative to GBD. This means use of standardized methodology, study instruments and reporting (see Chaps. 6 and 7). In particular, prevalences should be estimated for each age group by gender, and for definite and probable diagnoses of migraine and TTH. As important are good data on average frequency and duration of headache episodes for each diagnosis, to allow calculations of time spent with headache. Better diagnostic precision for the chronic headache disorders would allow them to be classified as migraine, TTH, MOH or, in a few cases, none of these, but this is a counsel of perfection.

9.5 Concluding Remarks

When GBD2010 was published, Steiner and co-workers drew attention to the project in the headache science community by authoring an editorial called "Migraine—the seventh disabler". This was published simultaneously in all three main scientific headache journals [35–37], after consultations with the three editors-in-chief, who thereby, presciently, endorsed the importance of GBD for their readers. In these papers, the following statement is found concerning the GBD reports: *"Few reports are likely to have more profound meaning for people with headache, or carry greater promise for a better future, than the seven papers ... that were presented [in GBD2010]".*

With GBD2016, we can now talk of migraine as the second disabler, and first in people under 50 [23]. With the increased relative importance of non-communicable diseases, the importance of headache for global public health is not likely to diminish in the future.

References

1. World Health Organization. The World Health Report 2001. Chapter 2. Burden of mental and behavioural disorders; 2001, pp 19–45. http://www.who.int/whr/2001/en/index.html.
2. Stovner LJ, Nichols E, Steiner TJ, Abd-Allah F, Abdelalim A, Al-Raddadi RM, Ansha MG, Barac A, Bensenor IM, Doan LP, Edessa D, Endres M, Foreman KJ, Gankpe FG, Gururaj G, Goulart AC, Gupta R, Hankey GJ, Hay SI, Hegazy MI, Hilawe EH, Kasaeian A, Kassa DH, Khalil I, Khang Y-H, Khubchandani J, Kim YJ, Kokubo Y, Mohammed MA, Moradi-Lakeh M, Nguyen HLT, Nirayo YL, Qorbani M, Ranta A, Roba KT, Safiri S, Santos IS, Satpathy M, Sawhney M, Shiferaw MS, Shiue I, Smith M, Szoeke CEI, Truong NT, Venketasubramanian N, Weldegwergs KG, Westerman R, Wijeratne T, Xuan Tran B, Yonemoto N, Feigin VL, Vos T, Murray CJL. Global, regional, and national burden of migraine and tension-type headache, 1990–2016: a systematic analysis for the Global Burden of Disease Study 2016. Lancet Neurol. 2018;17:954–76.

3. Murray CJ, Lopez AD, Jamison DT. The global burden of disease in 1990: summary results, sensitivity analysis and future directions. Bull World Health Organ. 1994;72:495–509.
4. Mather C, Bernard CS, Iburg KM, Inoue M, Fat DM, Shibuya K, Stein CM, Tomijima T, Xu H. Global burden of disease in 2002: data sources, methods and results. Global Programme on Evidence for Health Policy discussion paper no 54. Geneva: World Health Organization; 2004. https://www.who.int/healthinfo/paper54.pdf.
5. Leonardi M, Mathers C. Global burden of migraine in the Year 2000: summary of methods and data sources; 2000. http://www.who.int/healthinfo/statistics/bod_migraine.pdf.
6. Leonardi M, Steiner TJ, Scher AT, Lipton RB. The global burden of migraine: measuring disability in headache disorders with WHO's Classification of Functioning, Disability and Health (ICF). J Headache Pain. 2005;6:429–40.
7. Headache Classification Committee of the International Headache Society. Classification and diagnostic criteria for headache disorders, cranial neuralgias and facial pain. Cephalalgia. 1988;8(Suppl 7):1–96.
8. Murray CJ, Ezzati M, Flaxman AD, Lim S, Lozano R, Michaud C, Naghavi M, Salomon JA, Shibuya K, Vos T, Wikler D, Lopez AD. GBD 2010: design, definitions, and metrics. Lancet. 2012;380:2063–6.
9. Horton R. GBD 2010: understanding disease, injury, and risk. Lancet. 2012;380:2053–4.
10. Salomon JA, Vos T, Hogan DR, Gagnon M, Naghavi M, Mokdad A, Begum N, Shah R, Karyana M, Kosen S, Farje MR, Moncada G, Dutta A, Sazawal S, Dyer A, Seiler J, Aboyans V, Baker L, Baxter A, Benjamin EJ, Bhalla K, Bin Abdulhak A, Blyth F, Bourne R, Braithwaite T, Brooks P, Brugha TS, Bryan-Hancock C, Buchbinder R, Burney P, Calabria B, Chen H, Chugh SS, Cooley R, Criqui MH, et al. Common values in assessing health outcomes from disease and injury: disability weights measurement study for the Global Burden of Disease Study 2010. Lancet. 2012;380:2129–43.
11. Abduljabbar M, Ogunniyi A, Al Balla S, Alballaa S, Al-Dalaan A. Prevalence of primary headache syndrome in adults in the Qassim region of Saudi Arabia. Headache. 1996;36:385–8.
12. Stovner LJ, Hagen K, Jensen R, Katsarava Z, Lipton R, Scher A, Steiner T, Zwart JA. The global burden of headache: a documentation of headache prevalence and disability worldwide. Cephalalgia. 2007;27:193–210.
13. Stovner LJ, Al Jumah M, Birbeck GL, Gururaj G, Jensen R, Katsarava Z, Queiroz LP, Scher AI, Tekle-Haimanot R, Wang SJ, Steiner TJ. The methodology of population surveys of headache prevalence, burden and cost: principles and recommendations from the Global Campaign against Headache. J Headache Pain. 2014;15:5.
14. Steiner TJ. *Lifting The Burden*: the global campaign against headache. Lancet Neurol. 2004;3:204–5.
15. Ayzenberg I, Katsarava Z, Sborowski A, Chernysh M, Osipova V, Tabeeva G, Yakhno N, Steiner TJ. The prevalence of primary headache disorders in Russia: a countrywide survey. Cephalalgia. 2012;32:373–81.
16. Yu S, Liu R, Zhao G, Yang X, Qiao X, Feng J, Fang Y, Cao X, He M, Steiner T. The prevalence and burden of primary headaches in China: a population-based door-to-door survey. Headache. 2012;52:582–91.
17. Yu S, He M, Liu R, Feng J, Qiao X, Yang X, Cao X, Zhao G, Fang Y, Steiner TJ. Headache yesterday in China: a new approach to estimating the burden of headache, applied in a general-population survey in China. Cephalalgia. 2013;33:1211–7.
18. Rao GN, Kulkarni GB, Gururaj G, Rajesh K, Subbakrishna DK, Steiner TJ, Stovner LJ. The burden of headache disorders in India: methodology and questionnaire validation for a community-based survey in Karnataka state. J Headache Pain. 2012;13:543–50.
19. Vos T, Abajobir AA, Abate KH, Abbafati C, Abbas KM, Abd-Allah F, Abdulkader RS, Abdulle AM, Abebo TA, Abera SF, Aboyans V, Abu-Raddad LJ, Ackerman IN, Adamu AA, Adetokunboh O, Afarideh M, Afshin A, Agarwal SK, Aggarwal R, Agrawal A, Agrawal S, Ahmadieh H, Ahmed MB, Aichour MTE, Aichour AN, Aichour I, Aiyar S, Akinyemi RO, Akseer N, Al Lami FH, Alahdab F, Al-Aly Z, Alam K, Alam N, Alam T, et al. Global, regional,

and national incidence, prevalence, and years lived with disability for 328 diseases and injuries for 195 countries, 1990-2016: a systematic analysis for the Global Burden of Disease Study 2016. Lancet. 2017;390:1211–59.
20. Jonsson P, Hedenrud T, Linde M. Epidemiology of medication overuse headache in the general Swedish population. Cephalalgia. 2011;31:1015–22.
21. Katsarava Z, Muessig M, Dzagnidze A, Fritsche G, Diener HC, Limmroth V. Medication overuse headache: rates and predictors for relapse in a 4-year prospective study. Cephalalgia. 2005;25:12–5.
22. Salomon JA, Haagsma JA, Davis A, de Noordhout CM, Polinder S, Havelaar AH, Cassini A, Devleesschauwer B, Kretzschmar M, Speybroeck N, Murray CJ, Vos T. Disability weights for the Global Burden of Disease 2013 study. Lancet Glob Health. 2015;3:e712–23.
23. Steiner TJ, Stovner LJ, Vos T, Jensen R, Katsarava Z. Migraine is first cause of disability in under 50s: will health politicians now take notice? J Headache Pain. 2018;19:17.
24. Murray CJL, Lopez AD. Measuring global health: motivation and evolution of the Global Burden of Disease Study. Lancet. 2017;390:1460–4.
25. Zebenigus M, Tekle-Haimanot R, Worku DK, Thomas H, Steiner TJ. The burden of headache disorders in Ethiopia: national estimates from a population-based door-to-door survey. J Headache Pain. 2017;18:58.
26. Mbewe E, Zairemthiama P, Paul R, Birbeck GL, Steiner TJ. The burden of primary headache disorders in Zambia: national estimates from a population-based door-to-door survey. J Headache Pain. 2015;16:36.
27. Steiner TJ, Rao GN, Kulkarni GB, Gururaj G, Stovner LJ. Headache yesterday in Karnataka state, India: prevalence, impact and cost. J Headache Pain. 2016;17:74.
28. Manandhar K, Risal A, Linde M, Steiner TJ. The burden of headache disorders in Nepal: estimates from a population-based survey. J Headache Pain. 2015;17:3.
29. Kim BK, Chung YK, Kim JM, Lee KS, Chu MK. Prevalence, clinical characteristics and disability of migraine and probable migraine: a nationwide population-based survey in Korea. Cephalalgia. 2013;33:1106–16.
30. Lanteri-Minet M, Valade D, Geraud G, Chautard MH, Lucas C. Migraine and probable migraine—results of FRAMIG 3, a French nationwide survey carried out according to the 2004 IHS classification. Cephalalgia. 2005;25:1146–58.
31. Arruda MA, Guidetti V, Galli F, Albuquerque RC, Bigal ME. Primary headaches in childhood—a population-based study. Cephalalgia. 2010;30:1056–64.
32. Hagen K, Vatten L, Stovner LJ, Zwart JA, Krokstad S, Bovim G. Low socio-economic status is associated with increased risk of frequent headache: a prospective study of 22718 adults in Norway. Cephalalgia. 2002;22:672–9.
33. Lipton RB, Bigal ME. The epidemiology of migraine. Am J Med. 2005;118(Suppl 1):3S–10S.
34. Gururaj G, Kulkarni GB, Rao GN, Subbakrishna DK, Stovner LJ, Steiner TJ. Prevalence and sociodemographic correlates of primary headache disorders: results of a population-based survey from Bangalore, India. Indian J Public Health. 2014;58:241–8.
35. Steiner TJ, Stovner LJ, Birbeck GL. Migraine: the seventh disabler. Cephalalgia. 2013;33:289–90.
36. Steiner TJ, Stovner LJ, Birbeck GL. Migraine: the seventh disabler. J Headache Pain. 2013;14:1.
37. Steiner TJ, Stovner LJ, Birbeck GL. Migraine: the seventh disabler. Headache. 2013;53:227–9.

Chapter 10
Headache in the HUNT Study: Analytical Headache Epidemiology as a Source of Added Knowledge

Knut Hagen and Lars Jacob Stovner

10.1 Introduction

Most epidemiological studies on headache disorders until now have been singular ("stand-alone") studies [1], performed only once in a country or community, with headache as their main focus and aiming to describe prevalence and attributed burden. Such studies have been essential for the recognition of headache as a major public-health issue. However, since most of these studies concern only headaches, they can only to a limited degree put headaches into the context of other diseases and health problems. Also, the vast majority are not repeated and offer no means of measuring secular trends (change over time) in headache prevalence and burden.

For many disorders, epidemiological studies have been instrumental for detecting causes and risk factors, for example, regarding coronary heart disease. Epidemiological association between potential cause and effect is one of the main criteria of causality in medicine (the so-called Bradford-Hill criteria [2]). Demonstration of an epidemiological association requires good data on the disease under consideration and similarly good data on potential causes, usually in a large cohort of people. If such studies are performed only once, they can show a cross-sectional association between suspected risks and a disorder but, since both the disorder and the purported risk factor are recorded at the same point in time, it is unknown whether the putative cause preceded the disorder or not. Establishing a valid time sequence can be done only in studies where a large cohort is followed up. In these cohort studies, people at risk (i.e. those without the disease in the first study) are characterized according to whether or not they have been exposed to the

K. Hagen (✉) · L. J. Stovner
Department of Neuromedicine and Movement Science, NTNU Norwegian University of Science and Technology, Trondheim, Norway

Norwegian Advisory Unit on Headaches, Department of Neurology and Clinical Neurophysiology, St Olavs University Hospital, Trondheim, Norway
e-mail: knut.hagen@ntnu.no; lars.stovner@ntnu.no

T. J. Steiner, L. J. Stovner (eds.), *Societal Impact of Headache*, Headache,
https://doi.org/10.1007/978-3-030-24728-7_10

potential risk factor and then, in the follow-up study, assessed according to whether or not they have developed the disease. If, in the second study, the exposed group has a significantly higher prevalence of the disease, a causal link can be suspected. However, there may be other factors that differ between the exposed and the unexposed groups, which can explain the difference in the outcome. Such factors, referred to as confounders (e.g. age, gender, other diseases, other risk factors), must also be taken into consideration and corrected for. Hence, epidemiological studies on causal factors must also have data on all of these potential confounders.

Epidemiological studies aiming mainly to describe prevalence and incidence are often referred to as descriptive epidemiological studies, whereas those aiming to detect potential causes are called analytical. While there are a number of analytical studies in the fields of cardiovascular disease and cancer, very few exist for headaches. The International Classification of Headache Disorders (ICHD) contains many so-called secondary headache disorders, that is, headaches that can be attributed to a specific cause. For almost all of these, there is embarrassingly little actual evidence on the causal link. Mostly, causality is inferred from temporal association (the headache appears in temporal relation to the suspected cause), which is a weak and often misleading criterion of causation.

Actually, there is now more solid evidence about headache as a risk factor for other disorders. For example, migraine has been found to be associated with stroke, in particular migraine with aura occurring in combination with smoking and use of contraceptive pills [3]. Also, there have been studies showing headache as a cause of white matter hyperintensities on magnetic resonance imaging (MRI) [4].

The first large cohort with extensive information on headache, other disorders, several risk factors and repeated follow-up is the HUNT study (Helseundersøkelsen i Nord-Trøndelag - The Nord-Trøndelag Health Survey), now performed several times in the entire population of Nord-Trøndelag county in Norway. From 1 January 2018, this county was merged with Sør-Trøndelag county into a larger county, Trøndelag, but the last wave of the study is still performed in the same communities in the former Nord-Trøndelag.

In this chapter, we describe the HUNT surveys and give some principal results from these on headache. Our ultimate aim is to encourage inclusion of headache questions in other large health surveys all over the world, in order to establish a strong discipline of analytical headache epidemiology. We believe it is of utmost importance to set up such studies, which can, with robust methods, detect modifiable risk factors for a disorder that has been found to be the second most disabling for all ages, and the most disabling for those under 50 [5].

10.2 The HUNT Studies

Nord-Trøndelag was one of Norway's 19 counties until 2017. The region has approximately 127,000 inhabitants, living in both rural and industrial areas and showing relatively small socioeconomic differences. Although it lacks a large city, the county's inhabitants are considered to be fairly representative of the Norwegian population.

HUNT is a longitudinal cohort study in which all inhabitants aged 20 years or over in Nord-Trøndelag have been invited to participate. They have been investigated four times: 1984–1986 (HUNT1), 1995–1997 (HUNT2), 2006–2008 (HUNT3) and 2017–2019 (HUNT4) (see https://www.ntnu.edu/hunt).

In HUNT1, a total of 74,599 persons participated (participation proportion 88%). It focused mostly on cardiovascular risk factors and diabetes mellitus. The questionnaire did not include headache items, but 59,471 persons responded to a question on use of analgesics, and blood pressure was measured in all.

In HUNT2, 65,237 persons participated out of 93,898 invited (70%) and 51,856 (55%) indicated whether or not they suffered from headache [6]. Non-participants were described in a separate paper [7]. HUNT2 included a wide range of topics and collected more information from each participant in two questionnaires. The first questionnaire (Q1) was enclosed with the invitation letter and was completed at home and delivered during attendance at the health examination, which included measurements of blood pressure, height and weight, screening for asthma with spirometric methods and blood sampling. Q1 also collected information on education, smoking, physical activity, chronic musculoskeletal complaints (CMSCs), depression and anxiety (measured by the Hospital Anxiety and Depression Scale (HADS)), smoking and alcohol use (including a modified version in Norwegian of the CAGE alcohol screening questionnaire). The second questionnaire (Q2), which also included headache questions, was filled in after the examination and returned by mail. A number of blood analyses were performed, including a haemochromatosis screening of all participants and measurements of thyroid-stimulating hormone (TSH) in 28,058 subjects.

In HUNT3, 93,860 persons were invited, of whom 50,807 (54%) participated and 39,690 (42%) answered the headache questions [8]. Among the 65,237 persons who participated in HUNT2, 8545 had died and 4357 moved out of the county during the period before HUNT3. A total of 37,061 persons participated in both HUNT2 and HUNT3 and 26,197 participants answered questions regarding headache in both HUNT2 and HUNT3. Participants in HUNT3 underwent many of the same investigations as in HUNT2, but, in addition, there was a subgroup among them (n = 1006) who had participated in all three HUNT studies and had an MRI of the head taken some time after the questionnaires had been answered. Also, there were subgroups who were evaluated for physical fitness (peak oxygen uptake, n = 5633) and endothelial function (n = 4739).

HUNT4 was performed between September 2017 and March 2019. As in HUNT2 and HUNT3, the adult participants, aged 20 years and above, answered two questionnaires and under went a clinical examination.

10.2.1 Young-HUNT Studies

In HUNT2, there was a separate study including adolescents (Young-HUNT1), to which all students in junior high schools (aged 12–15 years) and high schools (aged 16–19 years) were invited. This also included headache questions and interviews

[9]. In total, 8984 (88%) participated of 10,202 invited. Those not participating were not in school on the day of the study, did not obtain consent from their parents or did not themselves wish to participate. The study followed the school year rather than the calendar year. As adolescents usually graduate from high school in the calendar year in which they turn 19, about half of the 19-year-olds had finished school and were not invited to participate in the study. Accordingly, the 19-year-old students in the study population were excluded ($n = 382$). In addition, all 12-year-old students in the first year of junior high school were excluded because of the low number ($n = 126$).

Participating students completed, during school hours, a self-administered questionnaire with more than 100 health-related questions. Within a month afterwards, a clinical examination, which included spirometry and weight, height and blood pressure measurements, was performed at school by a nurse. The students were also interviewed with respect to headache complaints. The intention was to interview the entire population in connection with the clinical examination, but the interviewers were not able to begin the interviews until February 1996; hence, the total interviewed study population within the age range 13–18 years was only 5847.

In the school years 1999–2000 and 2000–2001, a follow-up of Young-HUNT1 was performed (Young-HUNT2). All students in 2nd and 3rd grades in upper secondary school (aged 16–20 years), and all apprentices of the same age who participated in Young-HUNT1, were invited. A total of 2399 (77%) completed the questionnaire in Young-HUNT2 and 1665 (53% of those invited) underwent the headache interview.

10.2.2 Validation Studies of Headache Diagnoses in HUNT

The headache questions in HUNT2 and HUNT3 were designed mainly to determine whether participants suffered from headache and, if so, the frequency of headache, and to diagnose migraine and medication-overuse headache (MOH) [6, 8]. Both HUNT2 and HUNT3 questionnaires included the screening question: "Have you suffered from headache during the last 12 months?" In HUNT2, the question regarding headache frequency during the preceding year had three response options: less than 7 days/month, 7–14 days/month or more than 14 days/month. "Chronic headache" was defined as headache occurring on 15 or more days/month during the preceding year. In HUNT2, modified ICHD-I diagnostic criteria for migraine were used. Headache that did not satisfy the criteria for migraine was classified as non-migrainous headache, and diagnoses were mutually exclusive. MOH was defined as chronic headache occurring in association with use of analgesics daily or almost daily for 1 month or more during the previous 12 months (strictly this should be *probable* MOH (see Chap. 7)).

In HUNT3, the headache frequency question had four response options: in addition to those in HUNT2, there was a category of less than 1 day/month.

In all three adult HUNT studies collecting headache data (HUNT2, HUNT3 and HUNT4), validation studies were performed to evaluate the accuracy of headache diagnoses. In HUNT2, this was done by inviting a group of people who had participated in the questionnaire study with known headache, and another group without headache, to face-to-face interviews by headache specialists. Expert headache diagnoses were later compared with the diagnoses based on the HUNT questionnaires, both adult and youth [10, 11]. In HUNT3, validation studies were performed by selecting HUNT participants randomly, but stratified for age and gender, for face-to-face interviews with headache experts [12]. The same procedure has been followed in HUNT4 [13].

The validity of the diagnostic criteria used in HUNT2 and HUNT3 has been reported in separate publications. In HUNT2, the questionnaire-based diagnosis of chronic headache was made with a sensitivity of 38%, specificity of 97% and kappa value of 0.44 (95% CI: 0.21–0.67) [10]. For migraine, sensitivity was 69%, specificity 89% and kappa 0.59 (0.47–0.71), and for non-migraine headache, sensitivity was 61%, specificity 81% and kappa 0.43 (0.29–0.57). In the adult part of HUNT3, for any headache, sensitivity was 88%, specificity 86% and kappa 0.70. Chronic headache, chronic tension-type headache (TTH) and MOH were diagnosed with specificities of ≥99% and kappas of ≥0.73. Lower values were found for the diagnoses of migraine and TTH. For participants with headache on ≥1 days/month, migraine had a sensitivity of 58% and TTH of 96%, with specificities of 91% and 69% and kappa values of 0.54 and 0.44. The specificity for migraine with aura was 95% [12]. In HUNT4, partcipants with any headache on ≥1 days/month, sensitivity was 90%, specificity 80% and kappa 0.55 (0.41–0.69), migraine had a sensitivity of 50%, specificity of 94% and kappa 0.49 (0.41–0.69), and TTH had a sensitivity of 100%, specificity of 73%, and kappa 0.33 (0.17–0.49) [14].

In Young-HUNT1, the headache interviews were performed during school hours, along with the clinical examination. Nurses asked the students whether they had experienced recurring headaches that were not related to cold, fever or any other disease during the preceding 12 months. Two descriptions of typical symptoms, one for migraine and one for TTH, were read to students reporting headaches, who were asked to classify them according to one or other ("recognition-based diagnosis" (see Chap. 6)). They were also given a third option ("non-classifiable headache") when neither description resembled their own understanding of their headache. The average number of days with headache in the preceding 12 months was recorded in four categories: less than 1 day/month (less than monthly), 1–3 days/month (monthly), 1–5 days/week (weekly) or more than 5 days/week (daily).

The recognition-based diagnoses were validated against extensive semi-structured interviews by neurologists [11], showing an overall chance-corrected agreement (kappa) of 0.76 (95% CI: 0.66–0.86). For migraine, the positive and negative predictive values were 89% and 90% and kappa was 0.72 (0.58–0.87). For TTH, positive and negative predictive values were 83% and 91% and kappa was 0.74 (0.62–0.87).

All of these were good (kappa > 0.6) or moderate (kappa > 0.4).

10.3 Results

10.3.1 Descriptive Headache Epidemiology in HUNT

In HUNT2, among adults (aged 20 years or over), overall age-adjusted 1-year prevalence of headache was 37.7% (46% in women and 30% in men), of migraine 11.6% (16% in women and 8% in men) and of non-migrainous headache 26% (30% in women and 22% in men) [6]. For frequent headache (>6 days/month), for chronic headache (≥15 days/month) and MOH, prevalences were 8.0%, 2.3% and 1.0%, respectively.

In Young-HUNT1, 76.8% (n = 8984) reported headache during the preceding year (69.4% of boys and 84.2% of girls) [9]. Among those also interviewed (n = 5847), 29% reported recurrent headaches (21.0% of boys and 37% of girls) during the preceding year, and 7% of these had migraine, 18% TTH and 5% non-classifiable headache. Higher prevalences were found in girls in all age groups and all headache categories, and girls had significantly more frequent headaches than boys.

In HUNT3, among adults (aged 20 years or over), age-adjusted 1-year prevalence of headache was 37.4% and of chronic headache 2.5% (including MOH 1.0%, chronic migraine 0.3% and chronic TTH 1.0%). There was an apparent slight increase in prevalence of migraine from HUNT2 to HUNT3 (12.1% to 13.2% (estimates not age-adjusted); $p < 0.001$), due perhaps to slightly different use of diagnostic criteria or the lower participation proportion in HUNT3, or reflecting a real difference related to changes in lifestyle and general population health. The first of these is supported by an accompanying similar decrease in non-migrainous headache (26.0% to 24.2%; $p < 0.001$), while the other headache types remained essentially stable in this Norwegian county during this 11-year period.

In both HUNT2 and HUNT3, prevalences of migraine and non-migrainous headache followed a well-known pattern regarding age and gender. At all ages, headaches were more prevalent among females than males, particularly migraine, and in both men and women all headaches reached peak prevalence between 30 and 40 years of age.

In HUNT2, HUNT3 and HUNT4, the screening headache question was "Have you *suffered from* headache during the last year". HUNT3 investigated, in the validation study, the effect on estimated prevalences of this question compared with the more neutral "Have you *had* headache during the last year?" (emphasis added) [15]. It was substantial: during the preceding year, 74.1% reported that they had "had" headache, whereas only 31.0% stated that they had "suffered from" headache. With the neutral question, the 1-year prevalence of migraine was 17.2% and of TTH 51.9%. Migraine was ten times more likely among headache "sufferers" than among those who only "had" headache, while chronic TTH and MOH occurred only among the headache sufferers. Hence, in the large HUNT study, with many health-related items and limited space for headache questions, we concluded that "Have you suffered from headache?" is useful for screening when the goal is to identify most migraineurs and almost all with chronic headache even though it will underestimate the total prevalence and burden of headache. In addition, for the purpose of follow-up, it is preferable to have the same screening question in all the HUNT studies. However, if we were free to choose a screening question today, we might have chosen a neutral question in combination with one or two further questions about headache frequency and severity, as this would have enabled us to capture both those who "have" and those who "suffer from" headache.

10.3.2 Analytical Headache Epidemiology in HUNT

In HUNT2, we were able only to explore associations with potential risk factors in a cross-sectional design, that is, where both headache and potential risk factors were determined in the same study. In the cross-sectional analyses, we used multivariate logistic regression to estimate prevalence odds ratios (ORs) with 95% CIs. In HUNT3 and HUNT4, we can compare headache prevalences in the later study among those who were headache-free in the earlier study according to exposure or not to putative risk factors. Other types of multivariate analyses (e.g. modified Poison regression) are useful to estimate risk ratios (RRs). In the following, we focus on robust statistical findings without giving actual ORs or RRs. In all studies, adjustments for potential confounding factors have been made: always for age and gender, and, in addition, for factors deemed to be relevant for the association being investigated. In order to avoid over-correction, in many of the studies, analyses were performed first with adjustment only for age and gender (partly adjusted analyses) and then also for other factors (fully adjusted analyses).

Several HUNT studies have investigated the relation between headache and cardiovascular risk factors. In HUNT2, blood pressure was found to be inversely related to headache, that is, the higher the blood pressure, the lower the headache prevalence [16]. This was true for all headache types. A more thorough analysis revealed that the most consistent finding was between pulse pressure (difference between systolic and diastolic pressures), but the association was also true for systolic pressure [17]. This finding was confirmed in a HUNT3 population, where the inverse relation was most evident in the group not using blood pressure medication. Interestingly, the relation was evident also with blood pressures well within the normal range. It could also be demonstrated among adolescents in the Young-HUNT population [18]. These studies were cross-sectional, but it was also found, prospectively, that high pulse pressure, high systolic pressure and, to a lesser degree, high diastolic pressure at baseline in HUNT2 predicted significantly lower prevalences of all headache types in HUNT3 [19]. These findings have been discussed in relation to the well-known phenomenon of hypertension-associated hypalgesia [20]. The HUNT studies have shown that the inverse relation to blood pressure is true also for most other bodily pains [21].

As to other cardiovascular factors, the cross-sectional relation of headache to the Framingham risk score has been investigated in HUNT2 [22]. The score was somewhat elevated in non-migraine headache sufferers and migraineurs without aura, but most elevated among migraineurs with aura. The score increased with headache frequency. In migraine without aura and non-migrainous headache, the increased risk was accounted for by lifestyle factors such as smoking, high body mass index (BMI) and low physical activity, but this was not true for the elevated risk associated with migraine with aura. Hence, other mechanisms may underlie the elevated risk in migraine with aura.

In a follow-up study from HUNT2 to HUNT3, past or current smoking was found to increase the risk of migraine, whereas hard physical exercise (1–2 h/week) reduced the risk compared to inactivity. Among those who consumed alcohol, the risk of migraine was also lower than among abstainers. No associations were found between smoking, physical activity, alcohol use and risk of TTH [23]. The positive association between migraine and smoking, and negative with alcohol consumption, were also found in a previous cross-sectional study in HUNT2 [24].

As to physical exercise, a negative relation between peak oxygen uptake (VO_2) measured by ergospirometry and headache was found in 3899 participants in HUNT2. Among those aged 20–50 years, the prevalence of any headache increased with decreased peak VO_2 (apparent for migraine, TTH and unclassified headache). No significant association was found between peak VO_2 and headache in those aged 50 years or older [25].

Interestingly, and in contrast to what was found for other vascular risk factors, there was an inverse relationship between diabetes and headache prevalence (i.e. fewer with headache among diabetics) in cross-sectional analyses of HUNT2 and HUNT3 [26, 27]. In HUNT2, the relation was more pronounced among those who had had diabetes for a long period, and in HUNT3, it was seen only in those with diabetes type 1. In the prospective analysis (HUNT2 to HUNT3), diabetes type 1 in HUNT2 was associated with markedly lower headache prevalence in HUNT3: prevalence of any headache was reduced by 45% and of migraine by 53%. More recently, a nationwide cohort study using the Norwegian prescription database found that both type 1 and type 2 diabetes were significantly associated with a decreased risk of migraine [28]. Several mechanisms may account for this, for example, the (generally) more regular lifestyle of diabetic patients, or a (mostly) subclinical autonomic neuropathy.

Headaches have been related to several other disorders in the HUNT studies to elucidate potential comorbidities. In HUNT2, marked relations to anxiety and depression assessed by HADS have been shown, both in the adult HUNT and in Young-HUNT studies [29, 30]. Among adults, depression and anxiety disorders were significantly associated with migraine and non-migrainous headache in comparisons with headache-free individuals, anxiety disorders more strongly than depression. For both psychiatric disorders, headache frequency was more important than diagnostic category in these associations.

In Young-HUNT, recurrent headache was associated with symptoms of anxiety and depression in HUNT3 [30]. In the prospective study using data from Young-HUNT1 and Young-HUNT2, higher scores of anxiety and depressive symptoms at baseline were associated with recurrent headache at follow-up 4 years later, both for migraine and for non-classifiable headache, but not significantly for TTH [31]. Also, higher scores of anxiety and depressive symptoms at baseline were significantly associated with more frequent headache at follow-up.

Also, asthma, asthma-related symptoms, hay fever and chronic bronchitis were found to be approximately 1.5 times more likely among those with migraine or non-migrainous headache in HUNT2 (cross-sectional analysis), and the association increased with increasing headache frequency [32]. It is not known whether this association is due to some common biological factor, or can be related to medication, or whether the stress of having an intermittent and unpredictable disorder like headache or asthma can increase the likelihood of having the other disorder.

The relation of headache to sleep problems has been examined in prospectively in HUNT2 and HUNT3 [33]. Insomnia at baseline in HUNT2 was associated with a 40% increased risk for headache in HUNT3, and this was true for migraine, TTH and non-classified headache. Insomnia at baseline was also related to headache frequency at follow-up for both migraine and TTH.

As can be expected, headache is associated with musculoskeletal pain in other parts of the body. In HUNT2, both migraine and non-migrainous headache were strongly associated with musculoskeletal symptoms [34]. This was true for pain in all parts of the body, but neck pain was most strongly associated with headache. The frequency of headache had a higher impact than headache diagnosis on this association; hence, the prevalence of chronic headache was more than four times higher in those with musculoskeletal symptoms than in those without. A prospective analysis of data from HUNT2 and HUNT3 showed a bidirectional relationship between headache and chronic musculoskeletal complaints (CMSCs) [35]. A nearly twofold risk for developing chronic headache was found for those with CMSCs at baseline. Vice versa, a similarly elevated risk of CMSCs was found at follow-up among those with chronic headache at baseline. This bidirectional relationship may indicate a common underlying factor for headache and CMSCs.

In HUNT2, headache was also found to be related to gastrointestinal complaints: diarrhoea, constipation and nausea [36]. This was true both for non-migrainous headache and migraine, and again the association increased markedly with increasing headache frequency.

Some studies have investigated MOH specifically. An analysis of HUNT1 and HUNT2 data demonstrated an increased risk for having chronic pain at follow-up among those who had used analgesics at baseline in HUNT1 [37]. The risk was highest in those who used analgesics for chronic migraine, intermediate in those using them for chronic non-migrainous headaches and lowest in those using them for chronic neck or chronic low-back pain. In a prospective study using HUNT2 and HUNT3 data [38], the incidence of MOH was 0.72 per 1000 person-years (95% CI: 0.62–0.81). Multivariate analyses demonstrated a fivefold risk for developing MOH among those who at baseline reported regular use of analgesics or who had a combination of CMSCs, gastrointestinal complaints and HADS score of $\geq$11. Smoking and physical inactivity more than doubled the risk of MOH. Interestingly, these factors did not increase the risk of chronic headache without medication overuse, suggesting these headaches are pathogenetically distinct from MOH. Another study investigated the prognosis of chronic headache between HUNT-2 and HUNT-3, showing a remission rate of almost 75%. The proportion was almost identical in men and women, but the chance of remission was two to three times more likely among those without medication overuse or CMSCs in HUNT-2 [39].

Some HUNT studies have investigated the cross-sectional relation to blood analyses. In HUNT2, the blood haemoglobin and ferritin were measured in 2385 women between 20 and 55 years of age [40]. No association was found to ferritin, whereas somewhat unexpectedly there was a linear trend of decreasing headache prevalence with decreasing haemoglobin values. This finding may explain the headache related to polycythaemia and to altitude sickness. In a sample of HUNT2 participants, genotypes and phenotypes of hemochromatosis were determined. Phenotypic hemochromatosis and the C282Y/C282Y genotype were both associated with an 80% increase in headache prevalence. This was true only among women, which was surprising since phenotypical hemochromatosis is most prevalent among men [41].

One HUNT2 study related headache to thyroid function among more than 28,000 participants [42]. Generally, high TSH values were associated with low prevalence of headache. This was most evident in women with no history of thyroid dysfunction. Among these, headache was less probable when TSH was >10 mU/L than when it was in the normal range (0.2–4 mU/L). In all age groups between 40 and 80 years, TSH was lower among headache sufferers, especially migraineurs, than in those without headache complaints. Similar results were found for CMSCs [43].

Since headaches are to a large degree a women's disorder, several HUNT studies have looked at the relations to female hormonal factors and events in women's lives. In one study, headache (both migraine and non-migrainous) was found to be related to anticonception with oestrogen-containing drugs [44]. No relationship between headache and oestrogen dose in the oral contraceptives could be demonstrated, and no association was found between headache and contraceptives containing only gestagens. For hormone replacement therapy in post-menopausal women, there was also an association with headache, with both local and systemic applications [45], and for non-migrainous headache and migraine.

As to pregnancy and parity, in HUNT2 headache prevalence was lower among pregnant than among non-pregnant women [46]. The association between headache and pregnancy was significant for nulliparous women (never given birth) but not for primiparous (one child only) or multiparous (two or more children). This was evident for both migraine and non-migrainous headache. Among non-pregnant women, there was an increased headache prevalence among primiparous and multiparous women compared with nulliparous.

As to age at menarche, the relation to headache prevalence was investigated in both adult and youth parts of HUNT2 [47]. Headache was more prevalent in females with menarche before 12 years of age, both among adolescents and adults, evident for migraine and non-migrainous headache. Interestingly, headache prevalence was increased in those with early menarche even among women older than 60 years.

Headache has also been related to socioeconomic factors [48]. In a prospective analysis of data from HUNT1 and HUNT2, more than 22,000 adults not likely to suffer from headache because they did not use analgesics in HUNT1 were classified by socioeconomic status (SES) defined by educational level, occupation and income. Low SES was associated with increased risk of frequent and chronic headache at follow-up. The risk of both decreased with increasing individual income, but only among men. These findings were discussed in relation to both the social causation hypothesis (i.e. low SES causes headache) and the social selection hypothesis (people have lower SES because of their headache). The latter hypothesis may be corroborated by another HUNT2 study showing an increasing prevalence of sick leave with increasing frequency of migraine and non-migrainous headache, while sick leave lasting more than 8 weeks during the past year occurred much more often among those with chronic headache (20%) than in those without headache (6%) [49].

The HUNT studies are performed in a county where all citizens are treated in one of two local hospitals in the county, or in the regional university hospital. Thus, it is possible to link HUNT data to hospital diagnoses, which may be either exposures or endpoints. For headache, this has only been done for exposures. In one study, all HUNT3 participants who had been hospitalized during the last 20 years for intracranial infections (meningitis, encephalitis, abscess: $n = 43$) were compared to those without intracranial infections [50]. There was no significant increase in the prevalence of headache (migraine, TTH or chronic headache. However, there were far fewer with such infections than anticipated in the HUNT population, so the statistical power for detecting modest or small increases in headache prevalence was not very high. Another HUNT study looked in a similar way at those who had been hospitalized for head injuries ($n = 940$) since 1988 [51]. This showed that any head injury, more than one head injury and head injury during the last 10 years before HUNT3 were associated with significantly increased prevalence of any headache in comparisons with those not exposed to head injuries. A separate analysis among those who had had a head injury in the 11-year interval between HUNT2 and HUNT3 ($n = 294$) showed that these had a worse prognosis with regard to headache (i.e. more with new-onset headache, stable headache or lack of remission of headache) than those who had not been hospitalized for head injury [52]. This methodologically strong study, in which it was possible to correct for level of pre-traumatic headache, lends credibility to the diagnosis of post-traumatic headache.

The HUNT MRI study included a random sample of 1006 HUNT3 participants between 50 and 65 years of age who had participated in all three HUNT studies and had an MRI of the head, including MR angiography. The main aims of this study were to investigate the structure of the brain as an endpoint related to previous exposures and diseases reported in HUNT1, HUNT2 and HUNT3, and also in the future to explore later occurrence of dementia as an endpoint related to previous MRI findings. A methodological study looked at the representativeness of the HUNT MRI population and showed that they were somewhat healthier and better educated than the overall HUNT population [53].

For headache, the HUNT MRI study makes it possible to evaluate the relation between MRI findings and headache in a population-based sample, that is, without the potential selection biases that may be present in clinical patient samples. A separate paper on the findings in this population has been published [54]. Regarding headache, the study has shown that incidental findings at MRI scans were more common in headache sufferers (29%) than in headache-free individuals (22%), mostly white matter hyperintensities [55]. A separate analysis revealed that individuals with TTH or with new-onset headache were more likely to have extensive white matter hyperintensities than those without headache, whereas migraine and unclassified headache were not associated with such changes [56]. Another study has shown little difference between headache sufferers and non-sufferers with regard to presence of perivascular spaces, contrary to findings in some earlier clinic-based studies [57]. Yet another, on MRIs of the paranasal sinuses, found no significant association between headache, mucosal thickening, polyps/retention cysts and fluid in the sinuses [58].

Finally, a few studies have looked at headache as a risk factor for other disorders. One study found no influence of headache in HUNT2 on mortality in the following 20 years, either from all causes or from cardiovascular disorders [59]. In another study, HUNT2 data were linked to a dementia register in Nord-Trøndelag [60]. Among the 378 who had developed dementia, significantly more had headache in HUNT2. Interestingly, this was only true for vascular dementia and mixed dementia, but not for Alzheimer's disease. The results were confirmed in a later study when more participants had developed dementia (n = 746), and this study showed that the relation was true for all headache and non-migrainous headache but not for migraine [61].

10.4 Concluding Remarks

A wealth of data, potentially, derive from longitudinal surveys that are not available from cross-sectional studies. The HUNT studies have emphatically demonstrated this (although reservations must be noted).

Three HUNT studies have been performed since the mid-1980s, and the fourth is now being conducted. The last three (HUNT2, HUNT3 and HUNT4) have included validated questions on headache. The validation studies have shown the major influence the screening question has on the estimated headache prevalence. Since HUNT includes a wide range of other health-related items, and the HUNT cohort has been investigated several times with intervals of some years, it has been possible to evaluate both comorbidity and potential causal factors for headache, and headache as a cause for other disorders. Furthermore, it is also possible to evaluate predictors of remission of MOH and other types of frequent headache.

In epidemiology, as in other fields of medical research, it is probably true that, for a variety of reasons, most published research findings are false [62]. This may also be the case for many of the findings reported in the HUNT studies, and it is acknowledged that these studies are, in the main, only hypothesis generating. It would therefore be highly desirable if these hypotheses could be tested in other cohorts, by other groups and with different methods. Especially in analytical epidemiology, it has been pointed out that replication of results may be one of the best criteria for finding true causal relationships, even better than the strength of the association and biological gradient ("dose-response effect") [63]. Therefore, in order to be able to establish true causal factors for headaches, it is necessary to conduct many more studies in a similar way to the HUNT study, that is, including headache questions among many other health items, and with follow-up studies in the same cohorts. This should not be impossible or too costly, because there are many large population cohorts being followed around the world. Only in this way it will be possible to sift the results from the HUNT studies so that one can glean true causal associations that may give rise to public interventions or form the basis for better understanding of pathophysiology, thereby, ultimately, engendering better treatments. Many more groups must contribute to build a strong research discipline of analytical headache epidemiology. This will take some time and some costs, but, for a disorder of such large public-health importance as headache (see Chaps. 8 and 9), we believe this will prove a very good investment in health.

References

1. Stovner LJ, Al Jumah M, Birbeck GL, Gururaj G, Jensen R, Katsarava Z, Queiroz LP, Scher AI, Tekle-Haimanot R, Wang SJ, Steiner TJ. The methodology of population surveys of headache prevalence, burden and cost: principles and recommendations from the Global Campaign against Headache. J Headache Pain. 2014;15:5.
2. Bradford-Hill A. The environment and disease: association or causation? Proc Roy Soc Med. 1965;58:295–300.
3. Sheikh HU, Pavlovic J, Loder E, Burch R. Risk of stroke associated with use of estrogen containing contraceptives in women with migraine: a systematic review. Headache. 2018;58:5–21.
4. Monteith T, Gardener H, Rundek T, Dong C, Yoshita M, Elkind MS, DeCarli C, Sacco RL, Wright CB. Migraine, white matter hyperintensities, and subclinical brain infarction in a diverse community: the northern Manhattan study. Stroke. 2014;45:1830–2.
5. Steiner TJ, Stovner LJ, Vos T, Jensen R, Katsarava Z. Migraine is first cause of disability in under 50s: will health politicians now take notice? J Headache Pain. 2018;19:17.
6. Hagen K, Zwart JA, Vatten L, Stovner LJ, Bovim G. Prevalence of migraine and non-migrainous headache—head-HUNT, a large population-based study. Cephalalgia. 2000;20:900–6.
7. Holmen J, Midthjell K, Krüger Ø, Langhammer A, Holmen TL, Brattberg GH. The Nord-Trøndelag Health Study 1995–97 (HUNT 2): objectives, contents, methods and participation. Nor J Epidemiol. 2003;13:19–32.
8. Linde M, Stovner LJ, Zwart JA, Hagen K. Time trends in the prevalence of headache disorders. The Nord-Trondelag Health Studies (HUNT 2 and HUNT 3). Cephalalgia. 2011;31:585–96.
9. Zwart JA, Dyb G, Holmen TL, Stovner LJ, Sand T. The prevalence of migraine and tension-type headaches among adolescents in Norway. The Nord-Trondelag Health Study (Head-HUNT-Youth), a large population-based epidemiological study. Cephalalgia. 2004;24:373–9.
10. Hagen K, Zwart JA, Vatten L, Stovner LJ, Bovim G. Head-HUNT: validity and reliability of a headache questionnaire in a large population-based study in Norway. Cephalalgia. 2000;20:244–51.
11. Zwart JA, Dyb G, Stovner LJ, Sand T, Holmen TL. The validity of 'recognition-based' headache diagnoses in adolescents. Data from the Nord-Trondelag Health Study 1995–97, Head-HUNT-Youth. Cephalalgia. 2003;23:223–9.

12. Hagen K, Zwart JA, Aamodt AH, Nilsen KB, Brathen G, Helde G, Stjern M, Tronvik EA, Stovner LJ. The validity of questionnaire-based diagnoses: the third Nord-Trondelag Health Study 2006–2008. J Headache Pain. 2010;11:67–73.
13. Hagen K, Åsberg AN, Uhlig BL, Tronvik E, Brenner E, Stjern M, Helde G, Gravdahl GB, Sand T. The epidemiology of headache disorders: a face-to-face interview of participants in HUNT4. J Headache Pain. 2018;19:25.
14. Hagen K, Åsberg AN, Uhlig BL, Tronvik E, Brenner E, Sand T. The HUNT4 study: the validy of questionnaire-based diagnosis. J Headache Pain. 2019;20:70.
15. Hagen K, Zwart JA, Aamodt AH, Nilsen KB, Brathen G, Helde G, Stjern M, Tronvik EA, Stovner LJ. A face-to-face interview of participants in HUNT 3: the impact of the screening question on headache prevalence. J Headache Pain. 2008;9:289–94.
16. Hagen K, Stovner LJ, Vatten L, Holmen J, Zwart JA, Bovim G. Blood pressure and risk of headache: a prospective study of 22685 adults in Norway. J Neurol Neurosurg Psychiatry. 2002;72:463–6.
17. Tronvik E, Stovner LJ, Hagen K, Holmen J, Zwart JA. High pulse pressure protects against headache: prospective and cross-sectional data (HUNT study). Neurology. 2008;70:1329–36.
18. Tronvik E, Zwart JA, Hagen K, Dyb G, Holmen TL, Stovner LJ. Association between blood pressure measures and recurrent headache in adolescents: cross-sectional data from the HUNT-Youth study. J Headache Pain. 2011;12:347–53.
19. Fagernaes CF, Heuch I, Zwart JA, Winsvold BS, Linde M, Hagen K. Blood pressure as a risk factor for headache and migraine: a prospective population-based study. Eur J Neurol. 2015;22:156–62.
20. Stovner LJ, Hagen K. Hypertension-associated hypalgesia: a clue to the comorbidity of headache and other pain disorders. Acta Neurol Scand Suppl. 2009;189:46–50.
21. Hagen K, Zwart JA, Holmen J, Svebak S, Bovim G, Stovner LJ. Does hypertension protect against chronic musculoskeletal complaints? The Nord-Trondelag Health Study. Arch Intern Med. 2005;165:916–22.
22. Winsvold BS, Hagen K, Aamodt AH, Stovner LJ, Holmen J, Zwart JA. Headache, migraine and cardiovascular risk factors: the HUNT study. Eur J Neurol. 2011;18:504–11.
23. Hagen K, Asberg AN, Stovner L, Linde M, Zwart JA, Winsvold BS, Heuch I. Lifestyle factors and risk of migraine and tension-type headache. Follow-up data from the Nord-Trondelag Health Surveys 1995–1997 and 2006–2008. Cephalalgia. 2018;38:1919–26.
24. Aamodt AH, Stovner LJ, Hagen K, Brathen G, Zwart J. Headache prevalence related to smoking and alcohol use. The Head-HUNT study. Eur J Neurol. 2006;13:1233–8.
25. Hagen K, Wisloff U, Ellingsen O, Stovner LJ, Linde M. Headache and peak oxygen uptake: the HUNT3 study. Cephalalgia. 2016;36:437–44.
26. Hagen K, Asvold BO, Midthjell K, Stovner LJ, Zwart JA, Linde M. Inverse relationship between type 1 diabetes mellitus and migraine. Data from the Nord-Trondelag Health Surveys 1995–1997 and 2006–2008. Cephalalgia. 2017;38:417–26.
27. Aamodt AH, Stovner LJ, Midthjell K, Hagen K, Zwart JA. Headache prevalence related to diabetes mellitus. The Head-HUNT study. Eur J Neurol. 2007;14:738–44.
28. Antonazzo IC, Riise T, Cortese M, Berge LI, Engeland A, Bernt Fasmer O, Lund A, Joachim Odegaard K, Poluzzi E, Bjornevik K. Diabetes is associated with decreased migraine risk: a nationwide cohort study. Cephalalgia. 2018;38:1759–64.
29. Zwart JA, Dyb G, Hagen K, Odegard KJ, Dahl AA, Bovim G, Stovner LJ. Depression and anxiety disorders associated with headache frequency. The Nord-Trondelag Health Study. Eur J Neurol. 2003;20:147–52.
30. Blaauw BA, Dyb G, Hagen K, Holmen TL, Linde M, Wentzel-Larsen T, Zwart JA. Anxiety, depression and behavioral problems among adolescents with recurrent headache: the Young-HUNT study. J Headache Pain. 2014;15:38.
31. Blaauw BA, Dyb G, Hagen K, Holmen TL, Linde M, Wentzel-Larsen T, Zwart JA. The relationship of anxiety, depression and behavioral problems with recurrent headache in late adolescence—a Young-HUNT follow-up study. J Headache Pain. 2015;16:10.

32. Aamodt AH, Stovner LJ, Langhammer A, Hagen K, Zwart JA. Is headache related to asthma, hay fever, and chronic bronchitis? The Head-HUNT study. Headache. 2007;47:204–12.
33. Odegard SS, Sand T, Engstrom M, Stovner LJ, Zwart JA, Hagen K. The long-term effect of insomnia on primary headaches: a prospective population-based cohort study (HUNT-2 and HUNT-3). Headache. 2011;51:570–80.
34. Hagen K, Einarsen C, Zwart JA, Svebak S, Bovim G. The co-occurrence of headache and musculoskeletal symptoms amongst 51 050 adults in Norway. Eur J Neurol. 2002;9:527–33.
35. Hagen K, Linde M, Steiner TJ, Zwart JA, Stovner LJ. The relationship between headache and chronic musculoskeletal complaints: an 11-year follow-up in the Nord-Trondelag Health Study (HUNT). Eur J Neurol. 2012;19:1447–54.
36. Aamodt AH, Stovner LJ, Hagen K, Zwart JA. Comorbidity of headache and gastrointestinal complaints. The Head-HUNT study. Cephalalgia. 2008;28:144–51.
37. Zwart JA, Dyb G, Hagen K, Svebak S, Holmen J. Analgesic use: a predictor of chronic pain and medication overuse headache: the Head-HUNT study. Neurology. 2003;61:160–4.
38. Hagen K, Linde M, Steiner TJ, Stovner LJ, Zwart JA. Risk factors for medication-overuse headache: an 11-year follow-up study. The Nord-Trondelag Health Studies. Pain. 2012;153:56–61.
39. Hagen K, Kristoffersen ES, Winsvold BS, Stovner LJ, Zwart JA. Remission of chronic headache: an 11-year follow-up study. Data from the Nord-Trondelag Health Surveys 1995–1997 and 2006–2008. Cephalalgia. 2018;38:2026–34.
40. Aamodt AH, Borch-Iohnsen B, Hagen K, Stovner LJ, Asberg A, Zwart JA. Headache prevalence related to haemoglobin and ferritin. The HUNT study. Cephalalgia. 2004;24:758–62.
41. Hagen K, Stovner LJ, Asberg A, Thorstensen K, Bjerve KS, Hveem K. High headache prevalence among women with hemochromatosis: the Nord-Trøndelag health study. Ann Neurol. 2002;51:786–9.
42. Hagen K, Bjoro T, Zwart JA, Vatten L, Stovner LJ, Bovim G. Low headache prevalence amongst women with high TSH values. Eur J Neurol. 2001;8:693–9.
43. Hagen K, Bjoro T, Zwart JA, Svebak S, Bovim G, Stovner LJ. Do high TSH values protect against chronic musculoskeletal complaints? The Nord-Trondelag Health Study (HUNT). Pain. 2005;113:416–21.
44. Aegidius K, Zwart JA, Hagen K, Schei B, Stovner LJ. Oral contraceptives and increased headache prevalence: the Head-HUNT study. Neurology. 2006;66:349–53.
45. Aegidius KL, Zwart JA, Hagen K, Schei B, Stovner LJ. Hormone replacement therapy and headache prevalence in postmenopausal women. The Head-HUNT study. Eur J Neurol. 2007;14:73–8.
46. Aegidius K, Zwart JA, Hagen K, Stovner L. The effect of pregnancy and parity on headache prevalence: the Head-HUNT study. Headache. 2009;49:851–9.
47. Aegidius KL, Zwart JA, Hagen K, Dyb G, Holmen TL, Stovner LJ. Increased headache prevalence in female adolescents and adult women with early menarche. The Head-HUNT studies. Eur J Neurol. 2011;18:321–8.
48. Hagen K, Vatten L, Stovner LJ, Zwart JA, Krokstad S, Bovim G. Low socio-economic status is associated with increased risk of frequent headache: a prospective study of 22718 adults in Norway. Cephalalgia. 2002;22:672–9.
49. Fiane I, Haugland M, Stovner L, Zwart JA, Bovim G, Hagen K. Sick leave is related to frequencies of migraine and non-migrainous headache-The HUNT Study. Cephalalgia. 2006;26:960–7.
50. Linde M, Langnes HA, Hagen K, Bergh K, Stovner LJ. No increase in headache after previous intracranial infections: a historical cohort study (HUNT). Eur J Neurol. 2012;19:324–31.
51. Hoem Nordhaug L, Vik A, Hagen K, Stovner LJ, Pedersen T, Gravdahl GB, Linde M. Headaches in patients with previous head injuries: a population-based historical cohort study (HUNT). Cephalalgia. 2016;36:1009–19.
52. Nordhaug LH, Hagen K, Vik A, Stovner LJ, Follestad T, Pedersen T, Gravdahl GB, Linde M. Headache following head injury: a population-based longitudinal cohort study (HUNT). J Headache Pain. 2018;19:8.

53. Honningsvag LM, Linde M, Haberg A, Stovner LJ, Hagen K. Does health differ between participants and non-participants in the MRI-HUNT study, a population based neuroimaging study? The Nord-Trondelag health studies 1984–2009. BMC Med Imaging. 2012;12:23.
54. Haberg AK, Hammer TA, Kvistad KA, Rydland J, Muller TB, Eikenes L, Garseth M, Stovner LJ. Incidental intracranial findings and their clinical impact; the HUNT MRI study in a general population of 1006 participants between 50–66 years. PLoS One. 2016;11:e0151080.
55. Honningsvag LM, Hagen K, Haberg A, Stovner LJ, Linde M. Intracranial abnormalities and headache: a population-based imaging study (HUNT MRI). Cephalalgia. 2016;36:113–21.
56. Honningsvag LM, Haberg AK, Hagen K, Kvistad KA, Stovner LJ, Linde M. White matter hyperintensities and headache: a population-based imaging study (HUNT MRI). Cephalalgia. 2018;38:1927–39.
57. Husoy AK, Indergaard MK, Honningsvag LM, Haberg AK, Hagen K, Linde M, Garseth M, Stovner LJ. Perivascular spaces and headache: a population-based imaging study (HUNT-MRI). Cephalalgia. 2016;36:232–9.
58. Hansen AG, Stovner LJ, Hagen K, Helvik AS, Thorstensen WM, Nordgard S, Bugten V, Eggesbo HB. Paranasal sinus opacification in headache sufferers: a population-based imaging study (the HUNT study-MRI). Cephalalgia. 2017;37:509–16.
59. Asberg AN, Stovner LJ, Zwart JA, Winsvold BS, Heuch I, Hagen K. Migraine as a predictor of mortality: the HUNT study. Cephalalgia. 2016;36:351–7.
60. Hagen K, Stordal E, Linde M, Steiner TJ, Zwart JA, Stovner LJ. Headache as a risk factor for dementia: a prospective population-based study. Cephalalgia. 2014;34:327–35.
61. Rottereng AK, Bosnes O, Stordal E, Zwart JA, Linde M, Stovner LJ, Hagen K. Headache as a predictor for dementia: the HUNT study. J Headache Pain. 2015;16:89.
62. Ioannidis JP. Why most published research findings are false. PLoS Med. 2005;2:e124.
63. Ioannidis JP. Exposure-wide epidemiology: revisiting Bradford Hill. Stat Med. 2016;35:1749–62.

Chapter 11
Headache, Functional Impact and Environment

Timothy J. Steiner and Lars Jacob Stovner

11.1 Introduction

Headache disorders are very common, in particular migraine, tension-type headache (TTH) and medication-overuse headache (MOH). But it is because they limit function that they are responsible for so much public ill health and cost to society [1–5].

Recent improvements in the methodology of population-based studies have led not only to better estimates of prevalence but also to better, more inclusive descriptions of headache-attributed burden and impact (see Chaps. 6–9). Surveys conducted within the Global Campaign against Headache in Russia [6], China [7], India [8, 9], Pakistan [10], Zambia [11, 12], Ethiopia [13, 14] and Nepal [15, 16], and in Saudi Arabia, Morocco, Mongolia and Peru [not yet published], have adopted standardized methods of sampling and enquiry, which have formed the basis of guidelines and expert recommendations for burden-of-headache studies ([17]; also, Chap. 6). These developments are important; yet it is still not certain that existing methods and available instruments even recognize, let alone adequately describe, all the consequences of living with headache ([18, 19]; also, Chap. 7). A full account and quantitative descriptions of these are the necessary basis of healthcare needs

T. J. Steiner (✉)
Department of Neuromedicine and Movement Science, NTNU Norwegian University of Science and Technology, Trondheim, Norway

Division of Brain Sciences, Imperial College London, London, UK
e-mail: t.steiner@imperial.ac.uk

L. J. Stovner
Department of Neuromedicine and Movement Science, NTNU Norwegian University of Science and Technology, Trondheim, Norway

Norwegian Advisory Unit on Headaches, Department of Neurology and Clinical Neurophysiology, St Olavs University Hospital, Trondheim, Norway
e-mail: lars.stovner@ntnu.no

T. J. Steiner, L. J. Stovner (eds.), *Societal Impact of Headache*, Headache,
https://doi.org/10.1007/978-3-030-24728-7_11

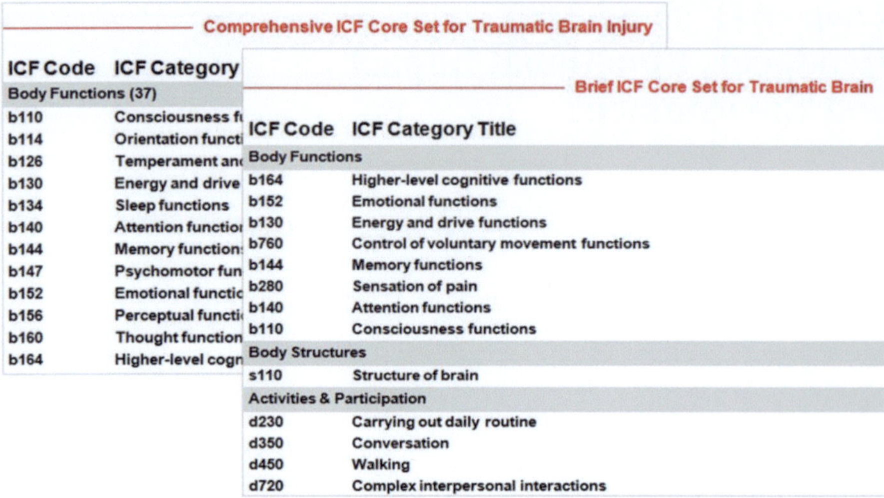

Fig. 11.1 Example: ICF Core Set for traumatic brain injury (from [25])

assessment and resource allocation, and people with headache will continue to be underserved by inadequate responses to their needs [2] while this account remains incomplete.

Against this background, the International Classification of Functioning, Disability and Health (ICF) [20–23] provides a framework to classify and describe the burden of living with a health condition. Approved by the World Health Assembly in 2001 [20], it is universally accepted. ICF provides comprehensive descriptions, at both individual and population levels, not only of disease-imposed difficulties in functioning but also of relevant environmental factors that may have impact—either as facilitators or barriers—upon these difficulties. It does this in a language standardized across diseases, and independently of specific assessment instruments [21] (Fig. 11.1).

Based on a biopsychosocial model, ICF organizes information in two parts (Fig. 11.2). The first, dealing with functioning and disability, has two components: *Body Functions and Structures*, and *Activities and Participation*. The second, covering contextual factors, also has two components of *Environmental Factors* and *Personal Factors.*[1] It is in these very areas—functioning and interaction with environmental factors—that the methodology for reporting the burden of living with a headache disorder appears most deficient. People with headache may be well served if headache disorders can be brought into the ICF framework [24], and this chapter considers how this might be done.

ICF is cumbersome, with more than 1400 categories [21]. *ICF Core Sets* [25–29] have a pragmatic purpose: by reducing its 1400 categories to far smaller, manageable numbers, they render the system useful in clinical practice and informative to

[1] Personal factors that potentially affect functioning include gender, race, ethnicity, age, social and educational background, past and current experiences and life events, character styles, behaviour patterns and psychological assets; they are not yet classified in ICF because of the large social and cultural variances associated with them, but may be annotated as free text.

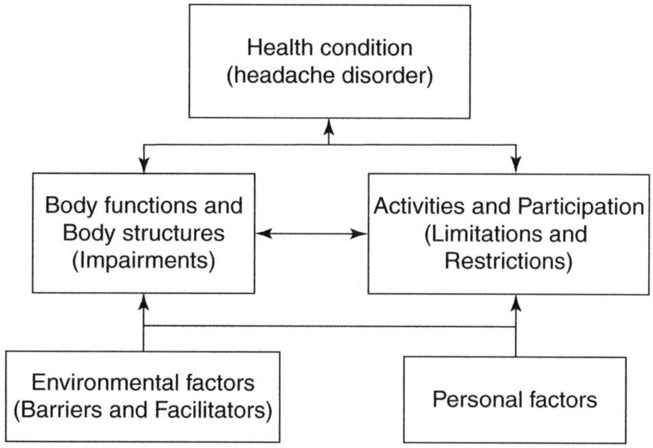

Fig. 11.2 ICF biopsychosocial model: interaction of components (adapted from [24])

Table 11.1 Three principal purposes of developing ICF Core Sets for headache disorders

1	To describe the full range of consequences of living with headache—that is, on a considerably broader basis than is currently achieved—using language that health professionals and researchers in all fields of medicine, policy makers, patients and patient organizations understand
2	To express more adequately the public-health consequences of headache in political arguments for healthcare priority and resource allocation
3	To support development of an instrument whereby clinicians and health professionals can better describe their patients' difficulties in functioning, and the environmental factors influencing these difficulties

needs-based health policy [30]. Careful selection, according to relevance to the disorders they describe, is the essence of development, with the methodology ensuring that "relevance" is not defined by the narrow view of any particular interest group [25, 29]. *Comprehensive ICF Core Sets* describe the full spectrum of functioning and health of individuals with a disorder. *Brief ICF Core Sets* list even smaller numbers of ICF categories, still descriptively sufficient but short enough to be useful in clinical studies (Fig. 11.1) [25].

ICF Core Sets have been developed for a large number of health conditions, including some neurological disorders [25], but not headache. Described here is methodology to develop ICF Core Sets for headache disorders, with the purposes shown in Table 11.1, informed by published guidance [25, 27–29]. It is assumed that single Core Sets (comprehensive and brief) can be applied to all headache disorders of public-health importance, but this must be tested during the development process.

11.2 Methodology for Developing ICF Core Sets for Headache

Four studies are needed in the preparatory phase [25, 29]. These capture the perspectives of people with headache, of healthcare providers (specialist and generalist) and of researchers in the field of headache, and they should involve academic and clinical collaborators from all world regions. They need not occur in sequence. A consensus conference, the next phase in development [25], should integrate the evidence from these preparatory studies, with final definition of the Core Set(s). These methodological stages are described in some detail below. The final phase is testing and validation in practice [25].

11.2.1 Systematic Literature Review

This review, to capture the researchers' perspective with two objectives (Table 11.2), should search the Medline and Embase databases from 1988 onwards (this year saw the first international classification of headache disorders [31], prior to which there were no universally accepted definitions). It should be results-driven (i.e. expanded or constrained according to the search output), with initial search terms ("headache" or "migraine" AND "impact" or "burden" or "cost" or "outcome" or "measure" or "questionnaire" AND NOT "clinical trial") that ensure inclusion of population- or patient-based studies or case-series of individuals with headache disorders, and studies and reviews of, and expert opinion papers on, outcome measures used in people with headache. Clinical trials generally have the narrow purpose of demonstrating efficacy of a drug in predefined terms, according to what it is expected that the drug will do; the legitimacy of this perspective to inform this development process is questionable [25].

The search methodology is standard. Two reviewers independently check the abstracts of retrieved studies for inclusion, resolving disagreements by discussion between themselves, with inclusion as the default option. From full manuscripts of all included studies, the two reviewers extract data independently into standardized data-capture forms, comparing their eventual results and resolving disagreements through discussion (consulting, when necessary, a third researcher).

Table 11.2 The specific objectives of the four preparatory studies

Systematic literature review	
1	To learn how the health states associated with headache disorders, and the consequences of living with them, are described in published studies
2	To identify the outcome measures and other instruments used to quantify these
Survey of experts	
To learn the views of health professionals with different healthcare backgrounds as to the health areas most relevant to individuals with headache disorders	
Focus groups with patients	
To identify whatever concepts of functioning and health are important to those who live with the different headache disorders	
Empirical cross-sectional multicentre study	
To describe the functioning and health of patients with headache disorders, and identify their most common problems	

This process should list all descriptors of the health states associated with headache disorders and the consequences of living with them, all outcome measures and all component items of questionnaires, with their underlying concepts. The reviewers decide whether any of these apply only to migraine, TTH or MOH rather than to all headache disorders; if so, separate lists are needed for each disorder.

Each listed item is then linked to ICF categories using the standardized linkage rules [32–34]. The protocol for linking requires two experts in the application of these rules, who first work separately and then compare their results, resolving disagreements (again, when necessary, by consultation with a third expert). Finally, absolute and relative frequencies of the items and their linked ICF categories are reported, in one or three lists.

11.2.2 Survey of Experts

An email-based survey captures the healthcare providers' perspective, with the objective described in Table 11.2. It is a three-round Delphi exercise [35, 36] for each headache disorder (migraine, TTH and MOH), conducted in English. It should include about 300 experts (physicians [whatever their speciality, and including general practitioners], psychologists, nurses or physical therapists, all with at least 5 years' specific training and practical experience [self-reported] in treating patients with headache disorders). Since ICF is intended to facilitate communication between different groups of people, and be used globally [20], these experts should come from all over the world, from different health professions and with different specializations, but all must be competent in the English language.

In the first round, background information, a description of the study objectives, a semi-structured questionnaire and an example from another health condition are sent to the experts. They are asked to list, in their own words, all the body functions, body structures, activities and participation and environmental factors that, in their opinions, are most relevant to and/or most typical for patients with each disorder. These lists are collated, and condensed as far as possible by eliminating duplications. Surviving items are then linked to ICF categories according to the same linkage rules and protocol [32–34].

In the second round, three lists (one for each headache disorder) are sent, setting out the ICF categories identified in the first round and the percentages of experts who considered each to be relevant and/or typical for patients with the disorder(s). Experts should then reconsider their own former responses, and indicate ("yes" or "no") which ICF categories they still believe are relevant and/or typical. The third round repeats this exercise.

Three lists of relevant ICF categories, and the frequency with which the experts endorsed each one, are then available, one for each headache disorder. These are scrutinized for differences. If these are negligible, the three lists should be merged into one, with frequencies averaged.

11.2.3 Focus Groups with Patients

These capture the perspective(s) of those who live with the different headache disorders (Table 11.2). This study should be conducted in at least two countries, at different income levels and from different world regions.

Patients consulting for headache participate in groups of up to seven. A moderator encourages interactions within each group in order to enrich the information generated [37, 38], using the local language of the group. These interactions may be inhibited, counterproductively, if, within groups, people are participating with widely different experiences (of different headache disorders, or on account of age or years affected). The maximum variation strategy [37] is therefore pursued *between* rather than within groups, with groups in each country constructed by convenience sampling:

(a) Patients with migraine
(b) Patients with TTH
(c) Patients with MOH
(d) Elderly patients (aged >65 years) with lifetime histories in excess of 40 years of any of these headache disorders
(e) Young patients (aged 16–18 years) with any of these headache disorders

All groups should include at least two people of each gender and be as diverse as possible with respect to occupation, socioeconomic level, marital status (excepting group (e)) and age (excepting groups (d) and (e)). The specific purpose of group (d) is to discover the views of those having lived a lifetime with headache, and experiencing its cumulative burden; group (e) acts as proxy for children, presenting the views of those affected by headache while at school.

Again, the methodology is standard. Each focus group is recorded, and the content of the discussion transcribed *verbatim* for analysis by the group moderator. First, it is divided into meaning units (specific units of text, either a few words or a few sentences, with a common dominating theme [38]). Meaning-unit division does not follow linguistic grammatical rules but breaks the text wherever the analyst discerns a shift in meaning [39]. Then the theme of each unit is determined, and the concept(s) contained in each theme identified. Finally, every concept is linked to ICF categories according to the same linkage rules and protocol [32–34].

Additional focus groups should be included until saturation is reached (the point during data collection when linking from two consecutive focus groups reveals no additional information with respect to previous focus groups).

11.2.4 Empirical Cross-Sectional Multicentre Study

This also captures the patients' perspective (Table 11.2), surveying patients consulting for headache in at least four countries: two high-income and two-low income, from different world regions.

For this study, physician-investigators in each country, fluent in the local language and English and trained in the core principles and model of ICF and the practical application of the case record form,[2] recruit patients by convenience sampling, as diverse as possible with respect to gender, age (in the range 18–65 years), occupation, socioeconomic level and marital status. Assuming an equal effects model (EEM), power (1-β) of 0.8 and significance level (α) of 0.05, a total sample of $N = 194$ (50 per country if four are included) is needed to determine frequencies with a precision of 10% [25, 29]. EEM does not take account of cluster effects, so interim analysis should test the sample's homogeneity; if relevant cluster effects are discovered, a larger sample may be needed.

Data collection, using a standardized form, begins with sociodemographic variables and main diagnoses. Functioning and health are judged from all available information, by direct interrogation and with reference when necessary to case records. The enquiry is driven by the standard extended ICF Checklist [29], a selection of 125 items (29 [25%] from *Body Functions*, 16 [29%] from *Body Structures*, 48 [41%] from *Activities and Participation* and 32 [43%] from *Environmental Factors*) from the 362 first- and second-level categories of the whole ICF classification system [20]. This relatively simple questionnaire, with guidelines and probes, enables classification of the most important ICF categories in clinical practice [25, 29]. Additional categories are added if identified as important by the literature review or any of the earlier enquiries.

Each category of *Body Functions*, *Body Structures* and *Activities and Participation* is graded 0 (no impairment or limitation) or 1 (some or total impairment or limitation) [25]. Those of *Environmental Factors* are graded +1 (facilitator), −1 (barrier) or 0 (neither). The qualifiers "8" indicate insufficient information and "9" not applicable (e.g. d760 *Family relationships* for a patient with no family). Problems associated with other health conditions than headache disorders are excluded from magnitude analysis by the qualifier "C" (for comorbidity).

For *Body Functions*, *Body Structures* and *Activities and Participation*, absolute and relative frequencies (prevalence) of impairments or limitations in the study population are computed, with 95% confidence intervals (CIs). For *Environmental Factors*, absolute and relative frequencies are calculated of persons regarding each specific category as either barrier or facilitator [25, 29].

11.2.5 Data Collation from the Preparatory Studies

All data—the lists and frequencies of ICF categories identified as relevant to the problems of living with headache disorder(s)—are collated into a single list, presenting the accumulated information in best-digestible form for the consensus conference [25, 29] (see below). If the assumption proves incorrect that a single list can cover all three headache disorders (migraine, TTH and MOH), plans for the consensus conference will require revision.

---

[2] Usually provided at the ICF Research Branch of the WHO Collaborating Centre of the Family of International Classifications.

11.2.6 Consensus Conference

The fifth and final stage of development seeks international consensus, informed by the preparatory stages, on this question:

> "Which ICF categories are the most relevant to be included in the ICF Core Set(s), and are adequate, for headache disorders?"

Participants will be specialists in the treatment of headache disorders or experts in the field of outcome measurement representing all world regions and high-, middle- and low-income countries. To balance these needs against practicality, a group of 21 might, for example, include

- Nine physicians practising as headache specialists
- Three general practitioners with a special interest in headache disorders
- Three psychologists specializing in the management of headache disorders
- Three nurses or clinical officers with a special interest in headache disorders
- Three specialists in outcome measurement

The conference should be held in a quiet place, distant from distractions [25, 29]. Initial training, in a half-day workshop, familiarizes participants with the ICF framework and classification, providing them with the ICF handbook describing the categories [21]. The summary list of ICF categories from the preparatory studies is made available, with an account of how it was developed (i.e. the designs of and evidence from these studies). The spectrum of problems generally encountered in individuals with headache disorders is identified, without comorbidities or medical complications. Finally, the ICF Core Set categories are agreed in an iterative decision-making process [25, 29] (Fig. 11.3).

Two kinds of session are distinguished during the consensus process: *Condition Group* (CG) sessions, in which all participants work together, and *Working Group* (WG) sessions, in which they are divided into groups working separately [25]. The main purpose of the WG sessions is to consider arguments for and against each ICF category, then vote on its selection. The CG sessions provide feedback from all participants on the arguments for and against controversial categories (those that are clearly relevant or clearly irrelevant, according to the pre-set decision rules depicted in Fig. 11.3, are not discussed in the CG).

The decision-making process is in two major parts [25, 29]. First, participants select ICF categories for the Comprehensive ICF Core Set, that is, the list of *all* ICF categories relevant to describing the spectrum of limitations in functioning and health of individuals with headache disorders. Up to and including CG session 2 (Fig. 11.3), participants decide on second-level categories. From WG session 3 to CG session 4, they decide "to dive or not to dive", that is, on third- and fourth-level categories to be included *only if* the additional specification yielded is *essential* to describing this spectrum [25, 29].

Second, participants reduce the second-level categories in the Comprehensive ICF Core Set to create a Brief ICF Core Set, short enough to be feasible in clinical studies while still sufficient for their purpose. This requires a two-round ranking exercise (Fig. 11.3). Working individually, participants rank the 15 most essential

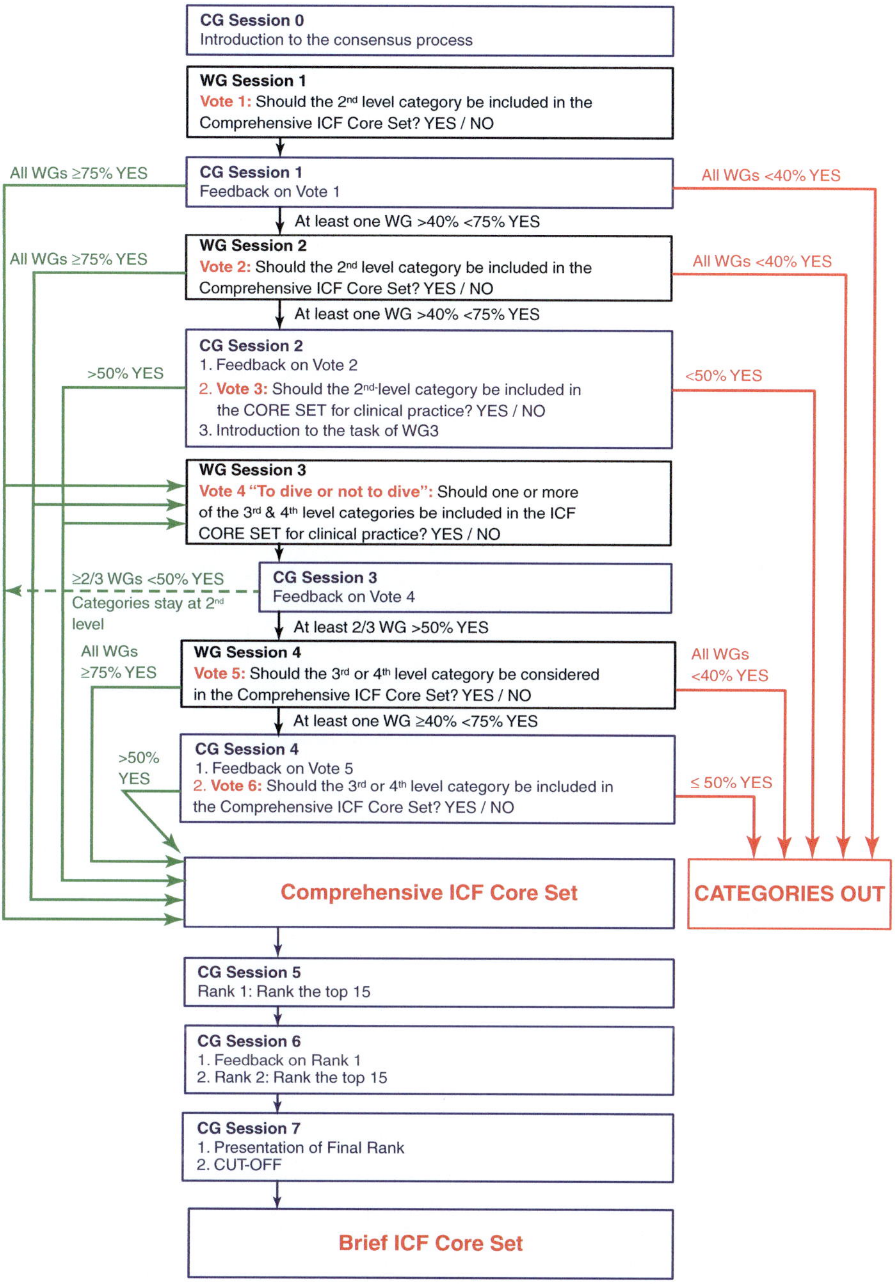

Fig. 11.3 Decision-making process at the ICF Core Set consensus conference (*CG* condition group, *WG* working group)

second-level categories in order of importance for each ICF component (*Body Functions, Body Structures; Activities and Participation; Environmental Factors*), repeating the exercise after feedback. Then participants each decide how many second-level ICF categories per ICF component they wish to include in the Brief ICF Core Set. In the last CG session, voting finalizes the Brief ICF Core Set for headache disorders.

11.3 Comment and Concluding Remarks

This methodology, based on a standard template [24, 29], is complex and resource-consuming, not to be undertaken without good reason. ICF Core Sets have so far been developed for 68 health conditions [25], which attests the importance attached by many to this system of classification. On a general level, the reasons, already enumerated, are clear:

1. It is a framework not only for classifying but also, and perhaps more importantly, for describing in full the burden of living with a health condition; no other system is so comprehensive.
2. It is universally accepted, having been approved by the World Health Assembly in 2001.
3. It operates at both individual and population levels.
4. Its language is standardized across diseases and independent of specific assessment instruments.

The key question here is: How might this benefit headache?

The two parts of ICF describe functioning and disability on the one hand and the relevant contextual (especially environmental) factors on the other, the very areas in which current methods and instruments for reporting the burden of headache are most deficient [18, 19]. An ICF Core Set for headache disorders, repairing this deficiency, will allow a better (more complete) account of the *societal impact* of headache disorders—the subject of this monograph—at the same time as headache disorders are brought fully into the International Classification of Diseases (ICD-11) [40, 41]. For this purpose, investment of considerable resources, as a one-off commitment, may be very worthwhile [24]. Much less clear is whether a more complete description of headache burden, in these terms, will lead to better management or the development of more useful *clinical* measures of headache [42, 43]. On the one hand, many such measures exist [19], on the other, comprehensiveness and ease of use are very much at odds, while the latter is likely only partly to be assured by developing ICF Core Sets.

Finally, inclusion of categories from the *ICF Generic Set* is recommended whenever an ICF Core Set is used [25]. This, it is argued, will widen applicability of collected data—for example, of data gathered for assessment purposes in a clinical setting to health statistics and service planning [25]. The ICF Generic Set has only a small number of ICF categories (seven second-level: Table 11.3); these are key

Table 11.3 Categories in the ICF Generic Set (from [25])

Body functions (physiological functions of body systems, including psychological functions)	
b130 Energy and drive functions	
	General mental functions of physiological and psychological mechanisms that cause the individual to move towards satisfying specific needs and general goals in a persistent manner *Inclusions: functions of energy level, motivation, appetite, craving (including craving for substances that can be abused) and impulse control* *Exclusions: consciousness functions (b110); temperament and personality functions (b126); sleep functions (b134); psychomotor functions (b147); emotional functions (b152)*
b152 Emotional functions	
	Specific mental functions related to the feeling and affective components of the processes of the mind *Inclusions: functions of appropriateness, regulation and range of emotion; affect; sadness, happiness, love, fear, anger, hate, tension, anxiety, joy, sorrow; lability of emotion; flattening of affect* *Exclusions: temperament and personality functions (b126); energy and drive functions (b130)*
b280 Sensation of pain	
	Sensation of unpleasant feeling indicating potential or actual damage to some body structure *Inclusions: sensations of generalized or localized pain in one or more body part, pain in a dermatome, stabbing pain, burning pain, dull pain, aching pain; impairments such as myalgia, analgesia and hyperalgesia*
Activities and participation(execution of a task or action by an individual and involvement in a life situation)	
d230 Carrying out daily routine	
	Carrying out simple or complex and coordinated actions in order to plan, manage and complete the requirements of day-to-day procedures or duties, such as budgeting time and making plans for separate activities throughout the day *Inclusions: managing and completing the daily routine; managing one's own activity level* *Exclusion: undertaking multiple tasks (d220)*
d450 Walking	
	Moving along a surface on foot, step by step, so that one foot is always on the ground, such as when strolling, sauntering, walking forwards, backwards or sideways *Inclusions: walking short or long distances; walking on different surfaces; walking around obstacles* *Exclusions: transferring oneself (d420); moving around (d455)*
d455 Moving around	
	Moving the whole body from one place to another by means other than walking, such as climbing over a rock or running down a street, skipping, scampering, jumping, somersaulting or running around obstacles *Inclusions: crawling, climbing, running, jogging, jumping and swimming* *Exclusions: transferring oneself (d420); walking (d450)*
d850 Remunerative employment	
	Engaging in all aspects of work, as an occupation, trade, profession or other form of employment, for payment, as an employee, full or part time, or self-employed, such as seeking employment and getting a job, doing the required tasks of the job, attending work on time as required, supervising other workers or being supervised, and performing required tasks alone or in groups *Inclusions: self-employment, part-time and full-time employment*

indicators of health and functioning, shown psychometrically to be most widely applicable [44, 45]. As a very brief description of functioning, able to compare health across health conditions, contexts, settings, population groups and countries, it may well have importance for health statistics and public health [25, 44, 45]. Whether it would help the description of living with headache disorders is not yet clear.

References

1. Stovner LJ, Hagen K, Jensen R, Katsarava Z, Lipton R, Scher A, Steiner TJ, Zwart JA. The global burden of headache: a documentation of headache prevalence and disability worldwide. Cephalalgia. 2007;27:193–210.
2. World Health Organization and *Lifting The Burden*. Atlas of headache disorders and resources in the world 2011. Geneva: WHO; 2011.
3. Linde M, Gustavsson A, Stovner LJ, Steiner TJ, Barré J, Katsarava Z, Lainez JM, Lampl C, Lantéri-Minet M, Rastenyte D, Ruiz de la Torre E, Tassorelli C, Andrée C. The cost of headache disorders in Europe: the Eurolight project. Eur J Neurol. 2012;19:703–11.
4. Vos T, Abajobir AA, Abate KH, Abbafati C, Abbas KM, Abd-Allah F, Abdulkader RS, Abdulle AM, Abebo TA, Abera SF, Aboyans V, Abu-Raddad LJ, Ackerman IN, Adamu AA, Adetokunboh O, Afarideh M, Afshin A, Agarwal SK, Aggarwal R, Agrawal A, Agrawal S, Ahmadieh H, Ahmed MB, Aichour MTE, Aichour AN, Aichour I, Aiyar S, Akinyemi RO, Akseer N, Al Lami FH, Alahdab F, Al-Aly Z, Alam K, Alam N, Alam T, et al. Global, regional, and national incidence, prevalence, and years lived with disability for 328 diseases and injuries for 195 countries, 1990–2016: a systematic analysis for the Global Burden of Disease Study 2016. Lancet. 2017;390:1211–59.
5. Steiner TJ, Stovner LJ, Vos T, Jensen R, Katsarava Z. Migraine is *first* cause of disability in under 50s: will health politicians now take notice? J Headache Pain. 2018;19:17.
6. Ayzenberg I, Katsarava Z, Sborowski A, Chernysh M, Osipova V, Tabeeva G, Yakhno N, Steiner TJ. The prevalence of primary headache disorders in Russia: a countrywide survey. Cephalalgia. 2012;32:373–81.
7. Yu S, Liu R, Zhao G, Yang X, Qiao X, Feng J, Fang Y, Cao X, He M, Steiner T. The prevalence and burden of primary headaches in China: a population-based door-to-door survey. Headache. 2012;52:582–91.
8. Kulkarni GB, Rao GN, Gururaj G, Stovner LJ, Steiner TJ. Headache disorders and public ill-health in India: prevalence estimates in Karnataka state. J Headache Pain. 2015;16:67.
9. Rao GN, Kulkarni GB, Gururaj G, Stovner LJ, Steiner TJ. The burden attributable to headache disorders in India: estimates from a community-based study in Karnataka state. J Headache Pain. 2015;16:94.
10. Herekar AA, Ahmad A, Uqaili UL, Ahmed B, Effendi J, Alvi SZ, Shahab MA, Javed U, Herekar AD, Khanani R, Steiner TJ. Primary headache disorders in the adult general population of Pakistan—a cross sectional nationwide prevalence survey. J Headache Pain. 2017;18:28.
11. Mbewe E, Zairemthiama P, Yeh H-H, Paul R, Birbeck GL, Steiner TJ. The epidemiology of primary headache disorders in Zambia: a population-based door-to-door survey. J Headache Pain. 2015;16:30.
12. Mbewe E, Zairemthiama P, Paul R, Birbeck GL, Steiner TJ. The burden of primary headache disorders in Zambia: national estimates from a population-based door-to-door survey. J Headache Pain. 2015;16:36.
13. Zebenigus M, Tekle-Haimanot R, Worku DK, Thomas H, Steiner TJ. The prevalence of primary headache disorders in Ethiopia. J Headache Pain. 2016;17:110.

14. Zebenigus M, Tekle-Haimanot R, Worku DK, Thomas H, Steiner TJ. The burden of headache disorders in Ethiopia: national estimates from a population-based door-to-door survey. J Headache Pain. 2017;18:58.
15. Manandhar K, Risal A, Steiner TJ, Holen A, Linde M. The prevalence of primary headache disorders in Nepal: a nationwide population-based study. J Headache Pain. 2015;16:95.
16. Manandhar K, Risal A, Linde M, Steiner TJ. The burden of headache disorders in Nepal: estimates from a population-based survey. J Headache Pain. 2016;17:3.
17. Stovner LJ, Al Jumah M, Birbeck GL, Gururaj G, Jensen R, Katsarava Z, Queiroz LP, Scher AI, Tekle-Haimanot R, Wang SJ, Steiner TJ. The methodology of population surveys of headache prevalence, burden and cost: principles and recommendations from the Global Campaign against Headache. J Headache Pain. 2014;15:5.
18. Steiner TJ, Gururaj G, Andrée C, Katsarava Z, Ayzenberg I, Yu SY, Al Jumah M, Tekle-Haimanot R, Birbeck GL, Herekar A, Linde M, Mbewe E, Manandhar K, Risal A, Jensen R, Queiroz LP, Scher AI, Wang SJ, Stovner LJ. Diagnosis, prevalence estimation and burden measurement in population surveys of headache: presenting the HARDSHIP questionnaire. J Headache Pain. 2014;15:3.
19. Buse DC, Sollars CM, Steiner TJ, Jensen RH, Al Jumah MA, Lipton RB. Why HURT? A review of clinical instruments for headache management. Curr Pain Headache Rep. 2012;16:237–54.
20. World Health Organization. International Classification of Functioning, Disability and Health ICF. Geneva: WHO; 2001.
21. World Health Organization. How to use the ICF: a practical manual for using the International Classification of Functioning, Disability and Health (ICF). Exposure draft for comment. Geneva: WHO; 2013.
22. Cieza A, Stucki G. The international classification of functioning disability and health: its development process and content validity. Eur J Phys Rehabil Med. 2008;44:303–13.
23. Stucki G, Kostanjsek N, Ustün B, Cieza A. ICF-based classification and measurement of functioning. Eur J Phys Rehabil Med. 2008;44:315–28.
24. Leonardi M, Steiner TJ, Scher AI, Lipton RB. The global burden of migraine: measuring disability in headache disorders with WHO's classification of functioning, disability and health (ICF). J Headache Pain. 2005;6:429–40.
25. ICF Research Branch. ICF Core Sets projects. At: https://www.icf-research-branch.org/icf-core-sets-projects2.
26. Üstün B, Chatterji S, Konstansjek N. Comments from WHO for the journal of rehabilitation medicine special supplement on ICF Core sets. J Rehabil Med. 2004;36(Suppl 44):7–8.
27. Cieza A, Ewert T, Üstün B, Chatterji S, Konstansjek N, Stucki G. Development of ICF core sets for patients with chronic conditions. J Rehabil Med. 2004;36(Suppl 44):9–11.
28. Grill E, Stucki G. Criteria for validating the comprehensive ICF Core sets and developing brief ICF Core set versions. J Rehabil Med. 2011;43:87–91.
29. Selb M, Escorpizo R, Kostanjsek N, Stucki G, Üstün TB, Cieza A. A guide on how to develop an international classification of functioning, disability and health core set. Eur J Phys Rehabil Med. 2014;51:105–17.
30. Avellanet M, Selb M, Stucki G, Cieza A. Utility of using the ICF Core sets in clinical practice. Rehabilitación. 2015;49:197–201.
31. Headache Classification Committee of the International Headache Society. Classification and diagnostic criteria for headache disorders, cranial neuralgia and facial pain. Cephalalgia. 1988;8:1–96.
32. Cieza A, Geyh S, Chatterji S, Kostanjsek N, Ustun B, Stucki G. ICF linking rules: an update based on lessons learned. J Rehabil Med. 2005;37:1–8.
33. Fayed N, Cieza A, Bickenbach JE. Linking health and health-related information to the ICF: a systematic review of the literature from 2001 to 2008. Disabil Rehabil. 2011;33:1941–51.
34. Cieza A, Fayed N, Bickenbach J, Prodinger B. Refinements of the ICF linking rules to strengthen their potential for establishing comparability of health information. Disabil Rehabil. 2016;41(5):574–83. https://doi.org/10.3109/09638288.2016.1145258.

35. Linstone HA, Turoff M. The Delphi method: techniques and applications. Reading: Addison-Wesley; 1975.
36. Weigl M, Cieza A, Andersen C, Kollerits B, Amann E, Stucki G. Identification of relevant ICF categories in patients with chronic health conditions: a Delphi exercise. J Rehabil Med. 2004;36(Suppl 44):12–21.
37. Clarke A. Focus group interviews in health-care research. Prof Nurse. 1999;14:395–7.
38. Parsons M, Greenwood J. A guide to the use of focus groups in health care research: part 1. Contemp Nurse. 2000;9:169–80.
39. Karlsson G. Psychological qualitative research from a phenomenological perspective. Stockholm: Almquist and Wirksell International; 1993.
40. Selb M, Kohler F, Robinson Nicol MM, Riberto M, Stucki G, Kennedy C, Üstün B. ICD-11: a comprehensive picture of health, an update on the ICD–ICF joint use initiative. J Rehabil Med. 2015;47:2–8.
41. World Health Organization. The 11th revision of the International Classification of Diseases (ICD-11) is due by 2018! 2018. http://www.who.int/classifications/icd/revision/en/.
42. Cieza A, Hilfiker R, Chatterji S, Kostanjsek N, Ustun BT, Stucki G. The international classification of functioning, disability, and health could be used to measure functioning. J Clin Epidemiol. 2009;62:899–911.
43. Kostansjek N, Rubinelli S, Escorpizo R, Cieza A, Kennedy C, Selb M, Stucki G, Üstün B. Assessing the impact of health conditions using the ICF. Disabil Rehabil. 2011;33:1475–82.
44. Cieza A, Geyh S, Chatterji S, Kostanjsek N, Ustun BT, Stucki G. Identification of candidate categories of the international classification of functioning disability and health (ICF) for a generic ICF core set based on regression modelling. BMC Med Res Methodol. 2006;6:36.
45. Cieza A, Oberhauser C, Bickenbach J, Chatterji S, Stucki G. Towards a minimal generic set of domains of functioning and health. BMC Public Health. 2014;14:218.

Chapter 12
The Financial Costs of Headache

Francesco Saverio Mennini and Lara Gitto

12.1 Introduction

During the last two decades, an understanding that headache has a major impact on public health and society as a whole has evolved (see Chaps. 8 and 9). In 2001, the World Health Organization (WHO) listed migraine among the 20 most disabling disorders. Later studies moved migraine, and headache disorders collectively, higher in the lists of disabling disorders. The Global Burden of Disease 2016 study (GBD2016), by the Institute for Health Metrics and Evaluation [1], ranked migraine the second most disabling disorder globally, and the most disabling in people under 50 years of age ([2]; also, Chap. 9).

GBD measures disease burden in time units (see Chap. 9). For headache disorders, an important aspect of disease burden is their cost, in economic terms. Good, comprehensive economic studies that take account of both individual and societal perspectives, which have come mostly during the last 2–3 decades, are important for several reasons. First, they inform the public, politicians and health service providers that headache not only imposes suffering and disability but also is an economic burden on individuals affected and on society as a whole. Second, knowledge about the different cost components (medicines, consultations, lost working capacity) are important for budgeting and planning health services for people with headache. Third, they make a very strong argument for allocation of more resources to health

F. S. Mennini (✉)
CEIS Economic Evaluation and HTA (EEHTA), and IGF Department, Faculty of Economics, University "Tor Vergata", Rome, Italy

Institute for Leadership and Management in Health, Kingston University, Kingston, UK
e-mail: f.mennini@uniroma2.it

L. Gitto
CEIS Economic Evaluation and HTA (EEHTA), Faculty of Economics, University "Tor Vergata", Rome, Italy
e-mail: gttlnc00@uniroma2.it

T. J. Steiner, L. J. Stovner (eds.), *Societal Impact of Headache*, Headache, https://doi.org/10.1007/978-3-030-24728-7_12

services for headache, particularly if it can be shown that part of the cost of treatment can be retrieved by reducing costs of hospital admissions or by improving productivity. Fourth, demonstration of substantial societal cost may be a strong argument for more resources for research on headache.

The aims of this chapter are to explain some principal aspects of the methodology of health economic studies on headache and then present the results of key studies.

12.2 Methodology of Headache Health-Economic Studies

12.2.1 Direct and Indirect Costs

Assessment of the economic burden of headache distinguishes between direct costs and indirect costs [3–5]. This is an important distinction. Most studies have focused on the direct costs, although it has been shown that the more relevant costs are the indirect costs [6].

Direct costs are all the healthcare costs caused by a disease, from diagnosis to treatment. For headache, the latter mostly concern the expenses of drugs, although these are not often assessed in an appropriate way. Expenses related to medical consultations, examinations (MRI, CT, etc.) and hospital admissions are also part of the direct costs.

Indirect costs have been estimated to depend mainly on lost productivity, from absence from work (*absenteeism*) and when working with headache (*presenteeism*). A large part of the indirect costs of migraine is driven by absenteeism, but loss of production capacity (so-called *debility*) may occur also when an ill person goes to work because he or she will not have the same level of productivity as a well person.

The Migraine Disability Assessment (MIDAS) instrument [7, 8], and its adaptation, the Headache-Attributed Lost Time (HALT) index [9], have proved extremely useful in estimating the reduced productivity burdens attributable to headache disorders, from both absenteeism and presenteeism.

While indirect costs are considered the more difficult to quantify, direct costs may also be underestimated, for several reasons. First, medical claims do not capture all migraine-related treatment costs, because the disease is often not treated with specific therapies. Second, it may be difficult to measure all over-the-counter medications and, when taken, preventative medications. Non-drug-related interventions for headache may be particularly difficult to measure. In the USA, an estimated 36% of people with migraine spend more than USD 1000 out-of-pocket every year on migraine treatments [10].

Most studies do not consider non-medical direct costs (e.g. the Eurolight study ([11]; and see below)). Further, direct costs may differ depending on who pays: the health service (national healthcare service, panel-based healthcare system or health insurance) on the one hand or patients themselves and their families on the other.

12.2.2 Top-Down Versus Bottom-Up Approaches

There are two fundamentally different approaches for calculating costs: top-down and bottom-up.

The former uses aggregate data (e.g. official data on medical expenses or sick leave) to estimate economic costs, whereas the bottom-up approach makes use of more detailed individual-level data (i.e. each person's use of medicines, consultations, sick leave, etc.) to compute estimates of costs. Generally, in public economics, a bottom-up approach is used to estimate the costs of service use, whereas top-down costing is more suitable when estimating societal-level costs, which are often intangible and for which data are scarce. Studies such as Eurolight ([11]; and see below) and the International Burden of Migraine Study ([12]; and see below), which have recently tried to summarize the evidence on the economic costs of headache, have employed the bottom-up approach.

12.2.3 How to Estimate the Burden of Disease: The Cost of Illness (COI) Approach

COI represents the economic evaluation methodology through which it is possible to determine the burden caused by illnesses on the population [13]. This approach is used to calculate the social and economic costs, considering also the loss of productivity caused by a disease.

Production losses, among the indirect costs of a disease, are not the only social costs. In a broad perspective, studies about costs may aim to focus on total costs and/or incremental costs. While total disease costs provide estimates of the total healthcare expenditure of people diagnosed with a disease, incremental costs estimate the increase in costs that is attributable solely to the presence of the disease. For both total disease cost and incremental cost methods, there are two general methodological approaches [14].

The *total cost approach* may calculate either the sum of all medical costs or the sum related only to a specific diagnosis. The former calculates costs by identifying all patients with the diagnosis of a disease and adding up all their health expenses, regardless of whether these healthcare costs directly relate to the disease of interest or not. The other approach considers only costs that are directly related to the disease of interest.

The *incremental cost approach* includes the "matched control" and "regression methods". These two methods consider a comparison group of people without the disease in estimating costs. The first identifies all patients with a diagnosis and sums the costs due to the disease, then the average cost of the sample (or, alternatively, the average cost of a matched cohort) is subtracted to find the incremental costs for a given treatment. In the regression analysis, instead, all patients with a diagnosis are identified and the individual β for each diagnosis is estimated.

As an example of the matched control approach, the costs of primary care for patients with headache have been estimated to be at least 87% more than those for their similar-age and same-gender counterparts without headache [15]. Hawkins et al. [16] compared the average annual indirect expenditures of a group of employees with migraine with those of a matched group of individuals without migraine: the burden of illness of migraine was defined as the difference in average indirect expenditures per person between migraine and control cohorts. Indirect-cost components were workplace absence, short-term disability and workers' compensation claims. The results of the first stage of the analysis were then employed in a regression analysis.

The crucial factor when performing a cost study on headache is that of identifying the most appropriate indicators to measure the loss of resources. Several indicators have been developed and applied in the economic evaluation studies [17], among which it is possible to mention:

- *Healthcare resource use*. This is the cost of healthcare resource utilization associated with migraine including inpatient, outpatient and prescription drug claims. This indicator has been considered recently, in works by Sanderson et al. [18], Steiner et al. [19] and Bonafede et al. [20].
- *Economic losses due to missed workdays*, used by Iigaya et al. [21], Lofland and Frick [22] and Burton et al. [23]. The total number of migraine-related missed workdays (TMWD) per year may be calculated for each age- and gender-specific stratum as follows:

  $$\text{TMWD} = \text{NMS} \times \text{MWD} \times \text{PWP} \times \text{WHW} / 40$$

  where NMS is the number of migraine sufferers, MWD is average migraine-related missed workdays per year, PWP is the percentage of the population working for pay (estimated at 73% for males and 57% for females) and WHW is the average working hours per week (most recently reported as 35 for both genders; by dividing by 40, working hours are converted into the standard full-time level of 8 working hours per day).
- *Impaired work performance*, applied, for example, by Holroyd et al. [24] and Smith [25], is a function of the number of workdays with migraine (NWDM) and reduced work efficiency during the attacks. NWDM may be calculated as follows:

  $$\text{NWDM} = \text{NMS} \times \text{WDM} \times \text{PWP} \times \text{WHW} / 40$$

  where NMS is the number of migraine sufferers, average number of workdays with migraine (WDM) per year is estimated according to patients' self-reporting, PWP is the percentage of the population working and WHW is the average working hours per week.
- *Lost workday equivalents* (LWDE) due to impaired work performance, used by Schwartz et al. [26] and Science Daily [27], are calculated as follows:

  $$\text{LWDE} = \text{NWDM} \times \left(1 - \text{EWM}\right)$$

where EWM is the average effectiveness at work with migraine.

- *Economic loss due to reduced productivity*, used, for example, by Burton et al. [23] and Serrano et al. [28]. The total employment lost due to migraine (TELM) in dollar terms, assuming 8 h for each working day, is

$$\text{TELM} = (\text{TMWD} + \text{LWDE}) \times \text{hourly salary} \times 8.$$

- Other indicators based on self-reporting are being developed, using a headache diary for example [29].

12.3 The Economic Cost of Headache Disorders: Results of Key Headache Health-Economic Studies

12.3.1 Direct and Indirect Costs

Virtually all studies that have assessed both direct and indirect costs of headache disorders have found the latter to be the greater. Hospital costs represent only a very small portion of total migraine management costs: in the USA, it has been calculated that the rate of hospitalization is usually less than 10%, varying between 2% and 7% [30, 31].

However, an exception is seen in a recent US study based on the "Truven Health Market Scan Research Databases" [20]. Here, direct healthcare costs accounted for 74% of the total annual mean costs due to headache, amounting to USD 6575 per patient. On the other hand, indirect costs accounted for only USD 2350 per patient, arising from an average of 8.9 more missed days of work by patients with migraine because of disease-related needs. This study employed "real world" data, and the evidence it reported requires comparison with that from other studies in order to verify whether its conclusions can be generalized. In its analysis, direct and indirect costs were assessed throughout a 12-month follow-up period [20]. Further, the study tried to compare the situations of patients with and without migraine: while the latter should be interested in receiving preventative treatment, patients with migraine need acute treatment. Two additional multivariable logistic regression analyses were aimed at taking into account the odds of having a short-term disability claim for both categories of patients. The conclusions of the study outlined that, compared to matched non-migraine patients, "migraine patients were more likely to have work loss and longer periods of work loss, leading to significantly higher indirect costs. Migraine patients also had higher levels of healthcare utilization".

In marked contrast, in European Union (EU) countries, according to a study carried out a decade ago, indirect (lost-productivity) costs greatly exceeded direct costs [11]. Working days lost as a result of migraine varied from 1.9 to 3.2 days per person affected per year. Reduced levels of effectiveness accounted for 70% of all work lost [11]. All studies agree that the majority of days lost are due not to absence but to presenteeism [32]. In some studies, presenteeism has been estimated to account for 76.5% of the headache-related lost productive time and 89% of the total cost burden [33, 34].

12.3.2 *The Eurolight Study and European Brain Council Reports*

Eurolight, launched in May 2007, was aimed at studying the prevalence and impact of headache disorders in Europe [35]. It was driven by the consideration that, until 2006–2007, only pharmaceutical companies had drawn-up economic evaluations on some parts of the global burden of headache, carrying out such analyses only for single countries. Since there were no data at European level on prevalence and global impact of headache, the project was the first data collection on headache at European level focusing on a patient-driven approach.

A cross-sectional survey was conducted in eight European countries (Austria, France, Germany, Italy, Lithuania, Luxembourg, Netherlands and Spain) representing 55% of the adult EU population from 2008 to 2009. Using a bottom-up methodology, direct costs, as medications, outpatient healthcare, hospitalization costs, etc., and indirect costs, such as work absenteeism and reduced productivity at work, were estimated per person per year. Prevalence data, simultaneously collected and, for migraine, also derived from a systematic literature review, were used to attribute correctly the levels of national costs.

In the EU, the total annual cost of headache among adults aged 18–65 years was calculated, according to the prevalence estimates, at EUR 173 billion, shared between the headache types as shown in Table 12.1 [11].

Eurolight applied a societal perspective, meaning that all costs, whether incurred by individuals, government or others, were taken into account. The economic value of productivity was estimated through the human capital approach; according to this methodology, the economic losses due to the headache were assumed to be equal to gross earnings in a well-functioning labour market, so that the more the days off from work because of headache, the higher the economic loss [36]. The human

Table 12.1 Eurolight estimates of total and per-person annual costs of headache disorders in Europe (from [11])

		Costs per-person affected (EUR)		
Headache type	Overall costs (EUR)	Total (EUR)	Direct (% of total)	Indirect (% of total)
All headache	173 billion			
Migraine	111 billion (64%)	1222	7	93
Tension-type headache	21 billion (12%)	303	8	92
Medication-overuse headache	37 billion (21%)	3561	8	92
Other headache	3 billion (2%)	253	18	82

capital approach is especially suitable for episodic headaches, where absences are mostly shorter than the time (and, consequently, the costs) required to replace the employee.

There were some weaknesses in the analysis carried out. For example, estimates were not adjusted for purchasing power parity (PPP), since the aim of the project was to show only actual costs of headache. This implied that the differences in price and wage levels did not allow comparisons across countries. However, this might be acceptable because the selected countries for the study were a diverse mix of European countries in terms of geographical location, population size, set-up of healthcare system and level of income.

Moreover, the estimates of costs per patient for the less common diagnoses (MOH and other headaches) were based on small samples for several countries, so that the differences across countries for these diagnoses were likely to have been caused by random variation, therefore being misleading.

The estimates of national total costs were the product of costs per patient and prevalence. However, Eurolight was not designed to estimate prevalence rates in all countries surveyed, so that the estimates employed in the analysis might be subject to errors arising from the low participation rate to the survey. This was countered by also deriving prevalence data from a systematic literature review.

All findings were also sensitive to assumptions made in the costing model, and to national statistics. For example, the numbers of drug doses administered to treat the headache were interpreted conservatively and, especially for prophylactic drugs, it was assumed that recommended quantities were used [37]. This simplifying hypothesis did not take account of non-adherence and eventual waste of resources.

Eurolight did not include direct non-medical costs, such as social-services support, disability adaptations and special transportation, which, anyway, are not common for headache. It also did not consider costs related to lost career advancement or early retirement. The cost estimates did not incorporate costs of disorders that might be secondary to headache, or of those sometimes consequential to its treatment (such as gastrointestinal, hepatic and renal damage caused by analgesic overuse and opioid addiction). Including these would increase total costs of headache even further.

Retrospective questionnaires were used to collect data on the impact of headache on work absence and productivity, although this method may introduce a "recall bias": as stressed in the report, respondents systematically underreport their absence at work, because of "the common inclination to perceive oneself favourably" [38].

Finally, the estimate of costs did not include the "intangible costs", such as the monetary values of pain and decreased enjoyment of life, the indirect costs of lost time for household duties and social enjoyment, or the time lost to caring for family members with migraine, all factors that are particularly difficult to be valued objectively.

The strength of this study relies on the choice of the bottom-up approach to calculate the costs. Prevalence and resource-use data were collected simultaneously in a field study, with the advantage that all drugs employed to treat headache were counted even when not licensed for the diagnosis, or when purchased over-the-counter rather than prescribed. Individuals who had not sought medical treatment, were unemployed, uninsured or not earlier diagnosed, were included in the study.

The results were not adjusted for age, gender or geographical area in some countries—Austria, France and Spain—because the samples in these countries were not population based. However, the external validity of the study, as stressed by the authors, is supported by relatively strong concordance with available previous European per-person estimates.

The European Brain Council (EBC) is a non-profit organization gathering patient associations and major brain-related professional societies as well as industries, whose mission is to promote brain research in order to improve the quality of life of people with brain disorders in Europe [39]. In a broader study than Eurolight, EBC considered the costs of the most common brain disorders. Their Report of 2006 presented, for the first time, overall estimates of annual costs for brain disorders in Europe [40]. Their Report of 2012 presented updated and more accurate and comprehensive estimates for 30 European countries and 19 brain disorders [41]. The 1-year prevalences and average annual costs per person were based on "best estimates" from the literature. EBC found about one-third of the European population were affected by brain disorders, although prevalence data were not available for all countries. Headache, in particular, affected 152.8 million people in the countries observed.

The cost model was populated with national statistics from Eurostat adjusted to 2010 values. All local currencies were converted to euros, and country estimates were aggregated according to PPP. For all groups of disorders in Europe, the aggregated cost of brain diseases was EUR 798 billion (data of 2010). The greater part of expenditures was for direct costs (60%), split into direct healthcare costs (EUR 296 billion) and direct non-medical costs (EUR 186 billion). Indirect costs (EUR 315 billion) constituted the remaining 40%. However, large variations in the distribution of cost categories across disorders were reported. Indirect costs were dependent on assumptions of lost production, which added to the uncertainties in the estimates. These generally ignored loss associated with presenteeism.

Regarding headache and its different types, EBC estimated that migraine affected almost 50 million people, with an overall cost of EUR 43.5 billion (Table 12.2). MOH affected 8.3 million people, with lower overall cost but substantially higher per-person costs (Table 12.2). TTH was most prevalent but least costly of the specific disorders (Table 12.2).

Table 12.2 European Brain Council estimates (aggregated according to purchasing power parity (PPP)) of total and per-person annual costs of headache disorders in Europe (from [40])

Headache type	People affected (N)	Overall costs (EUR)	Cost per-person affected (EUR)		
			Total	Direct	Indirect
Migraine	49.9 million	43.514 billion	370	84	286
Tension-type headache	84.4 million	5.433 billion	64	24	41
Medication-overuse headache	8.3 million	19.037 billion	2291	305	1986
Other headache	10.2 million	582 million	57	33	24

Table 12.3 European Brain Council and Eurolight estimates compared (from [11, 40])

	Total annual costs (EUR millions)		Individual annual costs (EUR)			
			Direct		Indirect	
Headache type	Eurolight	EBC	Eurolight	EBC	Eurolight	EBC
Migraine	111,000	43,514	86	84	1136	286
Tension-type headache	21,000	5433	24	24	279	41
Medication-overuse headache	37,000	19,037	285	305	3276	1986
Other headaches	3000	582	46	33	207	24

The analysis tried to avoid double counting, whenever people were affected by more than one disease. In general, the solution to this problem is to consider only representative populations who record disease-specific costs prospectively, although this is more time- and resource-consuming.

12.3.2.1 Eurolight and EBC Compared

An open issue concerns the real costs of headache in Europe, given that Eurolight and EBC provided different estimations (Table 12.3). Discrepancies in total costs were too large to be explained by the different prevalence rates calculated in the two reports. While direct individual costs did not differ significantly, indirect individual costs estimated within the two reports showed huge differences.

Several explanations are available. First, EBC estimated there were 152.8 million people suffering from headache when the investigation was carried out. This information was retrieved from the most relevant studies on the topic. Prevalence estimates in Eurolight were, instead, adjusted according to the national means for age and gender in Germany, Italy, Lithuania (age only), Luxembourg and the Netherlands, and also according to geographical area in Germany, Luxembourg and the Netherlands [11, 41]. Second, the human capital approach to costing, applied in the majority of studies, determines a considerable increase in indirect costs (in Eurolight, more than EUR 1100 for migraine and almost EUR 3300 for MOH ([11] and Table 12.3)). A regression analysis of the determinants of costs might be helpful in outlining the major cost drivers (e.g. age, comorbidities, lifestyle, field of activity), especially for indirect costs. Third, unlike Eurolight, EBC did not apply a bottom-up approach for all countries since, in some of the studies reviewed, only aggregate data or top-down estimates were available [40]. Fourth, and perhaps most importantly, Eurolight expressly included estimates of productivity losses associated with presenteeism [11] whereas EBC, in its broader enquiry, questioned the validity of this [40].

12.3.3 The International Burden of Migraine Study (IBMS)

IBMS used a web-based questionnaire to elicit data on several topics related to the burden of migraine, including health-resource utilization and productivity losses [12]. Potential survey participants were identified by Synovate Healthcare (Chicago,

USA) from a pool of registered panellists from various countries. The panellists were screened online to determine eligibility and to identify individuals with migraine (episodic (EM) or chronic (CM)), based on reported symptoms.

The first IBMS was a two-phase, web-based, cross-sectional panel survey conducted in ten countries (USA, Canada, France, Germany, Spain, United Kingdom, Australia, Italy, Taiwan and Brazil) between February and April 2009 [42]. It showed that there could be differences in costs across countries related to different medical approaches. For example, there was greater use of preventative medications in the US population than in the Canadian, especially for some types of preventative drugs (e.g. antidepressant and cardiovascular drugs). IBMS largely concerned itself with cost differentials between EM and CM, with the general finding that CM was associated with approximately three times higher healthcare costs, both in the USA and in Canada, than EM. Medication use accounted for much of the difference, although more US patients with CM were submitted to diagnostic testing than Canadian patients [42].

This study and its analyses are of limited interest because of the conflation in these studies of CM and MOH. Other important limitations have also to be considered. The analysis did not use a bottom-up approach but employed cost estimates derived from publicly available US and Canadian sources [42]. As a consequence, the results were subject to variation in the unit-cost estimates (although sensitivity analyses to account for variability in cost input parameters showed that estimates were robust against variations in the top three headache-related cost drivers: physician visits, diagnostic testing and medication use [42]). Further limitations concern the collection of data (by internet surveys) and the potential for bias due to unmeasured confounders (regional differences, both in the distribution of physicians and neurologists and in the distribution of responders to the survey). Finally, there is the possibility that costs were underestimated, since the study took a relatively conservative approach. For base case analyses, it considered the most conservative or lowest-cost estimates; at the same time, the most "expensive" patients were not considered because of questionably high values in the usage of some resources [42].

12.4 Comment and Concluding Remarks

Compared to other diseases with greater knowledge of the economic aspects of both the pathology-related costs and the likely benefits resulting from different therapeutic approaches, a full comprehension of all costs related to headache has still to be reached. There are still many unsolved problems in disease costing: the methods employed may lead to different outcomes, depending on the evaluation approach being used. Overall, the bottom-up approach, applied in Eurolight, seems the preferable and most comprehensive method to assess the societal burden of headache. However, a crucial factor is the attainment of a higher participation in the survey.

Given the social relevance of migraine, together with the assessment of therapeutic options, it is important to increase knowledge related to the economic consequences of prevention. Headache may damage the lives of millions of people but, when headache disorders become chronic (15 or more headache days per month), their impact and financial costs escalate rapidly.

There is no doubt that the implementation of good headache healthcare is likely to be cost-saving (see Chap. 15).

References

1. Institute for Health Metrics and Evaluation. The global burden of disease: generating evidence, guiding policy. 2010. http://www.healthdata.org/gbd.
2. GBD 2016 Disease and Injury Incidence and Prevalence Collaborators. Global, regional, and national incidence, prevalence, and years lived with disability for 328 diseases and injuries for 195 countries, 1990–2016: a systematic analysis for the Global Burden of Disease Study 2016. Lancet. 2017;390:1211–59.
3. Clarke CE, MacMillan L, Sondhi S, Wells NEJ. Economic and social impact of migraine. Quart J Med. 1996;89:77–84.
4. Rasmussen BK. Epidemiology and socio-economic impact of headache. Cephalalgia. 1999;19(Suppl 25):20–3.
5. Lanteri-Minet M. Economic burden and costs of chronic migraine. Curr Pain Headache Rep. 2014;18:385.
6. Solomon GD, Price KL. Burden of migraine. A review of its socioeconomic impact. PharmacoEconomics. 1997;11(Suppl 1):1–10.
7. Stewart WF, Lipton RB, Dowson AJ, Sawyer J. Development and testing of the Migraine Disability Assessment (MIDAS) Questionnaire to assess headache-related disability. Neurology. 2001;56:S20–8.
8. Stewart WF, Lipton RB, Kolodner K, Sawyer J, Lee C, Liberman JN. Validity of the Migraine Disability Assessment (MIDAS) score in comparison to a diary-based measure in a population sample of migraine sufferers. Pain. 2000;88:41–52.
9. Steiner TJ. Lipton RB on behalf of *Lifting The Burden*: the Global Campaign against Headache. The Headache-Attributed Lost Time (HALT) Indices: measures of burden for clinical management and population-based research. J Headache Pain. 2018;19:12.
10. Migraine in America. The hidden costs of migraine. 2016. https://migraine.com/infographic/the-hidden-cost-of-care.
11. Linde M, Gustavsson A, Stovner LJ, Steiner TJ, Barré J, Katsarava Z, et al. The cost of headache disorders in Europe: the Eurolight project. Eur J Neurol. 2012;19:703–43.
12. Payne KA, Varon SF, Kawatam AK, Yeomans K, Wilcox TK, Manack Adams A, et al. The International Burden of Migraine Study (IBMS): study design, methodology, and baseline cohort characteristics. Cephalalgia. 2011;31:1116–30.
13. Mennini FS, Gitto L, Martelletti P. Improving care through health economics analyses: cost of illness and headache. J Headache Pain. 2008;9:199–206.
14. Akobundu E, Ju J, Blatt L, Daniel Mullins C. Cost-of-illness studies. A review of current methods. PharmacoEconomics. 2006;24:869–90.
15. Fishman P, Von Korff M, Lozano P, Hecht J. Chronic care costs in managed care. Health Aff. 1997;16:239–47.
16. Hawkins K, Wang S, Rupnow MF. Indirect cost burden of migraine in the United States. J Occup Environ Med. 2007;49:368–74.

17. Mennini FS, Gitto L, Marcellusi A, Sakai F, Arakawa I. Economics of headache. In: Martelletti P, Steiner TJ, editors. Handbook of headache: practical management. Milan: Springer; 2011.
18. Sanderson JC, Devine EB, Lipton RB, Bloudek LM, Varon SF, Blumenfeld AM, et al. Headache-related health resource utilisation in chronic and episodic migraine across six countries. J Neurol Neurosurg Psychiatry. 2013;84:1309–17.
19. Steiner TJ, Gururaj G, Andrée C, Katsarava Z, Ayzenberg I, Yu SY, et al. Diagnosis, prevalence estimation and burden measurement in population surveys of headache: presenting the HARDSHIP questionnaire. J Headache Pain. 2014;15:3.
20. Bonafede M, Sapra S, Shah N, Tepper S, Cappell K, Desai P. Direct and indirect healthcare resource utilization and costs among migraine patients in the United States. Headache. 2018;58:700–14.
21. Iigaya M, Sakai F, Kolodner KB, Lipton RB, Stewart WF. Reliability and validity of the Japanese Migraine Disability Assessment (MIDAS) questionnaire. Headache. 2003;43:343–52.
22. Lofland JH, Frick KD. Workplace absenteeism and aspects of access to health care for individuals with migraine headache. Headache. 2006;46:563–76.
23. Burton WN, Landy SH, Downs KE, Runken MC. The impact of migraine and the effect of migraine treatment on workplace productivity in the United States and suggestions for future research. Mayo Clin Proc. 2009;84:436–45.
24. Holroyd KA, Stensland M, Lipchik GL, Hill KR, O'Donnell FS, Cordingley G. Psychosocial correlates and impact of chronic tension-type headaches. Headache. 2000;40:3–16.
25. Smith AP. Acute tension-type headaches are associated with impaired cognitive function and more negative mood. Front Neurol. 2016;7:42.
26. Schwartz BS, Stewart WF, Lipton RB. Lost workdays and decreased work effectiveness associated with headache in the workplace. J Occup Environ Med. 1997;39:320–7.
27. Science Daily. 86 million workdays lost to migraine in the UK every year. 2018. https://www.sciencedaily.com/releases/2018/04/180427144727.htm.
28. Serrano D, Manack A, Reed ML, Buse DC, Varon SF, Lipton RB. Cost and predictors of lost productive time in chronic migraine and episodic migraine: results from the American Migraine Prevalence and Prevention (AMPP) study. Value Health. 2013;16:31–8.
29. National Headache Foundation. https://headaches.org/resources/headache-diary-keeping-a-diary-can-help-your-doctor-help-you/. Accessed June 2018.
30. Hu XH, Markson LE, Lipton RB, Stewart WF, Berger ML. Burden of migraine in the United States: disability and economic costs. Arch Intern Med. 1999;159:813–8.
31. Barron R, Carlsen J, Duff SB, Burk C. Estimating the cost of an emergency room visit for migraine headache. J Med Econ. 2003;6:43–53.
32. Cerbo R, Pesare M, Aurilia C, Rondelli V, Barbanti P. Socio-economic costs of migraine. J Headache Pain. 2001;2:S15–9.
33. Goetzel RZ, Long SR, Ozminkowski RJ, Hawkins K, Wang S, Lynch W. Health, absence, disability, and presenteeism cost estimates of certain physical and mental health conditions affecting US employers. J Occup Environ Med. 2004;46:398–412.
34. Stewart WF, Wood GC, Razzaghi H, Reed ML, Lipton RB. Work impact of migraine headaches. J Occup Environ Med. 2008;50:736–45.
35. The Eurolight project. 2012. http://www.eurolight-online.eu.
36. Jönsson B. General principles of disease-costing. In: Olesen J, Steiner T, Lipton R, editors. Reducing the burden of headache. Oxford: Oxford University Press; 2003. p. 211–7.
37. Evers S, Afra J, Frese A, Goadsby PJ, Linde M, May A, et al. EFNS guideline on the drug treatment of migraine – revised report of an EFNS task force. Eur J Neurol. 2009;16:968–81.
38. Jones G. How often were you absent? A review of the use of self-reported absence data. J Appl Psychol. 1994;79:574–91.
39. Olesen J, Freund TF. European brain council: partnership to promote European and national brain research. Trends Neurosci. 2006;29:493–5.

40. Olesen J, Gustavsson A, Svensson M, Wittchen HU, Jönsson B on behalf of the CDBE2010 study group and the European Brain Council. The economic cost of brain disorders in Europe. Eur J Neurol. 2012;19:155–62.
41. Stovner LJ, Andrée C. Impact of headache in Europe: a review for the Eurolight project. J Headache Pain. 2008;9:139–46.
42. Stokes M, Becker WJ, Lipton RB, Sullivan SD, Wilcox TK, Wells L, et al. Cost of health care among patients with chronic and episodic migraine in Canada and the USA: results from the International Burden of Migraine Study (IBMS). Headache. 2011;51:1058–77.

Part III
Society's Response to Headache

Chapter 13
Barriers to Care

Timothy J. Steiner, Zaza Katsarava, and Jes Olesen

13.1 Introduction

Headache is one of the most frequent medical complaints. At least 40% of adults report it as a recurring nuisance, up to 30% are at least sometimes disabled by it, and 2–10% bear it—with varying levels of incapacity—on more days than not [1–5]. It might be assumed that disorders so highly prevalent, and with such adverse consequences for people and the societies they belong to, would be considered an important medical problem—by people affected by them, by healthcare providers and by health policy makers everywhere. Sadly, various studies tell a quite different story, [6–9], and describe something of a paradox.

For decades, headache has been reported as the most frequent cause of consultation in both primary care and neurological practice [6, 10, 11]. On top of this,

T. J. Steiner (✉)
Department of Neuromedicine and Movement Science, NTNU Norwegian University of Science and Technology, Trondheim, Norway

Division of Brain Sciences, Imperial College London, London, UK
e-mail: t.steiner@imperial.ac.uk

Z. Katsarava
Evangelical Hospital Unna, Unna, Germany

Department of Neurology, University of Duisburg-Essen, Essen, Germany

EVEX Medical Corporation, Tbilisi, Georgia

IM Sechenov First Moscow State Medical University (Sechenov University), Moscow, Russian Federation
e-mail: zaza.katsarava@uk-essen.de

J. Olesen
Department of Neurology, Danish Headache Centre, University of Copenhagen, Rigshospitalet Glostrup, Glostrup, Denmark
e-mail: jes.olesen@regionh.dk

T. J. Steiner, L. J. Stovner (eds.), *Societal Impact of Headache*, Headache,
https://doi.org/10.1007/978-3-030-24728-7_13

headache prompts many visits to internists, ENT specialists, ophthalmologists, dentists, orthopaedic surgeons, psychologists and the proponents of a wide variety of complementary and alternative medical practices, and is far from unknown as a presenting symptom in emergency departments [6]. Yet, very large numbers of people who need it do not receive effective healthcare for headache. Direct evidence collected over many years shows this in developed countries [6–9, 12–15], while people with headache are unlikely to fare better in areas where resources are more limited. A survey of 102 countries, conducted jointly by the World Health Organization (WHO) and *Lifting The Burden* (LTB), confirmed that headache disorders were ubiquitous, prevalent and disabling, but it found them under-recognized, underdiagnosed and undertreated: illness that could be relieved was not, and burdens, both individual and societal, persisted at high levels [6]. In summary, this survey illuminated "worldwide neglect of a major public-health problem, and … the inadequacies of responses to it in countries throughout the world."

Where economic constraints and social disparities mean that medical care is not freely accessible, deficiencies might be expected. But why in wealthy Germany, for example, with free access to medical care and almost any kind of necessary treatment, do people suffering from migraine not seek care, as has been reported [8]. And why are they apparently poorly served when they do [8]? Germany is not unique in this: other countries in Europe do no better [9]. In the USA, the world's wealthiest country, during the 10 years (1988–1998) that saw the launch and aggressive marketing of triptans as new, efficacious, prescription-only treatments for migraine, the percentage of the American population with migraine who received prescription medications rose barely from 37% to 41% [16]. "What is it about headache?" was the *cri de coeur* of Headache journal's editor, reflecting upon the lack of recognition and underfunding of headache in the USA [17].

This chapter explores this question. It describes barriers, not only to headache care but also to change for the better. They are social, clinical, economic and political, and largely artificial. It is hard to understand why they were ever there, and impossible to justify their continued existence.

13.2 Insouciance and Other Barriers

WHO's *Atlas of Headache Disorders and Resources in the World 2011* describes a world of enormous, largely remediable but mostly untreated public ill health [6]. Why does this persist? While ignorance and lack of will (insouciance) are high among the reasons, there is also a misdirection of the limited resources that *are* allocated to headache care.

Poor understanding of headache disorders is widespread, even among people directly affected by them. Headache disorders are not perceived as serious—presumably because they do not cause death and are not contagious. Among the general public, there is at best insouciance towards and at worst a joking disdain for headaches [18], which are often trivialized as "normal" (non-medical), a minor annoyance or, more tellingly, an excuse to avoid responsibility. This is coupled with a general disbelief that headache disorders have a biological basis or that they can genuinely be disabling or life-impairing. Rather, they are attributed to psychological factors and "stress", a notion reinforced in the public's mind by the fact that migraine is predominantly a female disorder and, worse in this style of thinking, clearly associated with menstruation. These are important *social barriers*, and they inhibit people who might otherwise seek professional help for what may be high levels of pain and disability. Alarm arises eventually, inducing consultation only after unnecessary suffering, when headache is out of control and management is more difficult.

So are people with headache themselves to blame? Failure to consult is a certain barrier to effective care, but the reasons for it need to be examined.

In Germany, people with lower levels of education were less likely to be diagnosed and effectively treated [8]. One-fifth of first-generation Turkish immigrants reported headache on 15 or more days per month, most of them overusing acute headache medications, but none had contacted a doctor for headache [19]. In Georgia, people with headache are keen to receive help, and even in this resource-poor country are willing to pay for it [20], but they are largely unaware of the possibility of effective treatment [4]. Doctors also characterize headache disorders as conditions of low importance, or undeserving, and do not commit the time needed to diagnose them, educate patients about them, give advice, initiate appropriate treatment and follow patients up to ensure best outcomes. This is highly discouraging to those who would seek care [6].

Are doctors therefore to blame? Again, the reasons require examination, with poor understanding once more at their heart.

Among doctors, this is a problem sewn in medical schools, and reaped as the principal *clinical barrier* to effective headache management. In WHO's survey, better professional education was called for by 75% of responding countries, ranking far above all other proposals for change [6]. Worldwide, only 4 h are committed to headache disorders in formal undergraduate medical training lasting 4–6 years, reflecting the low priority accorded to them. Doctors accordingly qualify with little knowledge of headache disorders and, therefore, little interest in them. Later, in postgraduate training, the primary headaches are rarely seen as hospital inpatients because they are virtually never a cause for hospital admission. Headache is frequently encountered as a symptom of other diseases [21], but the focus then is on the underlying disorders, and the headache often ignored. Migraine, cluster headache and medication-overuse headache (MOH) may be common in neurological outpatients, but present no neurological, imaging or laboratory abnormalities or other biomarkers to interest trainees in this specialty. Migraine and MOH, along with tension-type headache (TTH), occur in even larger numbers in primary care, where doctors untrained and unskilled in treating headache achieve poor outcomes and leave themselves and their patients dissatisfied.

Underlying these failures are *political barriers*. Most importantly, the resources that good management requires, for large numbers of needful patients, are simply not allocated. Of course, low levels of consultation encourage low levels of health-care provision and resource allocation, but the *economic barriers* put in place make little sense (see Chap. 15). WHO's survey found that, while effective drugs exist, access to them was restricted in rich countries as well as poor [6]. On the political level, responsiveness in supporting structures fit for the purpose of meeting headache-care needs is notably absent. The solution requires political recognition that the problem exists, acknowledgement of its scale and scope, and willingness to take the remedial action that these demand [22]. Many governments, even if aware of these issues, are more concerned that healthcare for large numbers of people with headache can come only at a considerable cost. This is true, but they fail to look at the whole picture: since the direct costs of headache (the resources sunk in treating it) are dwarfed by the indirect lost-productivity costs ([23–29]; also, Chap. 12), huge savings might be made from recovered lost work time if resources were allocated to treat headache disorders better ([6, 22]; also, Chap. 15). WHO's survey also revealed widespread wastage, for example, high usage of investigations [6], despite that few headache disorders require them for diagnosis or assessment. Better knowledge among doctors of how to diagnose and treat the small range of headache disorders that affect large numbers of people would avoid this, improve usage of available treatments, produce better outcomes, recover lost productivity and reduce overall costs [6].

Sadly, the low esteem granted to headache disorders is self-perpetuating. Few doctors are motivated to push for improvements in headache care, let alone for the structured headache services that WHO and LTB recommend ([6, 30]; also, Chap. 15). Policy makers responsible for healthcare, and granting authorities who effectively control research, are influenced by these factors, particularly the lack of public clamour for change; their decisions, made critically, invariably reflect them. For this, *insouciant* society has only itself to blame.

13.3 Headache Below the Horizon(s)

Why headache commands so little respect may never be fully explained, and it is very difficult to explain when headache disorders are the second highest cause, among all diseases, of disability worldwide ([31]; also, Chap. 9). As an example, major advances in the understanding and treatment of headache have been made in the last 30 years but, globally, none of these has touched the lives of more than 90% of people who might benefit from them. These people remain, in their ill health, unseen below the horizon—or, in reality, below a multiplicity of horizons.

First of these is the *priority horizon*, described above. In this world, now of over seven billion people, in which 80,000 among every million have need for care (Chap. 15), headache is considered unimportant and undeserving. There is a long queue competing for healthcare resources, and headache is lost in it: it is below the healthcare priority horizon.

Then there is the *migraine horizon*. The therapeutic advances just mentioned relate almost exclusively to migraine, on which research has focused strongly although TTH is more prevalent and the frequently recurring headaches including

MOH are generally more disabling. Migraine, affecting an estimated 15% of adults [31], may peek above the horizon, but other headache disorders, affecting 20%–25% ([2, 31]; also, Chap. 9), are largely unseen below it.

In each million of the population, some 67,000 adults and 13,000 children or adolescents would benefit from care, while *very* conservative assumptions support the calculation that 39 doctors, doing nothing but treat headache, are required to meet this amount of need (Chap. 15). No country achieves this, or anything like it, and the consequence is an *access horizon*. Further, organized headache services, when they exist at all, tend to be placed in specialist care. Here, the needs of only a small minority can be met, perhaps of those who can most benefit but rather more probably of those with the social advantages that enable them to obtain access to specialist care. More than 90%, the estimated proportion who cannot [30], remain below this access horizon.

These horizons are global [6]; others may be more localized and perhaps are less artificial. As noted, healthcare for headache is not cost-free. Costs can be contained, and moving services into primary care that properly belong there is one rational way of achieving this ([30, 32]; also, Chap. 15), but a *wealth horizon* is inevitable. Related to this, and just as inevitable, is a *developed-world horizon*. Epidemiological studies of headache conducted before 2007 largely excluded developing countries ([1]; also, Chap. 8), and little other research into headache had been conducted in low- and middle-income countries [33]. Of seven billion people in the world today, the 15% who live in developed countries control about 80% of global resources, while nearly six billion get by on the remaining 20% (an application of the Pareto principle noted by United Nations over 25 years ago [34]). In this unequal world, an enquiry pertinent to headache is "Who has access to triptans?" More than 10 years after their launch, even in wealthy countries, a mere 15% of those who might benefit from them had some access to them [14, 16, 35, 36], and after 20-plus years this has not changed [8, 9]. The restrictions that have caused this are largely cost-based, whatever might be said to the contrary. Calculations *pro rata*, according to resource levels, suggest that, among the nearly six billion people making do on 20% of global resources, fewer than 1% of those who might benefit gain access to triptans. The global average is about 3% ([{15∗1 bn} + {1∗6 bn}]/7 bn). Below the wealth and developed-world horizons are the other 97%.

13.4 The Failures of Advocacy

Headache disorders remain at the bottom of the heap, where they have always been. The principal reason why headache burden persists at high level is failure of health policy. It is not sufficient that efficacious therapies exist: resources must be allocated, and healthcare systems put in place, so that these therapies are delivered to everyone whose quality of life is spoiled by headache. This is not happening. The antidote to insouciance is *advocacy*. If this is evidence of a pressing need for advocacy, to speak for people with headache who stay hidden below these horizons [37–39], it is also evidence that advocacy has so far failed.

Sound data create a solid basis for advocacy for headache: the public-health messages are clear enough [37–39]. First, good healthcare can alleviate much of the symptom burden of most headache disorders, thereby mitigating both the humanitarian and the financial costs. Second, none of the five essential components of effective healthcare for headache is beyond the capabilities of primary care: awareness of the problem, correct recognition and diagnosis, avoidance of mismanagement, appropriate lifestyle modifications and informed use of cost-effective pharmaceutical remedies [30]. For the vast majority of those who need it, effective treatment requires no expensive equipment, tests or specialists. Third, therefore, structured headache services can be based in primary care ([30]; also, Chap. 15): provided at low-cost for this majority, with only the small proportion who truly need them managed in specialist services. These are WHO's recommended solution [6]. Fourth, as the economic studies show, the direct costs of headache are less than one tenth of the total costs ([23, 40]; also, Chap. 12). Greater advertent investment in headache care, expanding the use of effective treatments, will, predictably, not only improve public health but also be cost-saving at societal level ([6]; also, Chap. 15).

These are compelling messages, but they have not yet reached the consciousness of health policy makers. In Europe, where the funding of brain disorders has been estimated in relation to their costs, headache disorders were found to be the least funded of all neurological disorders [41]. In the USA, funding of headache by the National Institutes of Health (NIH) has been equally poor—far below that of other, less costly neurological disorders [7]. Paradoxically, the funding of headache disorders is dwarfed by marketing budgets for painkillers to treat headache.

Advocates have used these data and argued these messages throughout the world. In the Americas and Europe, but to a lesser extent in other world regions, both lay and professional headache organizations include advocacy among their purposes [6]. More than any other health authority, WHO has acknowledged the public-health importance of headache disorders, and acted as advocate for headache on a macro level ([6, 42–45]; also, Chap. 5). In this regard, nothing is more succinctly apt than WHO's message to all the Ministries of Health of the world [6]:

> "The facts and figures … illuminate the worldwide neglect of a major cause of public ill-health and reveal the inadequacies of responses to it in countries throughout the world."

Together with LTB, a UK-registered non-governmental organization, WHO launched the Global Campaign against Headache in 2004 ([46, 47]; also, Chap. 14). LTB was admitted into official relations with WHO in 2011 [48], a milestone event itself achieved through prolonged and persistent advocacy. At national level, examples include a group of charities in the UK (the Migraine Trust, the Organization for Understanding Cluster Headache [OUCH] and the British Association for the Study of Headache [BASH]) who lobby Parliament through the All-Party Parliamentary Group on Primary Headache Disorders [49]. But the most important output of this group, a publication pithily summarizing the problem (*Headache disorders—not respected, not resourced* [50]), has no more led to policy change than did the publication by BASH in 2000 of detailed and evidence-backed proposals for headache service organization. Elsewhere there have been successes. The Migraine Association of Ireland does much to raise awareness, and, with the country's President as their patron, has had some influence on policy. In Norway, the lay headache organization, among others, lobbied for a National Headache Competence Centre, which duly opened at St. Olavs Hospital and the Norwegian University of Science and Technology (NTNU) in Trondheim. The Danish Headache Centre in Copenhagen is accommodated in a new, specially designed building, made possible by a very large donation from a private foundation that was itself the fruit of concerted advocacy. These are important successes, but nonetheless limited: in none of these countries are there structured headache services in the form recommended by WHO [6]. In the Lombardy Region of Italy, legislative support for such services appears to be a unique triumph for advocacy in Europe. In the USA, Headache on the Hill (HOH) is an annual Congressional advocacy event co-sponsored by the American Headache Society, each year lobbying approximately 130 Members of Congress on behalf of those with disabling headache disorders [51]. A direct outcome of HOH in 2016 was the *Safe Treatments and Opportunities to Prevent Pain Act* ("STOP Pain Act") [52], signed into law. Congress now directs NIH to fund *pain* research to an extent commensurate with *pain's* societal burden. How this law will increase funding for research on headache disorders is yet to be seen. What is clear is that, if full benefit is to be had, *headache's* societal burden needs to be firmly quantified.

13.5 Recognition Dawns

Overall it is difficult to discern much in the way of substantial gains from all this advocacy effort. Perhaps the advocates have been too few in number, have failed to speak in unison, or are regarded in a world of limited resources merely as spokesmen for vested interests. Whatever the reasons, not only does headache research remain pitifully underfunded, but also care for headache patients is miserable in most countries [6].

But not all is in vain. The most effective medium for raising awareness of the burden of headache is the Global Burden of Disease (GBD) studies (see Chap. 9), which expressly dissociate themselves from vested interests [53]. Collaborating with many local investigators and with successive GBD studies, the Global Campaign informed the latter by conducting new population-based surveys—so far in Georgia, Russia, Lithuania, China, Mongolia, Nepal, India, Saudi Arabia, Pakistan, Zambia, Ethiopia, Benin, Cameroon, Morocco and Peru, with others planned ([47]; also, Chap. 5). This concerted data-collection effort supported increasingly accurate estimates, so that migraine ascended to second place (first in adults under 50 years) in the top specific causes of disability worldwide, and headache disorders also to second among groups of related disorders ([31]; also, Chap. 9). For the US Congress, and all other agencies that influence resource allocation to headache research or care, there is no longer any doubt regarding headache's societal burden.

13.5.1 Global Patient Advocacy Coalition

Meanwhile, in 2016, the International Headache Society (IHS) announced its adoption of an advocacy role [54]. During 2017/2018, it brought into alliance, now under the name "Global Patient Advocacy Coalition" (GPAC), all advocacy groups and those with related interests (including LTB), along with representatives of regulatory agencies and of pharmaceutical and biotechnology companies [55]. GPAC's aims are set out in the Vancouver Declaration [56]. It has turned its focus onto migraine rather than headache, arguing that migraine is better "branded" and generates more sympathy than headache. There is some truth in this, although it is something of a surrender to prejudice (and a manifestation of the migraine horizon described earlier). Adoption in its name of "patient" runs counter to two of the Global Campaign's key messages: that most people in the world disabled by headache (or migraine) are not and in the foreseeable future will not be patients, for want of access to care (see above); and that many should not seek to be *patients*, but still need help in some form (see Chap. 15).

GPAC appears not to speak for everyone. But it is true that migraine accounts for the largest share by far of the global headache-attributed burden (see Chap. 9), and especially true if those cases of MOH that arise from migraine (the majority) are considered part of the spectrum of migraine [31, 57]. This approach was sensibly adopted by GBD2016 ([31, 58]; also, Chap. 9).

13.6 Concluding Remarks

The barriers to effective headache care are high everywhere in the world and in many places insurmountable by the majority of those needing care. If advocacy—for more headache research and better headache care—is the means by which they will be dismantled, it has been largely in vain so far. Despite irrefutable evidence of the prevalence, burden and cost of headache disorders, it may be that results will come only after a very long haul. But it is crucially important that advocacy continues. The arguments for change are now uncontestable—but they have to be put to those who can make change happen. And, it appears, they will have to be repeated, again and again.

There are glimpses of light and small successes here and there, and these may help advocacy in other parts of the world. Actions at national levels must combine, in collaboration with WHO and the Global Campaign against Headache. GPAC, with the commitment of its many persuasive partners, will, hopefully, deliver on its promises [56]. If they work together, through these agencies, the many national and supranational professional and lay groups will find hitherto-closed doors are, at last, slowly opening.

References

1. Stovner LJ, Hagen K, Jensen R, Katsarava Z, Lipton R, Scher A, Steiner TJ, Zwart JA. The global burden of headache: a documentation of headache prevalence and disability worldwide. Cephalalgia. 2007;27:193–210.
2. Westergaard ML, Hansen EH, Glumer C, Olesen J, Jensen RH. Definitions of medication-overuse headache in population-based studies and their implications on prevalence estimates: a systematic review. Cephalalgia. 2014;34:409–25.
3. Ayzenberg I, Katsarava Z, Sborowski A, Chernysh M, Osipova V, Tabeeva G, Yakhno N, Steiner TJ. The prevalence of primary headache disorders in Russia: a countrywide survey. Cephalalgia. 2012;32:373–81.
4. Katsarava Z, Dzagnidze A, Kukava M, Mirvelashvili E, Djibuti M, Janelidze M, Jensen R, Stovner LJ, Steiner TJ. Primary headache disorders in the Republic of Georgia: prevalence and risk factors. Neurology. 2009;73:1796–803.
5. Mbewe E, Zairemthiama P, Yeh H-H, Paul R, Birbeck GL, Steiner TJ. The epidemiology of primary headache disorders in Zambia: a population-based door-to-door survey. J Headache Pain. 2015;16:30.
6. World Health Organization, *Lifting The Burden*. Atlas of headache disorders and resources in the world 2011. Geneva: WHO; 2011.
7. American Association for the Study of Headache, International Headache Society. Consensus statement on improving migraine management. Headache. 1998;38:736.
8. Radtke A, Neuhauser H. Prevalence and burden of headache and migraine in Germany. Headache. 2009;49:79–89.
9. Katsarava Z, Mania M, Lampl C, Herberhold J, Steiner TJ. Poor medical care for people with migraine in Europe—evidence from the Eurolight study. J Headache Pain. 2018;19:10.
10. Hopkins A, Menken M, DeFriese G. A record of patient encounters in neurological practice in the United Kingdom. J Neurol Neurosurg Psychiatry. 1989;52:436–8.
11. Wiles CM, Lindsay M. General practice referrals to a department of neurology. J Roy Coll Phys Lond. 1996;30:426–31.
12. Rasmussen BK, Jensen R, Olesen J. Impact of headache on sickness absence and utilisation of medical services: a Danish population study. J Epidemiol Community Health. 1992;46:443–6.
13. Dowson A, Jagger S. The UK migraine patient survey: quality of life and treatment. Curr Med Res Opin. 1999;15:241–53.
14. Lipton RB, Scher AI, Steiner TJ, Kolodner K, Liberman J, Stewart WF. Patterns of health care utilization for migraine in England and in the United States. Neurology. 2003;60:441–8.
15. Takeshima T, Ishizaki K, Fukuhara Y, Ijiri T, Kusumi M, Wakutani Y, Mori M, Kawashima M, Kowa H, Adachi Y, Urakami K, Nakashima K. Population-based door-to-door survey of migraine in Japan: the Daisen study. Headache. 2004;44:8–19.
16. Lipton RB, Diamond S, Reed M, Diamond M, Stewart WF. Migraine diagnosis and treatment: results from the American migraine study II. Headache. 2001;41:638–45.
17. Rothrock JF. What is it about headache? Headache. 2012;52:1052–3.
18. Katsarava Z, Steiner TJ. Neglected headache: ignorance, arrogance or insouciance? Cephalalgia. 2012;32:1019–20.
19. Kavuk I, Weimar C, Kim BT, Gueneyli G, Araz M, Klieser E, Limmroth V, Diener HC, Katsarava Z. One-year prevalence and socio-cultural aspects of chronic headache in Turkish immigrants and German natives. Cephalalgia. 2006;26:1177–81.
20. Lampl C, Steiner TJ, Mueller T, Mirvelashvili E, Djibuti M, Kukava M, Dzagnidze A, Jensen R, Stovner LJ, Katsarava Z. Will (or can) people pay for headache care in a poor country? J Headache Pain. 2012;13:67–74.
21. Headache Classification Committee of the International Headache Society. The international classification of headache disorders, 3rd edition. Cephalalgia. 2018;38:1–211.

22. Steiner TJ, Stovner LJ, Dua T, Birbeck GL, Jensen R, Katsarava Z, Martelletti P, Saxena S. Time to act on headache disorders. J Headache Pain. 2011;12:501–3.
23. Linde M, Gustavsson A, Stovner LJ, Steiner TJ, Barré J, Katsarava Z, Lainez JM, Lampl C, Lantéri-Minet M, Rastenyte D, Ruiz de la Torre E, Tassorelli C, Andrée C. The cost of headache disorders in Europe: the Eurolight project. Eur J Neurol. 2012;19:703–11.
24. Selekler MH, Gökmen G, Steiner TJ. Productivity impact of headache on a heavy-manufacturing workforce in Turkey. J Headache Pain. 2013;14:88.
25. Selekler HM, Gökmen G, Alvur TM, Steiner TJ. Productivity losses attributable to headache, and their attempted recovery, in a heavy-manufacturing workforce in Turkey: implications for employers and politicians. J Headache Pain. 2015;16:96.
26. Yu S, Liu R, Zhao G, Yang X, Qiao X, Feng J, Fang Y, Cao X, He M, Steiner T. The prevalence and burden of primary headaches in China: a population-based door-to-door survey. Headache. 2012;52:582–91.
27. Steiner TJ, Rao GN, Kulkarni GB, Gururaj G, Stovner LJ. Headache yesterday in Karnataka state, India: prevalence, impact and cost. J Headache Pain. 2016;17:74.
28. Mbewe E, Zairemthiama P, Paul R, Birbeck GL, Steiner TJ. The burden of primary headache disorders in Zambia: national estimates from a population-based door-to-door survey. J Headache Pain. 2015;16:36.
29. Zebenigus M, Tekle-Haimanot R, Worku DK, Thomas H, Steiner TJ. The burden of headache disorders in Ethiopia: national estimates from a population-based door-to-door survey. J Headache Pain. 2017;18:58.
30. Steiner TJ, Antonaci F, Jensen R, Lainez JMA, Lantéri-Minet M, Valade D. Recommendations for headache service organisation and delivery in Europe. J Headache Pain. 2011;12:419–26.
31. Vos T, Abajobir AA, Abate KH, Abbafati C, Abbas KM, Abd-Allah F, Abdulkader RS, Abdulle AM, Abebo TA, Abera SF, Aboyans V, Abu-Raddad LJ, Ackerman IN, Adamu AA, Adetokunboh O, Afarideh M, Afshin A, Agarwal SK, Aggarwal R, Agrawal A, Agrawal S, Ahmadieh H, Ahmed MB, Aichour MTE, Aichour AN, Aichour I, Aiyar S, Akinyemi RO, Akseer N, Al Lami FH, Alahdab F, Al-Aly Z, Alam K, Alam N, Alam T, et al. Global, regional, and national incidence, prevalence, and years lived with disability for 328 diseases and injuries for 195 countries, 1990-2016: a systematic analysis for the Global Burden of Disease Study 2016. Lancet. 2017;390:1211–59.
32. Coulter A. Shifting the balance from secondary to primary care. BMJ. 1995;311:1447–8.
33. Mateen FJ, Dua T, Steiner T, Saxena S. Headache disorders in developing countries: research over the past decade. Cephalalgia. 2008;28:1107–14.
34. United Nations Development Program. 1992 Human development report. New York: Oxford University Press; 1992.
35. Bigal ME, Kolodner KB, Lafata JE, Leotta C, Lipton RB. Patterns of medical diagnosis and treatment of migraine and probable migraine in a health plan. Cephalalgia. 2006;26:43–9.
36. Lohman JJHM, van der Kuy-de Ree MM. Patterns of specific antimigraine drug use—a study based on the records of 18 community pharmacies. Cephalalgia. 2004;25:214–8.
37. Steiner TJ, Stovner LJ, Birbeck GL. Migraine: the seventh disabler. J Headache Pain. 2013;14:1.
38. Steiner TJ, Stovner LJ, Birbeck GL. Migraine: the seventh disabler. Headache. 2013;53:227–9.
39. Steiner TJ, Stovner LJ, Birbeck GL. Migraine: the seventh disabler. Cephalalgia. 2013;33:289–90.
40. Hu XH, Markson LE, Lipton RB, Stewart WF, Berger ML. Burden of migraine in the United States: disability and economic costs. Arch Intern Med. 1999;159:813–8.
41. Sobocki P, Lekander I, Berwick S, Olesen J, Jönsson B. Resource allocation to brain research in Europe—a full report. Eur J Neurosci. 2006;24:2691–3.
42. World Health Organization. Headache disorders and public health. Education and management implications. Geneva: WHO (WHO/MSD/MBD/00.9); 2000.
43. World Health Organization. Headache disorders. Fact sheet no. 277. Geneva: WHO; 2003.
44. World Health Organization. Headache disorders. Ch 3.3 in: Neurological disorders: public health challenges. Geneva: WHO; 2007. p. 70–84.

45. Patel V, Chisholm D, Dua T, Laxminarayan R, Medina-Mora ME, editors. Mental, neurological, and substance use disorders. Disease control priorities, vol. 4. 3rd ed. Washington, DC: World Bank; 2015.
46. Steiner TJ. *Lifting The Burden*: the global campaign against headache. Lancet Neurol. 2004;3:204–5.
47. *Lifting The Burden*: the global campaign against headache. http://www.l-t-b.org.
48. Steiner TJ, Birbeck GL, Jensen R, Katsarava Z, Martelletti P, Stovner LJ. The Global Campaign, World Health Organization and *Lifting The Burden*: collaboration in action. J Headache Pain. 2011;12:273–4.
49. United Kingdom All-Party Parliamentary Group on Primary Headache Disorders. http://www.publications.parliament.uk/pa/cm/cmallparty/register/headache-disorders.htm.
50. United Kingdom All-Party Parliamentary Group on Primary Headache Disorders. Headache disorders—not respected, not resourced. A Report of the All-Party Parliamentary Group on Primary Headache Disorders (APPGPHD). Westminster: House of Commons; 2010.
51. Alliance for Headache Disorders Advocacy. Headache on the Hill. http://allianceforheadache-advocacy.org/headache-on-the-hill/.
52. United States Congress. https://www.congress.gov/bill/114th-congress/house-bill/5249/text.
53. Institute for Health Metrics and Evaluation. Global burden of disease (GBD). http://www.healthdata.org/gbd.
54. International Headache Society. IHS Newsletter Issue 14—August 2016. http://www.ihs-headache.org/binary_data/2796_ihs-newsletter-aug-2016.pdf.
55. International Headache Society. IHS Newsletter Issue 15—December 2016. http://www.ihs-headache.org/binary_data/2859_ihs-newsletter-dec-2016.pdf.
56. Dodick D, Edvinsson L, Makino T, Grisold W, Sakai F, Jensen R, Balch A, Ruiz de la Torre E, Henscheid-Lorenz D, Craven A, Ashina M on behalf of the International Headache Society Global Patient Advocacy Coalition. Vancouver Declaration on Global Headache Patient Advocacy 2018. Cephalalgia. 2018;38:1899–909.
57. GBD 2017 Disease and Injury Incidence and Prevalence Collaborators. Global, regional, and national incidence, prevalence, and years lived with disability for 354 diseases and injuries for 195 countries and territories, 1990–2017: a systematic analysis for the Global Burden of Disease Study 2017. Lancet. 2018;392:1789–858.
58. Steiner TJ, Stovner LJ, Vos T, Jensen R, Katsarava Z. Migraine is *first* cause of disability in under 50s: will health politicians now take notice? J Headache Pain. 2018;19:17.

Chapter 14
Dismantling the Barriers

Timothy J. Steiner, Rigmor Jensen, Paolo Martelletti, Lars Jacob Stovner, and Zaza Katsarava

T. J. Steiner (✉)
Department of Neuromedicine and Movement Science, NTNU Norwegian University of Science and Technology, Trondheim, Norway

Division of Brain Sciences, Imperial College London, London, UK
e-mail: t.steiner@imperial.ac.uk

R. Jensen
Department of Neurology, Danish Headache Centre, University of Copenhagen, Rigshospitalet Glostrup, Glostrup, Denmark
e-mail: rigmor.jensen@regionh.dk

P. Martelletti
Department of Clinical and Molecular Medicine, Sapienza University, Rome, Italy

Regional Referral Headache Centre, Sant'Andrea Hospital, Rome, Italy
e-mail: paolo.martelletti@uniroma1.it

L. J. Stovner
Department of Neuromedicine and Movement Science, NTNU Norwegian University of Science and Technology, Trondheim, Norway

Norwegian Advisory Unit on Headaches, Department of Neurology and Clinical Neurophysiology, St Olavs University Hospital, Trondheim, Norway
e-mail: lars.stovner@ntnu.no

Z. Katsarava
Evangelical Hospital Unna, Unna, Germany

Department of Neurology, University of Duisburg-Essen, Essen, Germany

EVEX Medical Corporation, Tbilisi, Georgia

IM Sechenov First Moscow State Medical University (Sechenov University), Moscow, Russian Federation
e-mail: zaza.katsarava@uk-essen.de

T. J. Steiner, L. J. Stovner (eds.), *Societal Impact of Headache*, Headache,
https://doi.org/10.1007/978-3-030-24728-7_14

14.1 Introduction

Chapter 13 described the barriers that stand in the way of effective headache care, high as they are, and insurmountable for many. They need dismantling. The task, addressed here, is not an easy one: the barriers are multiple and in many cases entrenched.

Advocacy has an important role (see Chap. 13), but it is supportive only: it cannot achieve much on its own. What is needed is a concerted programme of action, focused in its strategy, tactically coherent and demonstrably built on sound data. Also required is political will, and this needs credible partners to foster it.

14.2 WHO and the Global Campaign Against Headache

The World Health Organization's acknowledgement of headache disorders and its commitment to their better management have stood for 20 years [1–5]. Their global survey found major public-health challenges posed by headache, which were similar throughout the world ([4]; also, Chap. 5). So were the six actions needed, for which WHO set out a template, along with a series of messages aimed at the governments of the world [4].

The ingredients of this template are recognizable in the activities of the Global Campaign against Headache [6–10], described later.

14.2.1 Knowledge Gaps Must Be Filled

Knowledge to inform policy is incomplete, with large geographical gaps [4, 11]. Further well-conducted epidemiological studies, incorporating population-based measures of individual and societal burdens, are needed in many countries, and especially in those that are resource-poor [4].

14.2.2 Healthcare for Headache Disorders Must Be Improved

Worldwide, reportedly, about 50% of people with headache are primarily self-treating, without contact with health professionals [4].

Actually, this does not appear unreasonable: much tension-type headache (TTH) and some migraine manifests only as infrequent and/or mild attacks. On the other hand, this estimate almost certainly reflects biased reporting by professionals who see *patients* (usually at the bad end of the spectrum) rather than *people with headache*. If the proportion of people *diagnosed* is a better reflection of quality and reach of headache services, which is likely, there is much room for improvement in all world regions: at best it is 40%, meaning that a majority of people with headache disorders are disenfranchised [4]. For medication-overuse headache (MOH), a high cause of disability, the proportion is 10% (90% not) [4]. Since this disorder is both preventable and remediable, but unlikely to resolve without medical care, this is a catastrophic failure of healthcare, with major adverse health and economic consequences.

Guidelines for diagnosis and treatment support better management, particularly by non-experts in primary care. That many countries have none in place, especially low-income countries, is a low-cost opportunity for substantial service improvement [4]. Again worldwide, investigations are performed in high numbers to support diagnosis [4]. This is not expected, since headache disorders mostly do not require investigations, either for diagnosis or assessment. With guidance, substantial reductions are possible, and the resource savings (negative cost) can be channelled into better medical care.

Assessment of headache impact is an essential part of management, especially where resources are limited, allowing them to be directed efficiently. Existing instruments are easy to use [12–14], but employed in only a quarter of responding countries [4]. This also is a low-cost opportunity for improvement.

Many effective drugs exist for headache disorders [15], but countries in all income categories identify lack of access to them as a barrier to best management [4]. A highlighted point was that triptans ought to be more widely available, and used in preference to ergotamine, which, globally, they are not. Ergotamine is cheaper, but less effective, more toxic and more liable to accumulation and overuse [15]. Reimbursement of drug costs is, for many people, the key to better access to drugs. Reimbursement has obvious societal cost implications, but these must be considered in full: given the cost-effectiveness of most drugs for headache, wider reimbursement appears to be a sensible policy from a societal perspective.

14.2.3 Headache Services Must Be Organized

The headache disorders that cause most population ill health are migraine, TTH and MOH (see Chaps. 2 and 9). It is primarily for these disorders that headache services throughout the world must cater.

The numbers are central to the problem and largely dictate the response to it. In each million of the population, some 67,000 adults and 13,000 children or adolescents would benefit from care, while *very* conservative assumptions about uptake (people who will seek available care as a percentage of those who should), and about the time required per patient to deliver adequate care, lead to the calculation that 39 doctors, doing nothing but treat headache, are required to provide it (see Chap. 15). In the European Union, for example, almost 20,000 doctors must practise solely in the field of headache to meet the care needs of its 500 million people.

Daunting this may be, but it is a poor excuse for inaction. This simply ignores not only the problem but also, and more pertinently, its humanitarian and economic consequences.

Headache services need to be delivered efficiently, equitably and countrywide. Organization of services to achieve this is a challenge with, perhaps, no single, complete and universally appropriate solution, but the numbers again dictate: headache services *must* be based in primary care (see Chap. 15). Specialist services are required by only a very small minority and, importantly, should be reserved for these because they are costly: the proportion currently seen by specialists (10%) is far in excess of this [4]. Most headache diagnosis and management require no more than a basic knowledge of a relatively few very common disorders (see Chap. 2), along with standard clinical skills, which every physician should have; neither special investigations nor equipment are necessary. These are the criteria by which it is recognized that a particular area of clinical practice belongs in primary care. At the same time, primary care has long been acknowledged as where patients generally prefer to be treated [16], and furthermore, it is usually provided at lower cost [17]. A strong efficiency-based argument therefore exists for expanding primary-care management of headache disorders, and this is particularly so in countries where health-service reforms are, generally, shifting priority towards primary care [18–21].

14.2.4 Education Is a Central Pillar of Effective Headache Services

First among the contributors to poor care is that people with headache do not consult doctors: only a minority seek medical help, even where it is potentially available [4]. This seems strange, but the reasons for it (discussed in Chap. 13) include a lack of general awareness—complete, in many parts of the world—that headache disorders have a biological basis and *should* receive medical attention.

A second, reinforcing reason is that those who do seek help are likely to encounter doctors less than willing to treat them, and be sent away discouraged. This, too, has a number of causes, but chief among them, and self-perpetuating, is that doctors generally are not well trained to treat headache ([4]; also, Chap. 13). Low priority accorded to headache disorders, despite increasingly clear evidence that this is wrong—both from a public-health perspective and in view of the serious economic consequences (see Chaps. 4 and 12)—means they are given little emphasis in medical training (worldwide, just 4 h in courses lasting 4–6 years [4]). *Educational failures* cause this evidence to be unseen or ignored.

Poor training translates later into misdiagnosis, mismanagement and poor outcomes, which waste healthcare resources while tending to make the initial problem worse. Doctors as well as patients find this discouraging.

Even doctors trained and genuinely interested in headache are commonly constrained because resources are not allocated to its management. But under-resourcing for whatever reason, while a factor in undertreatment, is not a complete explanation of it. The diffusion of triptans worldwide may be slow because of their cost, but good headache management is not achieved merely by prescribing triptans [15] and rarely entirely dependent upon access to this class of drug.

Lack of education—at all levels—was seen in WHO's survey as the key issue impeding good management of headache [4].

Better *professional education* ranked far above all other proposals for change (75% of countries that responded to the enquiry) [4]. Professional education needs to impart knowledge of only the few headache disorders of public-health importance to minimize the risk of failed or delayed diagnosis, which occurs too often, and to support early and appropriate therapeutic intervention. Professional education improves usage of available treatments, with better outcomes and avoidance of wastage [22, 23], and encourages follow-up, so often omitted but crucial to good outcomes. Because most headache should be treated in primary care, the emphasis in professional education should first be on undergraduate training, in medical schools, requiring changes to the undergraduate curriculum. Secondly, it should be on continuing medical education for general practitioners.

Limited-access and suboptimal professional care bring the certainty of self-treatment. Worldwide, at least 50% of people with headache are primarily self-treating, without any contact with health professionals [4] (the true proportion is probably much higher, since the survey depended largely on contact with professionals and was conducted only in countries where this was possible). Therefore, *education of people with headache*—about how to self-treat their headaches effectively and efficiently, and how and when (and when not) to engage with professional care—is of similar importance [4].

14.2.5 National Professional Organizations Should Be Supported

National professional headache organizations for headache disorders exist in two thirds of countries that responded, with a very marked difference between high- and upper middle-income (71–76%) and low-income countries (16%) [4]. The true proportions may be much lower, since respondents were much more readily identified in countries with such organizations.

Where they exist, these organizations have clear roles in promoting education, in producing locally relevant management aids including guidelines, and in importing knowledge and international standards through links to international groups. Support for the establishment and maintenance of these organizations appears highly worthwhile [4].

14.2.6 Political Will and Public-Health Policy

For all of these steps, there is a need for political recognition—firstly that the problem exists and secondly that it demands remedial action. WHO's report [4] should leave no doubt in the minds of health policy makers that headache disorders command their attention and can no longer be regarded as simple inconveniences undeserving of medical care. Apart from the humanitarian burden of pain and debility and the public ill health arising from headache, the financial costs of headache disorders to society through lost productivity are enormous ([24–30]; also, Chap. 12) (and far in excess of healthcare expenditure on headache [24, 31]). The arguments for investment in well-organized headache services, supported by education, are irrefutable.

Governments, say WHO very clearly, need to take note [4].

14.3 The Response

The problem then resolves into this: how to get the many people with headache to knowledgeable and equipped primary-care physicians, backed up by specialist care when needed, everywhere in the world?

Over 20 years ago, these arguments were put to WHO: that headache disorders were ubiquitous, prevalent and disabling, and mostly treatable; that barriers to care maintained large gaps between need for treatment and its provision; that heavy burdens persisted that could be alleviated; and that these arguments established headache as a global public-health priority, which WHO itself ought to take action upon. WHO's initial response, quite reasonably, was to this effect: "If you believe that headache disorders should be among our priorities, prove to us that they should be".

That proof came from the Global Burden of Disease Study 2000 (GBD2000), published in *World Health Report* 2001 ([32]; also, Chap. 9). Migraine was included, and on the collated evidence then available shown to be in the top 20 causes of disability worldwide (19th overall, and 12th in women). WHO's ultimate response, coming 2 years later, was the launch of the Global Campaign against Headache [6].

Initially the Global Campaign operated as a partnership between WHO, International Headache Society (IHS), European Headache Federation (EHF) and World Headache Alliance (WHA), all co-signatories to a Memorandum of Understanding. *Lifting The Burden* (LTB) was created to direct the Campaign in 2009, a legal entity in its own right, incorporated in the UK [11]. Two years later, LTB was invited into official relations with WHO [10]—a marker of considerable success in its formative years. More broadly based now, the Global Campaign is best described as a collaboration between WHO, international non-governmental organizations, academic institutions and many willing individuals around the world. Its academic base at the Norwegian University of Science and Technology (NTNU) is enthusiastically embraced within NTNU's interests and research priorities of headache and global public health [33].

It is important to be clear about what the Global Campaign is not. Firstly, it is *not* an advocacy campaign: advocacy is only one, albeit important, part of its scope. Secondly, it is *not* aimed solely at developing countries. It is true that most people with headache live in developing countries, and true also that, in many of these countries, headache is not even recognized to be a medical disorder. But in all *developed* countries, headache is both underdiagnosed and undertreated, and there are unmet needs in these as well [34–37].

14.4 Activities of the Global Campaign

As originally conceived, the Campaign defined three objectives, the culminations in turn of three "stages" [6, 7]. The first, and LTB's priority since the Campaign launch, was to know the nature and size of the burden of headache in all regions of the world ("knowledge for action"). For this purpose, it would gather the data upon which successful advocacy must be mounted, and to understand the scope and scale of the problem to be solved. The second objective ("awareness for action") would use this knowledge, to show policy makers and other change agents that they needed to act. While LTB is not an advocacy organization, it recognizes advocacy as a necessary intermediate step in achieving its third and ultimate objective: to reduce the burden of headache worldwide ("action for beneficial change") [6–10].

As the Campaign proceeded, the three stages resolved into two interdependent themes, with a common ultimate purpose [33]:

- Headache-related healthcare needs assessment (globally and locally);
- Formulation of an adaptable model for intervention.

14.4.1 Headache-Related Healthcare Needs Assessment

The necessary steps in healthcare needs assessment for headache disorders are, first, the recognition and description of those that contribute to public ill health and disability and, second, measurement of the burdens these impose.

14.4.1.1 Classifying Headache

A systematic classification of the types of headache (over 200 are listed in the International Classification of Headache Disorders (ICHD-3) [38]) underpins the recognition, description and measurement of those that contribute to public ill health and disability. The classification system promoted by WHO, and adopted globally, is the International Classification of Diseases (ICD).

The 11th edition of ICD (ICD-11), published in 2018 [39], not only has a separate section on headache disorders for the first time but also aligns with ICHD-3. LTB played three roles in creating this new section: it reviewed and commented upon the linear structure of the headache classification in order to maintain this alignment; it provided descriptions of the headache disorders included; and it helped develop the methodology for field-testing of the section.

14.4.1.2 Describing the Burden of Headache

To know the nature and size (scope and scale) of the burden of headache in all regions of the world required two major steps. The first, completed in 2007, was to bring together all evidence then published of this burden worldwide [11]. The second, still ongoing, was to set up new studies in those parts of the world where the evidence was (in some cases, is) lacking or of poor quality.

There was need for this. Even up to 2007, very little was known of the prevalence or burden of any headache disorder for more than half the people of the world: those living in most of the Western Pacific Region, including China, all of South East Asia including India, all of Eastern Europe including Russia, most of the Eastern Mediterranean Region and most of Africa [11].

Before starting, there were methodological issues to be addressed [40]. In published burden-of-headache studies, the methodology had been variable, hindering comparisons, and not always adequate, hindering interpretation. For this second step, therefore, better—and standardized—methodology was needed, especially for application in developing countries with relatively inaccessible populations. This project itself had three parts, with three outputs: (a) review of the literature and a discussion of the headache-specific epidemiological issues [40]; (b) formulation of practical methodological guidelines, by convening an expert consensus group (who met at NTNU) and undertaking wide consultation ([41]; also, Chap. 6); (c) development of a survey instrument (the HARDSHIP questionnaire) based on expert opinion and worldwide empirical field testing ([42]; also, Chap. 7).

Then, collaborating with many local investigators and, crucially, with successive GBD studies (see Chap. 9), the Global Campaign informed the latter by conducting new population-based surveys—16 completed or planned so far, in adults, focusing on the major geographical knowledge gaps. In the African Region, large and diverse, little was known of the burden of headache anywhere. Studies are completed in Zambia [29, 43] and Ethiopia [30, 44], and two are starting in Benin and Cameroon. In the Region of the Americas, the burden of headache is well-documented in the USA, but published burden data are of questionable quality in Central and South America. New studies are underway in Peru and planned in Brazil. In Eastern Mediterranean Region, the very sparse data have been supplemented by studies in Pakistan [45] and in Saudi Arabia and Morocco (both in analysis). In the European Region, the former USSR was a high priority because little knowledge of headache burden existed in this very large area. Studies have been completed in Russia [46–48], Georgia [49] and Lithuania [50]. The Eurolight project, an activity supported by a grant of the EC Public Health Executive Agency, harvested information in Austria, France, Germany, Ireland, Italy, Lithuania, Luxembourg, the Netherlands, Spain and the UK, showing the total annual cost of all headache in the European Union to be an astronomical €155 billion [24]. Throughout the large and diverse South East Asia Region, no data existed on the prevalence or burden of headache. A study has been completed in Karnataka State [51, 52] but, since extrapolation to all India from an enumerated population of about 12,000 within one State may not be appropriate, another study is underway around Delhi. A nationwide survey in Nepal, funded through NTNU and the Central Norway Regional Health Authority, has shown very high headache burden in this very poor country, and a strong association between migraine and altitude of dwelling [53, 54]. Finally, in the Western Pacific Region, with relatively little known of the burden of headache, studies are completed in China [27] and Mongolia (in analysis).

Many of these studies have been summarized ([55]; also, Chap. 8), and all have contributed to iterations of GBD. GBD studies translate prevalence data into burden, quantified as years lived with disability (YLDs). They do this by applying disability weights (DWs) for the many and various health states generated by living with disease (see Chap. 9). LTB's concerted data-collection effort allowed replacement of many of the assumptions of earlier GBD studies with empirical data, so supporting increasingly accurate estimates. Thus, by GBD2016, migraine had ascended to second place (first in adults under 50 years) in the top specific causes of disability worldwide ([56, 57]; also, Chap. 9). MOH was ranked 18th in GBD2013 [58], and both GBD2016 and GBD2017 established headache disorders, collectively, as second among the groups of related disorders [56, 59].

In addition to these adult studies, LTB developed methods for school-based studies of child and adolescent headache burden, testing them in a pilot study in Austria and Turkey [60], and applying them, so far, in nine national studies in Turkey [61], Serbia, Lithuania, Zambia and Ethiopia (all in analysis), and in Iran, Benin, Cameroon and Mongolia (in progress).

A key component of the burden of headache, of enormous socioeconomic and therefore political importance, is the very substantial lost productivity among the workforce affected by headache. Work impact studies in Turkey have provided direct empirical evidence of this [25, 26].

The Campaign's second objective ("awareness for action"), to persuade governments and other health-service policy makers, healthcare providers, people directly affected by headache and the general population that headache must have higher healthcare priority, has been largely achieved by LTB's collaboration with GBD. For the US Congress [62], and all other questioning agencies that influence resource allocation to headache research or care, there can be no further doubt regarding the scale of headache's societal burden. Even in 2011, in a joint publication with LTB, WHO had sent this message to all the Ministries of Health of the world:

> "The facts and figures … illuminate the worldwide neglect of a major cause of public ill-health and reveal the inadequacies of responses to it in countries throughout the world" [2].

Nothing more succinctly apt could, or can, be said.

14.4.2 *Healthcare Interventions*

The Campaign's third objective reflected what was and is its ultimate purpose [6, 7, 10]: effective intervention ("action for beneficial change"), to be achieved by working with local policy makers and principal stakeholders. The planning, implementation and evaluation of healthcare services for headache as the solution to headache are forms of health-services research, backed by scientific method. The solution is necessarily adapted to the needs, infrastructure and resources of the country in which intervention occurs.

Global Campaign activities here are on five fronts, involving empirical, health-services and action research.

14.4.2.1 Development of Practical Management Aids

These are needed to support interventions [15], aimed at general practitioners (GPs) and other non-experts in primary care, where, it is expected, interventions will largely be based (see below).

They include diagnostic aids based on ICHD-3 [38], assessment aids [12], management principles and recommendations [15], an outcome measure to guide follow-up [13, 14], information leaflets for patients [15], and translation protocols so that all of these, developed in English, can be rendered useful to non-English speakers [63–65].

14.4.2.2 Proposals for Headache Service Organization and Delivery

These proposals describe structured headache services ([66, 67]; also, Chap. 15).

Healthcare solutions to the problem of headache must recognize the problem as it exists locally. They often depend upon the planning and implementation of new headache services rather than improvement of those that currently exist—because, in many countries, none do on any formal basis. There are key questions to be answered: how should headache services be structured, organized and delivered: where, to whom, by whom, how much and with what objectives? The answers often depend upon resource availability, but there is a general agreement (see above) that headache services must be based in primary care [4].

LTB has, with the European Headache Federation (EHF), developed an organizational model on three levels: primary care, an intermediate level, and specialist headache care reserved for the quite small proportion of people (maybe 1%) who need it (see Chap. 15). While the model is for Europe, it is very adaptable for less well-resourced countries (the focus of LTB's work).

14.4.2.3 Effectiveness of GP Education

Educational failures are often the root cause of headache-care failures [4], with headache disorders not well understood or recognized, and commonly misdiagnosed and mismanaged. Education of GPs and other primary healthcare providers in good headache management, according to a basic syllabus, and instruction in the effective use of what are often limited resources, are therefore an integral part of intervention, an essential pillar upon which success depends [4, 66].

But it is not sufficient merely to educate: education must be shown to achieve its purpose. Enquiry into and demonstration of the effectiveness of GP education are the aims of a project begun in Estonia [22, 23].

14.4.2.4 Service-Quality Evaluation (SQE)

SQE is explored further in Chap. 16. While healthcare solutions to headache, as it exists locally, should self-evidently be the best possible, there had been no agreement on the meaning of "best" in this context. Consequently, there was no established methodology for evaluating headache services, or standard against which to evaluate them. Two key questions identified themselves: how is "quality" defined in the context of headache services, and from whose perspective(s), and, in the light of a definition of quality, by what means should headache services be evaluated?

Through a worldwide process of consultation, LTB, again in collaboration with EHF, has produced answers to these questions, developing both a definition and a set of quality indicators coupled with methods to apply them [68, 69]. These are being empirically validated in various countries, in specialist centres [70–72] and in primary care (in progress).

14.4.2.5 Implementation and Evaluation of Actual Interventions in Selected Countries

The tactical approach to effective intervention first and absolutely requires local champions. Secondly, it requires agreement upon the desired and achievable objectives—which should be based on local needs assessment—and upon local priorities.

LTB is collaboratively involved in projects in Georgia, setting up a headache service in a country where none existed, and where there was little infrastructure to build upon [73]; in Russia (in Sverdlovsk Oblast, centred in Yekaterinburg), implementing a 3-level service delivery model [74]; and in China, integrating headache services within the ongoing healthcare reform, with service provision mainly in primary care but supported by 31 specialist headache centres throughout the country [75, 76].

Quality—its meaning and measurement—is the subject of Chap. 16. Assessing the *effect* of interventions is methodologically challenging, but necessary. Ideally it is done in terms of outcomes (reductions in population burden attributable to headache), but this is especially difficult. The final step in any intervention, if evaluation indicates this to be necessary, is to revise and re-apply the modified interventions in plan-do-study-act cycles, using standard management-of-change methodology (see Chap. 16).

One of WHO's messages in 2011 was "Poor knowledge and understanding of headache lead to misdiagnosis, mismanagement and poor outcomes which, often, not only waste health-care resources but also make the initial problem worse—adding to headache-related burden" [4]. Through more efficient use and avoidance of this wastage, resources already allocated to headache can be made to go further, achieving quite a lot more than they do. But the major cost-benefit opportunity comes through reduction in the consequential financial costs of headache.

In a direct collaboration with WHO, LTB has assessed *cost-effectiveness* of structured headache services supported by educational initiatives aimed at both healthcare providers and people with headache (the public) ([77]; also, Chap. 15). More detailed cost-effectiveness analyses are underway. More is said about these in Chap. 15, but they confirm, as WHO predicted [4], that intervention in the form of structured headache services has the potential to be cost-*saving*. This is a crucial demonstration. Thought must obviously be given to paying for what the Campaign seeks to achieve: beneficial change, in a world of competing demands and scarce resources. These analyses show that it can be done.

14.4.3 Building Research Capacity

Research experience and capacity are often very limited, especially in low-income countries where many Global Campaign initiatives are undertaken [78]. Training in the research methods involved in implementing and testing new headache services is also, therefore, an integral part of any interventional project.

LTB provides such training through its many collaborations with local investigators.

14.5 Concluding Remarks

Dismantling the multiple, substantial and often entrenched barriers that stand in the way of effective headache care is not an easy task. The Global Campaign against Headache is a structured, coherent stepwise action programme, undertaken in response to a clear and measured global need, with the ultimate objective of reducing the burden of headache worldwide. Its many activities involve many partners—including WHO—in more than 35 countries.

References

1. World Health Organization. Headache disorders and public health. Education and management implications. Geneva: WHO (WHO/MSD/MBD/00.9); 2000.
2. World Health Organization. Headache disorders. Fact sheet no. 277. Geneva: WHO; 2003.
3. World Health Organization. Headache disorders. Ch 3.3 in: Neurological disorders: public health challenges. Geneva: WHO; 2007. p. 70–84.
4. World Health Organization and *Lifting The Burden*. Atlas of headache disorders and resources in the world 2011. Geneva: WHO; 2011. http://www.who.int/mental_health/management/atlas_headache_disorders/en/2011.
5. Patel V, Chisholm D, Dua T, Laxminarayan R, Medina-Mora ME, editors. Mental, neurological, and substance use disorders. Disease control priorities, third edition, volume 4. Washington, DC: World Bank; 2015.
6. Steiner TJ. *Lifting The Burden*: the global campaign against headache. Lancet Neurol. 2004;3:204–5.
7. Steiner TJ. *Lifting The Burden*: the global campaign to reduce the burden of headache worldwide. J Headache Pain. 2005;6:373–7.
8. Steiner TJ, Birbeck GL, Jensen R, Katsarava Z, Martelletti P, Stovner LJ. *Lifting The Burden*: the first 7 years. J Headache Pain. 2010;11:451–5.
9. Steiner TJ, Birbeck GL, Jensen R, Katsarava Z, Martelletti P, Stovner LJ. The global campaign, World Health Organization and *Lifting The Burden*: collaboration in action. J Headache Pain. 2011;12:273–4.
10. *Lifting The Burden*. The global campaign against headache. http://www.l-t-b.org.
11. Stovner LJ, Hagen K, Jensen R, Katsarava Z, Lipton R, Scher AI, Steiner TJ, Zwart J-A. The global burden of headache: a documentation of headache prevalence and disability worldwide. Cephalalgia. 2007;27:193–210.
12. Steiner TJ, Lipton RB on behalf of *Lifting The Burden*: The Global Campaign against Headache. The Headache-Attributed Lost Time (HALT) Indices: measures of burden for clinical management and population-based research. J Headache Pain. 2018;19:12.
13. Steiner TJ, Buse DC, Al Jumah M, Westergaard ML, Jensen RH, Reed ML, Prilipko L, Mennini FS, Láinez MJA, Ravishankar K, Sakai F, Yu S-Y, Fontebasso M, Al Khathami A, MacGregor EA, Antonaci F, Tassorelli C, Lipton RB on behalf of *Lifting The Burden*: The Global Campaign against Headache. The headache under-response to treatment (HURT) questionnaire, an outcome measure to guide follow-up in primary care: development, psychometric evaluation and assessment of utility. J Headache Pain. 2018;19:15.
14. Buse DC, Sollars CM, Steiner TJ, Jensen RH, Al Jumah MA, Lipton RB. Why HURT? A review of clinical instruments for headache management. Curr Pain Headache Rep. 2012;16:237–54.
15. Steiner TJ, Jensen R, Katsarava Z, Linde M, MacGregor EA, Osipova V, Paemeleire K, Olesen J, Peters M, Martelletti P on behalf of the European Headache Federation and *Lifting The Burden*: the Global Campaign against Headache. Aids to management of headache disorders in primary care (2nd edition). J Headache Pain. 2019;20:57.
16. Mainous AG, Baker R, Love MM, Gray DP, Gill JM. Continuity of care and trust in one's physician: evidence from primary care in the United States and the United Kingdom. Fam Med. 2001;33:22–7.
17. Van Weel C. Primary care: political favourite or scientific discipline? Lancet. 1996;348:1431–2.
18. World Health Organization International Conference on Primary Health Care. Declaration of Alma-Ata. Geneva: WHO; 1978.
19. Tarino E, Webster EG. Primary health care concepts and challenges in a changing world. Alma-Ata revisited. Geneva: WHO; 1995.
20. Walley J, Lawn JE, Tinker A, de Francisco A, Chopra M, Rudan I, Bhutta ZA, Black RE and the Lancet Alma-Ata Working Group. Primary health care: making Alma-Ata a reality. Lancet. 2008;372:1001–7.

21. World Health Organization and United Nations Children's Fund (UNICEF) Global Conference on Primary Health Care. Declaration of Astana. From Alma-Ata towards universal health coverage and the Sustainable Development Goals. Astana, Kazakhstan: WHO/UNICEF; 2018.
22. Braschinsky M, Haldre S, Kals M, Iofik A, Kivisild A, Korjas J, Koljal S, Katsarava Z, Steiner TJ. Structured education can improve primary-care management of headache: the first empirical evidence, from a controlled interventional study. J Headache Pain. 2016;17:24.
23. Braschinsky M, Haldre S, Kals M, Arge M, Saar B, Niibek M, Katsarava Z, Steiner TJ. Structured education to improve primary-care management of headache: how long do the benefits last? A follow-up observational study. Eur J Neurol. 2018;25:497–502.
24. Linde M, Gustavsson A, Stovner LJ, Steiner TJ, Barré J, Katsarava Z, Lainez JM, Lampl C, Lantéri-Minet M, Rastenyte D, Ruiz de la Torre E, Tassorelli C, Andrée C. The cost of headache disorders in Europe: the Eurolight project. Eur J Neurol. 2012;19:703–11.
25. Selekler MH, Gökmen G, Steiner TJ. Productivity impact of headache on a heavy-manufacturing workforce in Turkey. J Headache Pain. 2013;14:88.
26. Selekler HM, Gökmen G, Alvur TM, Steiner TJ. Productivity losses attributable to headache, and their attempted recovery, in a heavy-manufacturing workforce in Turkey: implications for employers and politicians. J Headache Pain. 2015;16:96.
27. Yu S, Liu R, Zhao G, Yang X, Qiao X, Feng J, Fang Y, Cao X, He M, Steiner T. The prevalence and burden of primary headaches in China: a population-based door-to-door survey. Headache. 2012;52:582–91.
28. Steiner TJ, Rao GN, Kulkarni GB, Gururaj G, Stovner LJ. Headache yesterday in Karnataka state, India: prevalence, impact and cost. J Headache Pain. 2016;17:74.
29. Mbewe E, Zairemthiama P, Paul R, Birbeck GL, Steiner TJ. The burden of primary headache disorders in Zambia: national estimates from a population-based door-to-door survey. J Headache Pain. 2015;16:36.
30. Zebenigus M, Tekle-Haimanot R, Worku DK, Thomas H, Steiner TJ. The burden of headache disorders in Ethiopia: national estimates from a population-based door-to-door survey. J Headache Pain. 2017;18:58.
31. Hu XH, Markson LE, Lipton RB, Stewart WF, Berger ML. Burden of migraine in the United States: disability and economic costs. Arch Intern Med. 1999;159:813–8.
32. World Health Organization. World health report 2001. Geneva: WHO; 2001. p. 22–4.
33. Norwegian University of Science and Technology. Headache disorders. https://www.ntnu.edu/inb/headache-disorder.
34. American Association for the Study of Headache, International Headache Society. Consensus statement on improving migraine management. Headache. 1998;38:736.
35. Steiner TJ, Scher AI, Stewart WF, Kolodner K, Liberman J, Lipton RB. The prevalence and disability burden of adult migraine in England and their relationships to age, gender and ethnicity. Cephalalgia. 2003;23:519–27.
36. Lipton RB, Scher AI, Steiner TJ, Bigal ME, Kolodner K, Liberman JN, Stewart WF. Patterns of health care utilization for migraine in England and in the United States. Neurology. 2003;60:441–8.
37. Katsarava Z, Mania M, Lampl C, Herberhold J, Steiner TJ. Poor medical care for people with migraine in Europe—evidence from the Eurolight study. J Headache Pain. 2018;19:10.
38. Headache Classification Committee of the International Headache Society. The international classification of headache disorders, 3rd edition. Cephalalgia. 2018;38:1–211.
39. World Health Organization. International Classification of Diseases 11th Revision. The global standard for diagnostic health information. 2018. https://icd.who.int.
40. Steiner TJ, Stovner LJ, Al Jumah M, Birbeck GL, Gururaj G, Jensen R, Katsarava Z, Queiroz LP, Scher AI, Tekle-Haimanot R, Wang S-J, Martelletti P, Dua T, Chatterji S. Improving quality in population surveys of headache prevalence, burden and cost: key methodological considerations. J Headache Pain. 2013;14:87.
41. Stovner LJ, Al Jumah M, Birbeck GL, Gururaj G, Jensen R, Katsarava Z, Queiroz LP, Scher AI, Tekle-Haimanot R, Wang SJ, Steiner TJ. The methodology of population surveys of head-

ache prevalence, burden and cost: principles and recommendations from the global campaign against headache. J Headache Pain. 2014;15:5.
42. Steiner TJ, Gururaj G, Andrée C, Katsarava Z, Ayzenberg I, Yu SY, Al Jumah M, Tekle-Haimanot R, Birbeck GL, Herekar A, Linde M, Mbewe E, Manandhar K, Risal A, Jensen R, Queiroz LP, Scher AI, Wang SJ, Stovner LJ. Diagnosis, prevalence estimation and burden measurement in population surveys of headache: presenting the HARDSHIP questionnaire. J Headache Pain. 2014;15:3.
43. Mbewe E, Zairemthiama P, Yeh H-H, Paul R, Birbeck GL, Steiner TJ. The epidemiology of primary headache disorders in Zambia: a population-based door-to-door survey. J Headache Pain. 2015;16:30.
44. Zebenigus M, Tekle-Haimanot R, Worku DK, Thomas H, Steiner TJ. The prevalence of primary headache disorders in Ethiopia. J Headache Pain. 2016;17:110.
45. Herekar AA, Ahmad A, Uqaili UL, Ahmed B, Effendi J, Alvi SZ, Shahab MA, Javed U, Herekar AD, Khanani R, Steiner TJ. Primary headache disorders in the adult general population of Pakistan—a cross sectional nationwide prevalence survey. J Headache Pain. 2017;18:28.
46. Ayzenberg I, Katsarava Z, Sborowski A, Chernysh M, Osipova V, Tabeeva G, Yakhno N, Steiner TJ. The prevalence of primary headache disorders in Russia: a countrywide survey. Cephalalgia. 2012;32:373–81.
47. Ayzenberg I, Katsarava Z, Sborowski A, Chernysh M, Osipova V, Tabeeva G, Steiner TJ. Headache-attributed burden and its impact on productivity and quality of life in Russia: structured healthcare for headache is urgently needed. Eur J Neurol. 2014;21:758–65.
48. Ayzenberg I, Katsarava Z, Sborowski A, Obermann M, Chernysh M, Osipova V, Tabeeva G, Steiner TJ. Headache yesterday in Russia: its prevalence and impact, and their application in estimating the national burden attributable to headache disorders. J Headache Pain. 2015;16:7.
49. Katsarava Z, Dzagnidze A, Kukava M, Mirvelashvili E, Djibuti M, Janelidze M, Jensen R, Stovner LJ, Steiner TJ. Primary headache disorders in the republic of Georgia: prevalence and risk factors. Neurology. 2009;73:1796–803.
50. Rastenytė D, Mickevičienė D, Stovner LJ, Thomas H, Andrée C, Steiner TJ. Prevalence and burden of headache disorders in Lithuania and their public-health and policy implications: a population-based study within the Eurolight Project. J Headache Pain. 2017;18:53.
51. Kulkarni GB, Rao GN, Gururaj G, Stovner LJ, Steiner TJ. Headache disorders and public ill-health in India: prevalence estimates in Karnataka State. J Headache Pain. 2015;16:67.
52. Rao GN, Kulkarni GB, Gururaj G, Stovner LJ, Steiner TJ. The burden attributable to headache disorders in India: estimates from a community-based study in Karnataka state. J Headache Pain. 2015;16:94.
53. Manandhar K, Risal A, Steiner TJ, Holen A, Linde M. The prevalence of primary headache disorders in Nepal: a nationwide population-based study. J Headache Pain. 2015;16:95.
54. Manandhar K, Risal A, Linde M, Steiner TJ. The burden of headache disorders in Nepal: estimates from a population-based survey. J Headache Pain. 2016;17:3.
55. Saylor D, Steiner TJ. The global burden of headache. Semin Neurol. 2018;38:182–90.
56. Vos T, Abajobir AA, Abate KH, Abbafati C, Abbas KM, Abd-Allah F, Abdulkader RS, Abdulle AM, Abebo TA, Abera SF, Aboyans V, Abu-Raddad LJ, Ackerman IN, Adamu AA, Adetokunboh O, Afarideh M, Afshin A, Agarwal SK, Aggarwal R, Agrawal A, Agrawal S, Ahmadieh H, Ahmed MB, Aichour MTE, Aichour AN, Aichour I, Aiyar S, Akinyemi RO, Akseer N, Al Lami FH, Alahdab F, Al-Aly Z, Alam K, Alam N, Alam T, et al. Global, regional, and national incidence, prevalence, and years lived with disability for 328 diseases and injuries for 195 countries, 1990–2016: a systematic analysis for the Global Burden of Disease Study 2016. Lancet. 2017;390:1211–59.
57. Steiner TJ, Stovner LJ, Vos T, Jensen R, Katsarava Z. Migraine is *first* cause of disability in under 50s: will health politicians now take notice? J Headache Pain. 2018;19:17.
58. Vos T, Barber RM, Bell B, Bertozzi-Villa A, Biryukov S, Bolliger I, Charlson F, Davis A, Degenhardt L, Dicker D, Duan L, Erskine H, Feigin VL, Ferrari AJ, Fitzmaurice C, Fleming T, Graetz N, Guinovart C, Haagsma J, Hansen GM, Hanson SW, Heuton KR, Higashi H,

Kassebaum N, Kyu H, Laurie E, Liang X, Lofgren K, Lozano R, MacIntyre MF, Moradi-Lakeh M, Naghavi M, Nguyen G, Odell S, Ortblad K, et al. Global, regional, and national incidence, prevalence, and years lived with disability for 301 acute and chronic diseases and injuries in 188 countries, 1990–2013: a systematic analysis for the Global Burden of Disease Study 2013. Lancet. 2015;386:743–800.

59. GBD 2017 Disease and Injury Incidence and Prevalence Collaborators. Global, regional, and national incidence, prevalence, and years lived with disability for 354 diseases and injuries for 195 countries and territories, 1990–2017: a systematic analysis for the Global Burden of Disease Study 2017. Lancet. 2018;392:1789–858.
60. Wöber-Bingöl C, Wöber C, Uluduz D, Uygunoğlu U, Aslan TS, Kernmayer M, Zesch H-E, Gerges NTA, Wagner G, Siva A, Steiner TJ. The global burden of headache in children and adolescents—developing a questionnaire and methodology for a global study. J Headache Pain. 2014;15:86.
61. Wöber C, Wöber-Bingöl C, Uluduz D, Aslan TS, Uygunoglu U, Tüfekçi A, Alp SI, Duman T, Sürgün F, Emir GK, Demir CF, Balgetir F, Özdemir YB, Auer T, Siva A, Steiner TJ. Undifferentiated headache: broadening the approach to headache in children and adolescents, with supporting evidence from a nationwide school-based cross-sectional survey in Turkey. J Headache Pain. 2018;19:18.
62. United States Congress. https://www.congress.gov/bill/114th-congress/house-bill/5249/text.
63. Peters M, Bertolote JM, Houchin C, Kandoura T, Steiner TJ. Translation protocol for technical documents. J Headache Pain. 2007;8(Suppl 1):S41–2.
64. Peters M, Bertolote JM, Houchin C, Kandoura T, Steiner TJ. Translation protocol for lay documents. J Headache Pain. 2007;8(Suppl 1):S43–4.
65. Peters M, Bertolote JM, Houchin C, Kandoura T, Steiner TJ. Translation protocol for hybrid documents. J Headache Pain. 2007;8(Suppl 1):S45–7.
66. Antonaci F, Valade D, Lanteri-Minet M, Láinez JM, Jensen J, Steiner TJ. Proposals for the organisation of headache services in Europe. Intern Emerg Med. 2008;3:S25–8.
67. Steiner TJ, Antonaci F, Jensen R, Lainez MJ, Lanteri-Minet M, Valade D. Recommendations for headache service organisation and delivery in Europe. J Headache Pain. 2011;12:419–26.
68. Peters M, Perera S, Loder E, Jenkinson C, Gil Gouveia R, Jensen R, Katsarava Z, Steiner TJ. Quality in the provision of headache care. 1: systematic review of the literature and commentary. J Headache Pain. 2012;13:437–47.
69. Peters M, Jenkinson C, Perera S, Loder E, Jensen R, Katsarava Z, Gil Gouveia R, Broner S, Steiner T. Quality in the provision of headache care. 2: defining quality and its indicators. J Headache Pain. 2012;13:449–57.
70. Katsarava Z, Gil Gouveia R, Jensen R, Gaul C, Schramm S, Schoppe A, Steiner TJ. Evaluation of headache service quality indicators: pilot implementation in two specialist-care centres. J Headache Pain. 2015;16:53.
71. Schramm S, Uluduz D, Gil Gouveia R, Jensen R, Siva A, Uygunoglu U, Gvantsa G, Mania M, Braschinsky M, Filatova E, Latysheva N, Osipova V, Skorobogatykh K, Azimova J, Straube A, Emre Eren O, Martelletti P, De Angelis V, Negro A, Linde M, Hagen K, Radojicic A, Zidverc-Trajkovic J, Podgorac A, Paemeleire K, De Pue A, Lampl C, Steiner TJ, Katsarava Z. Headache service quality: evaluation of quality indicators in 14 specialist-care centres. J Headache Pain. 2016;17:111.
72. Pellesi L, Benemei S, Favoni V, Lupi C, Mampreso E, Negro A, Paolucci M, Steiner TJ, Ulivi M, Cevoli S, Guerzoni S. Quality indicators in headache care: an implementation study in six Italian specialist-care centres. J Headache Pain. 2017;18:55.
73. Giorgadze G, Mania M, Kukava M, Dzagnidze A, Mirvelashvili E, Steiner TJ, Katsarava Z. Implementation of effective, self-sustaining headache services in the Republic of Georgia: evaluation of their impact on headache-related disability and quality of life of people with headache. Cephalalgia. 2018;38:639–45.

74. Lebedeva ER, Olesen J, Osipova VV, Volkova LI, Tabeeva GR, Steiner TJ. The Yekaterinburg headache initiative: an interventional project, within the Global Campaign against Headache, to reduce the burden of headache in Russia. J Headache Pain. 2013;14:101.
75. Steiner TJ. *Lifting The Burden*: WHO's Global Campaign against Headache, and headache services in China. Chin J Pain Med. 2010;16(S):3–4.
76. Yu S, Steiner TJ. Lifting the burden of headache in China: managing migraine in a SMART way. J Headache Pain. 2017;18:79.
77. Linde M, Steiner TJ, Chisholm D. Cost-effectiveness analysis of interventions for migraine in four low- and middle-income countries. J Headache Pain. 2015;16:15.
78. Mateen FJ, Dua T, Steiner T, Saxena S. Headache disorders in developing countries: research over the past decade. Cephalalgia. 2008;28:1107–14.

Chapter 15
The Healthcare Solution to Headache

Timothy J. Steiner, Rigmor Jensen, Zaza Katsarava, Derya Uluduz, Michela Tinelli, Hallie Thomas, and Lars Jacob Stovner

T. J. Steiner (✉)
Department of Neuromedicine and Movement Science, NTNU Norwegian University of Science and Technology, Trondheim, Norway

Division of Brain Sciences, Imperial College London, London, UK
e-mail: t.steiner@imperial.ac.uk

R. Jensen
Department of Neurology, Danish Headache Centre, University of Copenhagen, Rigshospitalet Glostrup, Glostrup, Denmark
e-mail: rigmor.jensen@regionh.dk

Z. Katsarava
Evangelical Hospital Unna, Unna, Germany

Department of Neurology, University of Duisburg-Essen, Essen, Germany

EVEX Medical Corporation, Tbilisi, Georgia

IM Sechenov First Moscow State Medical University (Sechenov University), Moscow, Russian Federation
e-mail: zaza.katsarava@uk-essen.de

D. Uluduz
Neurology Department, Cerrahpaşa School of Medicine, Istanbul University, Istanbul, Turkey

M. Tinelli
Personal Social Services Research Unit, The London School of Economics and Political Science, London, UK
e-mail: m.tinelli@lse.ac.uk

H. Thomas
Department of Neuromedicine and Movement Science, NTNU Norwegian University of Science and Technology, Trondheim, Norway

L. J. Stovner
Department of Neuromedicine and Movement Science, NTNU Norwegian University of Science and Technology, Trondheim, Norway

Norwegian Advisory Unit on Headaches, Department of Neurology and Clinical Neurophysiology, St Olavs University Hospital, Trondheim, Norway
e-mail: lars.stovner@ntnu.no

T. J. Steiner, L. J. Stovner (eds.), *Societal Impact of Headache*, Headache,
https://doi.org/10.1007/978-3-030-24728-7_15

15.1 Introduction

Earlier chapters have described the societal impact of headache disorders (Chaps. 4, 8 and 9), and their recognition by the World Health Organization (WHO) from 2000 onwards as a high-priority public-health concern ([1–4]; also, Chap. 5). Over this period, headache disorders have come to be acknowledged as the second highest cause of disability in the world ([5–7]; also, Chap. 9). Three only of the more than 200 headache disorders classified by the International Headache Society [8]—migraine, tension-type headache (TTH) and medication-overuse headache (MOH)—account for almost all headache-attributed burden ([5–7]; also, Chaps. 2–4, 8 and 9): These disorders are common and in many cases lifelong conditions (Chap. 2), associated with recognizable and substantial burdens that include personal suffering, disability, impaired quality of life and financial cost ([9]; also, Chaps. 4 and 12). Their impact extends beyond those immediately affected ([9]; also, Chaps. 4 and 8–12).

Not surprisingly, in countries where data are available, large numbers of people with headache are seen by physicians [10, 11]. For example, in a United Kingdom (UK) study based in primary care 20 years ago, 17% of registered patients aged 16–65 years had consulted a general practitioner (GP) because of headache, and a large proportion (9%) were referred to secondary care [12]. Since, in the UK, virtually everyone is registered with a local GP, these are closely indicative of population-based statistics. As a consequence, neurologists, who received by far the most of these referrals, reported that up to a third of all their patients consulted for headache, more than for any other neurological condition [10].

Despite this, everywhere in the world, headache care reaches only a minority of those who might be considered to need it ([4, 13–18]; also, Chap. 13). Chapter 14 proposed the solution: structured headache services [4, 19, 20].

Of course, fully developed health services for headache, delivering care equitably and nationwide to large numbers of people, will consume significant healthcare resources. But what this means is *not* that their priority should be questioned; this is established beyond doubt (see Chap. 14). Rather, it means that their organization calls for efficiency and attention to cost-effectiveness. Here, the service model, adaptable and supported by educational initiatives, is described in detail.

15.2 The Status Quo: Inefficient and Failing, and Not Only in Low-Income Countries

There is a worldwide context, identified 20 years ago, of low priority accorded to headache disorders in the queue for healthcare resources [21]. Thirteen years later, WHO's *Atlas of Headache Disorders and Resources in the World 2011* described a world of enormous, largely remediable but mostly untreated public ill health attributed to headache ([4]; also, Chap. 5).

Studies in wealthy countries such as the United States of America (USA) and UK found that only two thirds of adults with migraine were correctly diagnosed, only half were consulting healthcare providers, yet over 60% of those not consulting exhibited high migraine-related disability [15]. The Eurolight study in ten countries of the European Union (EU) [22, 23] included indicators of adequacy of medical care [18]. With the focus again on migraine, the findings were depressing. Among 1175 participants in the ten countries reporting frequent migraine—on more than 5 days per month, indicating unambiguous need for preventative medication—fewer than 20% had seen a healthcare professional (GP or specialist). In most countries, fewer than 10% were receiving what might be considered adequate acute treatment, and even smaller proportions had the preventative medication for which they were clearly eligible. In other words, the authors of this report concluded, in wealthy Europe, too few people with migraine consult physicians, and migraine-specific medications are used inadequately even among those who do [18]. Is there hope at all for people with headache in less well-resourced countries?

In Russia, population-based data showed that only 15% of people with headache were consulting, one third of these—far too high a proportion—going directly to neurologists [24, 25]. In Estonia, with better-developed primary care and referral systems, the proportion sent by GPs to neurologists (prior to an educational intervention) was a similar 39.5% [26]. In Nepal, almost three fifths (58%) of participants with headache in a population-based survey had consulted a professional healthcare provider (HCP) in the previous year, and 8% had seen a specialist of some sort [27]. These findings, in a low-income country, suggest better availability of healthcare than in many other, wealthier countries: for example, in Japan [13] and Taiwan [28], in EU countries [15, 18, 29] and in North America [15, 30, 31].

But, of course, all was not as it seemed. The survey in Nepal included a very wide range of HCPs in the count of "medical consultations", some with no counterparts in many other countries, or who would not be accredited as health professionals [27]. When pharmacist consultations (15%) were excluded, the consultation proportion fell to 43% [27], similar to the 47% in China [32]. When consultations only with physicians were considered, probably the most salient comparison, the proportion (less than 19%: GPs 11%, specialists 8% [27]) was much lower than those elsewhere [13, 15, 18, 29–32]—except for Russia [24, 25]. Further, Nepal has no headache specialists, and few neurologists or neurosurgeons, so "specialist" consultations were most likely with ophthalmologists, ENT specialists or psychiatrists [27]. In other words, these findings reflected high demand without indicating good care: on the contrary, headache-attributed burden in Nepal remains egregiously high [33].

These Nepalese findings are given emphasis for a reason relevant to what follows in this chapter. The authors took a positive view: over half of survey participants with headache had engaged at some level with professional healthcare [28], a proportion well in line with international recommendations for headache service organization and delivery ([20]; and see estimates below). This indicated that capacity was available within the health services of even this low-income country that could be built upon in a programme aimed at improvement [27].

15.3 Proposals for Change

So to the solution: nationwide, educationally supported, structured headache services, integrated within a country's healthcare system, efficiently, effectively and equitably mitigating the personal and societal burdens of headache.

Their focus should be on migraine, TTH and MOH. Other headaches, although generally much less common, are nonetheless important, since they may be symptoms of underlying disorders that threaten health and wellbeing. These secondary headaches [8] require both correct and timely diagnosis and effective treatment, sometimes urgently in order to prevent serious consequences (see Chap. 2). *Management* of these is, essentially, treatment of the causative disorders and outside the ambit of headache services. On the other hand, their *recognition* must be the responsibility of the services to which affected patients present—most likely to be headache services when headache is the symptom. So adequate provision is needed for this also.

Proposals for change must build on the health services that exist, in whichever country, wherever it is in the world, accepting that these are differently structured and usually inadequately resourced. In the face of very high levels of need for headache-related healthcare (see below), they must be readily adaptable, as well as efficient, effective and equitable, to match what is achievable in any country while making best use of resources that are available. They should formulate a basic model of healthcare organization rationally spread across primary and secondary healthcare sectors, with due regard for the different skills and levels of expertise in these sectors.

15.3.1 Headache-Related Healthcare Needs Assessment

Existence of a health disorder does not translate directly into need for professional healthcare. *Need* is generally defined with regard to potential for benefit (there is no need for something that will not in some way be helpful). The proposal that everyone with headache would gain benefit from professional headache care might be arguable, but the suggestion that they all have a *need* for care must be constrained in a resource-limited world. Need predicated on anticipated benefit must rise above a *threshold of benefit* and be judged with due regard to benefits achievable by other means. These stipulations are at the heart of health economics and policy, and dictate constraints to whatever is proposed.

Thresholds are hard to set objectively, although needs assessments are highly sensitive to them. With regard to headache, many people treat themselves, some through necessity, others from choice. Those who do so are not only those who are less severely affected [15]; many choose self-management when they expect the marginal benefit of professional involvement in their care to be small (subthreshold benefit negates need). Here is a problem, because expectations are quite often unrealistic—too high or sometimes too low—so that needs assessments based on *what people currently do* [10–18, 24, 25, 27–32] have very questionable validity. This is more so when service improvement is planned: a better service—if "better" means delivering enhanced benefit—should see greater usage than a poor service it replaces (*discovered* need). While planning must factor this in, it is difficult to estimate.

Aside from these consumer-driven issues, another is also threshold-dependent. Cash-limited health services seek *value for money*: they will discount assessed needs, however great, whenever utility gain per unit of healthcare resource consumption will be low. In headache medicine, the potential for benefit from professional healthcare is generally greatest among those worst affected, so that health policy might reasonably focus on these. Further, both migraine and MOH, in most cases, can be effectively treated at rather low cost ([34]; and see below).

The approach in this chapter to needs assessment—estimating how much professional care should be provided—is conservative: it will underestimate rather than overestimate need. Any other approach would be unhelpful—as will become apparent.

A first assumption is that *only those with disabling headache are in need of professional care*. The implication that others can adequately look after themselves is possibly unfair, but the assumption respects a reasonable view of priority. About two thirds (66%) of the world's population are aged 15–64 years [35], these being the years during which headache disorders tend to be particularly troublesome. About 25% are aged 14 or under [36]. With regional variations, in every million people living in the world, there are 660,000 and 250,000 in these age groups, respectively. Primary headache is less common, and less troublesome, in older people [7].

Best epidemiological evidence ([7]; also, Chaps. 8 and 9) suggests about 15% of adults aged 15–64 have migraine. This number is a global average, still based on incomplete data (see Chap. 9): population-based studies in many countries have found adult prevalences well in excess of 20% ([37]; also, Chap. 8). Some 80% of these (i.e. 12% of adults) are significantly disabled through severe pain and/or debilitating associated symptoms [38]. Perhaps another 25%, although again there are wide variations, have occasional other headaches, mostly episodic TTH (see Chap. 8), which generally is not regarded as significantly disabling ([39]; also, Chaps. 2 and 9). About 1.5% (the proportion varies greatly from country to country) [40] are highly disabled by MOH. In other words, in every million people in the world, there are approximately 80,000 adults disabled at least to some extent by migraine (660,000 adults $*$ 0.15 [prevalence] $*$ 0.8 [proportion disabled]), and therefore in need of headache care, and a minimum of 10,000 with MOH (660,000 adults $*$ 0.015 [prevalence]), all of whom need care because this disorder will not otherwise resolve. Note that the total (90,000 out of 660,000 [13.6%]), which effectively ignores TTH, is of the order only of one third of the estimated prevalence of headache including TTH ([5]; also, Chap. 9), which, arguably, is overconservative.

Needs arise in the child and adolescent populations also but are more difficult to quantify because there are fewer data. Headache is apparently as common in children as in adults, with an estimated 1-year prevalence in excess of 50% (based on rather sparse data) [41]. But it has different characteristics (see Chap. 3). It is clear that *migraine* prevalence is lower in children [41], dependent upon age and reaching adult levels during the course of adolescence, but *undifferentiated headache* largely fills its place, albeit with less disabling consequences (Chap. 3). In the absence of better data, a conservative but reasonable working basis is that headache care needs in these age groups are, per head, half those of adults [20]: another 17,000 in each million of the population (250,000 children/adolescents $*$ 0.136/2 [half adult need]).

15.3.2 Service Provision Requirement

Upon these statistics, with some further assumptions (Table 15.1), it is possible to make estimates of service requirements (Table 15.2).

First, *need* for care is distinguished from *demand*. The two overlap, but they are not the same—each can exist without the other. Need for professional headache care, defined as above, becomes demand only in those who seek care (which is not everyone with need (see Chap. 13)). Complex factors, not all well understood, govern healthcare utilization by people with headache [15]. Unavailability of good care is one, and self-perpetuating, since demand is sensitive to this, suppressed regardless of need. Evidence suggests that demand for headache care is expressed by only

Table 15.1 Assumptions in estimating service requirements to meet headache-related healthcare demand in a population

Assumption	Argument
The average consultation need per adult patient is 1.25 h per 2 years	This average is within a wide range of variation, mostly according to diagnosis but also subject to level within the healthcare system: consultations in specialist care are usually longer, reflecting case complexity. In most cases, a longer first consultation, with diagnostic enquiry and impact assessment (up to 45 min in specialist care), will be followed by 1–3 shorter review appointments in the first 2 years
The average consultation need per child or adolescent patient is greater: 2 h per 2 years	Expert opinion cites the need for additional enquiry into family dynamics, schooling and peer relationships as issues relevant to management success
No wastage occurs through failures by patients to attend appointments	This assumption appears manifestly false, but wastage of this sort is very difficult to predict in the context of proposals for service improvement. At present, it is commonly discounted by overbooking
Each full-time healthcare provider (HCP) is available for 1380 h/year of consultation time	One day per week is assumed for non-clinical work (administration, audit and continuing professional development); each week therefore allows 4 days, each of 7.5 h, of patient contact time. Only 46 weeks are worked per year

Table 15.2 Estimated service requirements to meet headache-related healthcare demand in a population of one million

	Expected demand	
Estimated numbers expressing demand[a]	Hours/year of medical consultation time required	Full-time equivalent (FTE) health-care providers[b] required to deliver
Adults: 67,500	42,200[c]	30[e]
Children and adolescents: 12,750	12,750[d]	9[e]

[a]Assuming 75% of those with need (90,000 adults and 17,000 children/adolescents (see text))
[b]One FTE provider does not necessarily imply one provider engaged full-time; it could, for example, be two engaged half-time or ten working 10% of full time
[c](67,500∗1.25 h)/2 years (see text and Table 15.1)
[d](12,750∗2.0 h)/2 years (see text and Table 15.1)
[e](hours/year of time required)/(1380 h/year per healthcare provider) (see Table 15.1)

50% of those who might be considered in need [12, 13, 15, 42], but the assumption is made here that better and more accessible services will increase this to 75% (still leaving 25% of need unmet).

Second are a range of assumptions about time. Inpatient management is ignored: the need for it in the management of primary headache is very low. Admission is sometimes good practice, because of comorbidities, or for detoxication in MOH, but only in a tiny percentage of all presenting patients. The multiple assumptions relating to time allocations therefore consider only ambulatory care. They are based on expert views of requirement [20], again tempered with conservatism.

Despite this deep conservatism pervading the assumptions, Table 15.2 sets out very challenging estimates of service requirement. While they may be imprecise, two conclusions follow.

15.3.3 Structured Headache Services

First of these is that headache services must be formally organized and integrated within the structure of local health services. If they merely develop *ad hoc*, as is now the case in most countries providing any service at all, they can be neither efficient nor equitable. In the context of failing headache services described earlier, systems or practice that lead to large numbers of headache referrals to neurologists [4, 10–12, 24–26] must be questioned. On the other hand, if headache service provision is envisaged only in the form of headache centres—national or regional—large numbers of referrals are inevitable.

Second, inexorably, is that headache services *cannot* in any case be provided, in the main, in specialist care. The very limited capacity in specialist care offers no chance of needs being met—or even a substantial part of them.

This is not a bad thing, for two reasons.

First, and of specific relevance to headache, most diagnosis and management of headache disorders requires no more than a basic knowledge of a relatively few very common disorders (see Chap. 2), which ought to be very familiar to primary-care providers. Only standard clinical skills need be applied, and no special investigations or equipment are usually necessary. In other words, there is no *clinical* objection to locating most headache services in primarycare [20].

Second, wherever healthcare reform is in progress, there is emphasis on strengthening primary care [43–47]. There are good reasons for this, recognized since WHO's Alma-Ata declaration of 40 years ago [43], which characterized primary healthcare as "the first level of contact of individuals, the family and community with the national health system bringing healthcare as close as possible to where people live and work". While models of healthcare vary throughout the world, whatever the overarching system of care (assuming there is one), primary care has a recognized and important role nearly everywhere. In highly rural regions, those of sub-Saharan Africa, for example, primary care is the *only* point of contact for most patients. Among advanced systems, some provide free, subsidized or reimbursed care, supported by insurance-based financial structures operated by the State or in which the State is a controlling intermediary; others levy fees for service, which patients may or may not recover through private or employer-provided insurance. All of these can accommodate primary care as the first port of call [45].

There are other reasons, too, which have to do with efficiency and cost-saving. These are discussed later.

15.3.4 A Model of Headache-Service Organization

Recognizing these arguments, the fundamental purpose of headache-service organization is to divide service provision rationally between primary and secondary (specialist) care. Within a structured system, management of patients at the lowest level commensurate with good care makes most efficient use of allocated resources and is the means by which effective care can reach more who need it. How this is best done practically depends on the local health-service structure and resources allocated.

The model described below (Table 15.3; Fig. 15.1) provides a general guide and template, adaptable as necessary. Its essential elements are organization on three interdependent levels, with facilitated but nonetheless controlled pathways between them, and expansion of the contribution from primary care.

Table 15.3 Headache services organized on three levels

Level 1: General primary care	• Front-line headache services (accessible first contact for most people with headache) • Ambulatory care delivered by primary healthcare providers (physicians, clinical officers, nurses and/or pharmacists)
• Referring when necessary and acting as gatekeeper[a], to:	
Level 2: Special-interest headache care	• Ambulatory care delivered by trained physicians, clinical officers or nurses with a special interest in headache, in primary or secondary care
• Referring when necessary to:	
Level 3: Specialized headache centres	• Advanced multidisciplinary care delivered by headache specialists in hospital-based centres

[a]More is said below about the gatekeeper role of level 1 (see Sect. 15.3.4.5).

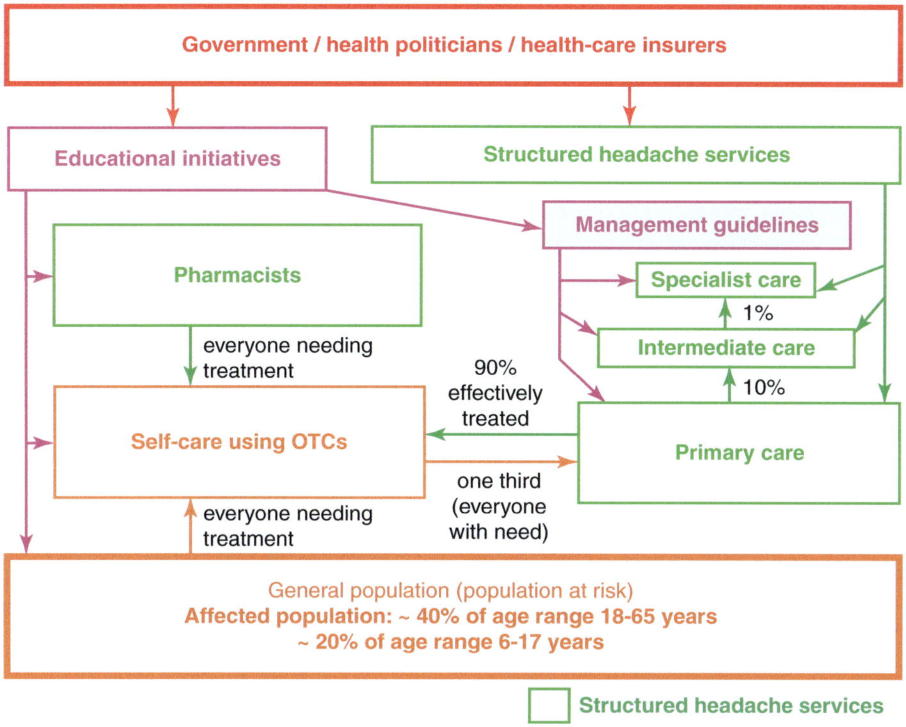

Fig. 15.1 Template for structured headache services supported by educational initiatives and expected patient flows (see text for explanation)

15.3.4.1 Level 1: General Primary Care

Primary care, with the benefit to patients of being available locally, should be the accessible front line for almost all people needing care for a headache disorder. This is not everyone with headache: an estimated two thirds should, with advice from public education and guidance from pharmacists, be able adequately to manage themselves (see Sect. 15.3.1).

At this level, nonspecialist HCPs—with some training in headache—should meet the needs of the great majority of people consulting for headache [1], controlling flow to higher levels. They may be primary-care physicians (GPs), but this is not essential in a healthcare system that relies more on clinical officers, nurses or pharmacists. Whatever their background, many HCPs at this level will need better knowledge of headache for this purpose, but the model does not require *every* HCP in primary care to offer headache services if they can share caseload between themselves according to their skills and interests.

Most cases of migraine and TTH should be competently diagnosed and managed at level 1 [48].

Cluster headache, medication-overuse headache (MOH) and some other common secondary headache disorders listed in Table 15.4 should be recognized but not necessarily managed; red-flag warnings of serious secondary

Table 15.4 ICDH-3 diagnoses [8] to be recognized at level 1

Primary headache disorders		Secondary headache disorders	
1.1	Migraine without aura[a]	5.2.1	Chronic post-traumatic headache attributed to moderate or severe head injury
1.2	Migraine with aura[a]		
1.2.3	Typical aura without headache[a]	6.2.2	Headache attributed to subarachnoid haemorrhage
		6.4.1	Headache attributed to giant cell arteritis
2.1	Infrequent episodic tension-type headache[a]	7.4.1	Headache attributed to increased intracranial pressure or hydrocephalus caused by neoplasm
2.2	Frequent episodic tension-type headache[a]	8.2	Medication-overuse headache (and subtypes)[a]
		9.1	Headache attributed to intracranial infection
2.3	Chronic tension-type headache	10.3	Headache attributed to arterial hypertension
		11.3.1	Headache attributed to acute glaucoma
3.1.1	Episodic cluster headache	13.1.1	Classical trigeminal neuralgia
3.1.2	Chronic cluster headache		

[a]Management of most of these should be within the competence of level 1

headaches (see Chap. 2) should also be recognized and duly acted upon [48]. Referral channels to levels 2 and 3, urgent when necessary, should be in place for these cases and for other patients who are diagnostically complex or difficult to manage [20].

This level should also continue the long-term care of patients discharged with treatment plans from levels 2 or 3 [20].

15.3.4.2 Level 2: Special-Interest Headache Care

Level 2 may, in some countries, be in primary care, provided by GPs with a special interest and additional training in headache. In others it is more likely to be offered in polyclinics or district hospitals by neurologists, also with additional training in headache [20].

HCPs at this level, usually physicians, should provide more skilled ambulatory care to the small proportion of patients referred upwards from level 1 (Fig. 15.1), who require greater expertise. Their competence should embrace the diagnosis and management of more difficult cases of primary headache and some secondary headache disorders, but not those that are very rare [20]. To fulfil their role, they need access to other services such as neuroimaging, psychology and physiotherapy.

For a minority of their patients—those outside their competence—they require a referral channel to level 3 (Table 15.5) [20].

15.3.4.3 Level 3: Specialized Headache Centres

Specialized headache centres sit at the apex of structured headache services. In many countries, they remain an unfulfilled aspiration; in others, they exist—disadvantageously—without the lower levels in place. They have four important roles (Table 15.6).

First and foremost, specialized headache centres are tertiary referral centres. They manage the very few patients with primary or secondary headache disorders

Table 15.5 Patients likely to be referred to level 3 within optimally structured headache services (adapted from [20])

Patients with: • Refractory disabling headache of any type • Cluster headache and other trigeminal autonomic cephalalgias, at first presentation • Medication-overuse headache involving drugs of dependence, where personality mitigates against withdrawal of medication or where withdrawal attempts have failed • High and low CSF pressure headaches • Trigeminal and other cranial neuralgias or painful lesions of the cranial nerves • Rare primary or secondary headaches • Headaches with severe physical and/or psychological comorbidities
Cases: • Of persisting diagnostic uncertainty • Where risk of serious underlying disorders demands specialist investigation • Of other probable or certain serious secondary headache
Patients who may participate in specific level-3 research projects (including clinical trials)

Table 15.6 Four roles of specialized headache centres within structured headache services

1. To provide best possible level-3 clinical care for adults and/or children, having regard to the resources locally available
2. To support levels 1 and 2 through clinical advice and training and by contributing to the development, periodic review and updating of national management guidelines
3. To conduct research into headache appropriate to the needs of the local community
4. To provide empirical evidence in support of their existence

Table 15.7 Other disciplines to which specialized headache centres need access

• Neurology • Neuroradiology • Neurosurgery • Psychiatry	• Ophthalmology • Otorhinolaryngology • Dentistry	• Paediatrics • Gynaecology	• Cardiology • Rheumatology • Endocrinology • Infectious diseases • Orthopaedics • Trauma

that are difficult to diagnose or treat, refractory, or for other reasons require specialist intervention [20, 49–53] (Fig. 15.1; Table 15.5). They concentrate experience in the rare primary and secondary headache disorders and cranial neuralgias. For this role, they employ accredited headache specialists and/or neurologists and provide full-time inpatient facilities, multidisciplinary management and access to equipment and specialists in other disciplines (Table 15.7) for the diagnosis and management of the underlying causes of all secondary headache disorders. Specialized headache centres are therefore closely affiliated to a university or other major hospital.

In their second role (Table 15.6), specialized headache centres support nonspecialists at levels 1 and 2 through direct clinical advice, training and development of national management guidelines. This is a symbiotic relationship: demand at level 3 is controllable only when levels 1 and 2 are in place and functioning well. In this role, level 3 not only maintains standards throughout the system but also protects its ability to perform in its first role.

The third role is research (Table 15.6), focused on the other roles. Research may seem a luxury in some countries, but it improves understanding of needs in the local community, what and where they are and how best to meet them. Research thereby helps to control demand while maintaining or improving quality of care.

Finally, specialized centres need to justify their continued existence. Historically, few centres have documented their activities and the outcomes achieved in their intended roles [49–52, 54–56]. In truth this is not easy, but empirical evidence of efficient achievement of desired outcomes justifies investment in the continued existence of specialized centres and appropriate expansion in their number.

15.3.4.4 Division of Caseload

The model, a broad-based pyramid with a narrow apex, reflects the proportion of presenting patients whose healthcare needs cannot be met at primary care level because of diagnostic or management complexity. Quantitative estimates are necessary. While these are largely based on expert opinion [20], there is some empirical support from a large UK general practice for presuming that about 10% of presenting patients might appropriately be treated at a higher level [12]. Accordingly, level 1 should be able to meet the needs of 90% of people consulting for headache [20] (Fig. 15.1).

On this estimate, and the earlier assumptions about consultation times (Table 15.1), one full-time HCP can provide headache care at level 1 for a population no larger than 30,000 (33 HCPs per million).

Not all of the remaining 10% require the highest (level-3) expertise. In most countries, specialized centres are few and would be overwhelmed even by this proportion. This is the justification for level 2, which should provide care to most patients referred upwards from level 1 (Fig. 15.1). Again on this estimate, and the assumptions about consultation times (Table 15.1), one full-time HCP can provide headache care at level 2 for a population no larger than 200,000 (5 HCPs per million).

At level 3, capacity should match needs at that level: more would simply consume resources that lower levels could use better (i.e. more cost-effectively). When levels 1 and 2 are adequately set up also, demand at level 3 should be limited to no more than 1% of all headache patients (Fig. 15.1). Relieved of the other 99%, specialized headache centres can cover relatively large geographical catchment areas and populations (one full-time specialist per two million people (0.5 per million)). For inpatients, a recommended minimum is two beds per million population [20].

Equitable distribution is a likely challenge, well exemplified by a survey in Brazil. Of 243 "headache specialists" in 2004/2005 (more than twice the number needed in a well-functioning three-level model for Brazil's 198 million people [57]), the south-east region had 68% for 42.6% of the country's population, the north-east had only 12.4% for 28.1% of the population, and five of Brazil's 27 States had none at all [58].

15.3.4.5 The Gatekeeper Role Within the Model

One of the model's essential purposes is to shift demand from secondary care services into primary care—a move which is not only appropriate from a clinical viewpoint but also, in general, cost-saving [43–47] (see Sect. 15.5). The *gatekeeper* role of primary care is a key organizational issue [44, 59].

More needs to be said on this, because it is somewhat controversial [59–61]. Patients cannot be blamed for seeking access directly to those whom they perceive to be experts, and gatekeeping is not a norm in many countries' health systems. Ostensibly, where it is in place, gatekeeping guides patients efficiently and in their best interests through the health system according to their needs, not their demands [59]—a somewhat paternalistic but well-intentioned aim. In reality, it is the principal means of preventing overload in specialist services, which would deny access to some who really need it—a more crucial consideration. Whatever its supposed purpose, gatekeeping contributes—and perhaps is essential—to cost containment, because unrestricted access to specialists induces demand for costly and sometimes unnecessary services.

The effectiveness of this model [60], and the equity of it, rely on efficiency at the interfaces between levels, seams in service continuity where breakdowns can occur readily, and detrimentally to patients [61]. There should not be undue system-created delays or other barriers set against those who *do* need specialist care—an equally crucial consideration (see Chap. 13). Efficient interfaces between the levels are matters of implementation, best determined in the context of local health services. Importantly, if the model is implemented well, with appropriate provision at each level, *demand within the three levels is likely to be self-regulating*, effectively governed by waiting lists.

15.3.4.6 Flexibility of the Model

Much depends on this. How this model might be implemented in a country (or in a regional or district pilot) depends on two principal factors: the resources allocated to headache services (which, as a matter of sensible policy, should match the priority due to them) and the general structure of the health service within which these services are accommodated.

National modifications may therefore be demanded, but the model has considerable flexibility, in a number of ways, that allows adaptation without altering its intrinsic structure (Table 15.8).

15.3.5 Educational Implications

Education has two major roles in better headache services.

Table 15.8 Adaptability of the model according to local requirements and resources

Requirement	Adaptation
Doctors vs. other healthcare providers (HCPs)	Many countries, as policy, are expanding the healthcare roles of HCPs other than doctors. Systems in some countries may require service delivery at level 1, and perhaps level 2 also, by nurses or clinical officers. This is the way forward, supported by training (see below), when the alternative is nothing
Primary vs. secondary care	Level 1 must be in primary care; the arguments are expressed earlier. Level 2, on the other hand, can be in primary or secondary care. Options include neurologists, trained (but nonspecialist) physicians in district hospital outpatient departments or polyclinics, GPs with a special interest in headache working in primary care (a development in the UK [62], initially popular but later fading) and clinical officers or nurses in community-based outreach centres. Essential in all cases is a special interest in headache
Two-level systems	Level-3 centres must be in secondary care (or tertiary care in countries that make this distinction). It is therefore costly and may be unaffordable. When level 3 cannot be fully implemented within this model, or at all, this need and should not detract from the benefits that can be provided to the great majority by levels 1 and 2
Combined levels	There is no intrinsic reason why one centre cannot provide both level-2 and level-3 care. This should not replace any part of level 2 with level 3, which would result in loss of efficiency Level 1, by its nature, is community-based. It is possible nonetheless, and may be appropriate, for certain level-2 centres to offer, additionally, local level-1 care
Division of caseload	The 90:9:1% split between levels 1, 2 and 3 are estimates of need, based on expert opinion. Throughout the world, there are variations in prevalence and characteristics of the common headache disorders (see Chaps. 2–4), particularly in the frequency of MOH [40]. The division of caseload between levels may need adjustment in particular countries, along with capacity at each level, ideally based on locally gathered empirical data. The model will accommodate this without fundamental change

On the one hand, *public education* needs to improve people's understanding of headache and of the appropriate use of services. It needs to change their behaviour, not only with regard to seeking healthcare but also, and necessarily, to promote better adherence [63, 64]. On the other hand, *professional education* must ensure that the expertise necessary at levels 1 and 2 is available. Limited but better knowledge of headache, coupled with the use of evidence-based guidelines in primary care [48], can keep the great majority of patients at level 1, reducing unnecessary demand upon specialist care [26, 65]. A somewhat enhanced but still limited knowledge requirement exists at level 2 [20].

There are, however, major political and logistic implications here. The start is to give more emphasis to headache diagnosis and management in the medical school undergraduate curriculum, ensuring that newly qualified doctors will have at least some understanding of a set of burdensome and very common disorders—which is often not the case now. This is far from easily achieved and will itself involve a battle of priorities in an already overfilled curriculum. But much more is needed, and more quickly. Far-reaching training initiatives, at national level, must be part and parcel of effective headache service reform. The educational challenge is greatest at level 1, because of the weight of numbers of HCPs who need training.

Within the three-level care system proposed, a training role for each higher level to the level below can be envisaged. It is likely that the entire structure will depend upon these roles being developed.

15.4 Political Will

The expectations of successful implementation embrace improved headache services, achieved in a number of complementary ways: greater community-based availability, reduced delivery costs by pulling inappropriate demand in secondary care back into primary care, freed resources to discover and meet unrecognized headache-related healthcare needs in the community, and mitigated lost productivity and its detriment to gross domestic product ([66–73]; also, Chap. 12). All of these outcomes are *politically* desirable [4]: there should be political will to achieve them.

Distorted priorities may lie at the heart of the current inadequacies. It is likely to be argued that the creation of a better headache-care structure, and the delivery of more effective care, will stimulate demand—with unaffordable results. There is probable truth in this, but it should be recognized that, if this occurs, it is simply unmasking need that is there already, not creating it. In counter-argument, the humanitarian symptom-based burden (see Chaps. 4 and 8) causing substantial public ill health ([4]; also, Chap. 9) must be seen as unacceptable, as is the financial penalty of inaction.

15.5 The Cost of Doing Nothing

Chapter 12 lays out the high financial cost of headache as it is—imperfectly treated. Global Campaign studies around the world have estimated massive lost-productivity costs: of up to 2% of gross domestic product [66, 68–73]. These, enormous though they may be, are not the sole cost of doing nothing.

While major improvements to services may require substantial up-front investment, there is promise—if even a small part of the lost productivity can be recovered—for even greater savings to offset it [4]. These savings, foregone, are also part of the *financial penalty of inaction.*

Cost-effectiveness of the structured headache services model was analysed by *Lifting The Burden* (LTB) in collaboration with WHO [34]. The enquiry, including only migraine (because better data were available), asked what monetary investment would yield what amount of population-level disability reduction. The focus was not on individual drugs, although costs and effects of these must be included, but on the means by and extent to which these would reach and be used by people likely to benefit from them. *Effect estimation* used clinical trial evidence of drug efficacy (first-line acute and prophylactic) and assumed that structured services, when implemented and supported by educational initiatives, would improve both coverage (the proportion of people needing treatment to whom it was made available) and adherence (the proportion actually taking it as intended) [34]. *Estimated costs* included those of running the services, those of increased treatment uptake and those of the educational initiatives, aimed at both HCPs and people with headache (the public). Epidemiological data were those supplied by LTB to the Global Burden of Disease Study 2010 (GBD2010) ([74]; also, Chap. 9), from population-based surveys in China [32, 68], India [72, 75, 76], Russia [24, 25, 77] and Zambia [71, 78], the countries included. In the analytical WHO-CHOICE model [79], disability weights were also taken from GBD2010 [39].

The analysis found that self-management with simple analgesics, generating a healthy life year (HLY) for less than USD 100, was a very highly, and by far the most, cost-effective strategy for migraine treatment [34]. Adding a triptan, in a stepped-care treatment paradigm [48], required management within headache services and incurred an incremental cost of over USD 10,000 per extra HLY: still cost-effective and an efficient use of health resources in low- and middle-income countries. Consumer education and provider training were also economically attractive, accelerating progress towards desired levels of coverage and adherence while costing relatively little to implement [34].

However, this analysis was limited in scope: it did not include other headache disorders than migraine, and, crucially, it ignored the indirect costs of lost work productivity (absenteeism because of headache and reduced working effectiveness of those at work despite headache ([66–73]; also, Chap. 12)).

In a further collaboration, between LTB, European Headache Federation (EHF), European Brain Council (EBC) and London School of Economics, wider-ranging analyses are underway (not yet formally published). These similarly estimate cost-effectiveness of structured services delivering appropriate treatments with known efficacy. They compare baseline (current care) with a target scenario in which implemented services, provider training and consumer education improve both coverage and adherence. They include migraine, TTH and MOH. The perspectives are those of provider and society, so analyses include not only direct costs (resources sunk into healthcare provision) per HLY gained but also direct costs invested versus indirect costs saved. Because of the European interests of EHF and EBC, the analyses were of Russia, Spain and Luxembourg, European countries for which LTB had population-based data [22–25, 27].

The findings, when published, may vary slightly from those in Table 15.9, but the preliminary analyses confirm, as predicted in 2011 by WHO ([4]; also, Chap. 5), that intervention in the form of structured headache services is not only cost-effective but also likely to be cost-*saving*. The far-right column of Table 15.9 bears witness to the *magnitude* of the financial penalty of inaction: EUR 6.7 billion per year of unrealized potential savings (in addition to the public-health penalty of 215,000 unrecovered HLYs).

Table 15.9 Cost-effectiveness analysis of structured headache services: Spain as an example (timeframe, 1 year)

	Migraine	Tension-type headache	Medication-overuse headache	Totals
Provider perspective				
Numbers of patients treated	10,772,263	7,850,265	2,128,185	21 million people treated
Additional costs (EUR)	90,077,116	98,760,746	33,185,022	EUR 222 million spent
HLYs gained	97,311	3146	114,829	215,000 HLYs gained
EUR spent for each HLY gained	926	31,392	289	
Societal perspective (indirect costs included)				
Costs saved (EUR)	2,421,187,601	624,717,880	3,674,177,951	EUR 6.7 billion saved

EUR euro, *HLY* healthy life year

This is a crucial demonstration. The question looms large of how to pay for what the Global Campaign seeks to achieve—beneficial change, in a world of competing demands and scarce resources—but these analyses emphatically provide the answer. While avoidance of wastage is a likely benefit of effective intervention [4], the anticipated benefit of recovered work-productivity losses is greater by far [66–73]. If it is proven that untreated headache costs society more, in total, than treated headache, paying for change should no longer be an issue, at least in more industrialized nations.

On the face of it, governments should urgently want to know this. Perhaps this is the highest priority of all.

But it still has to be empirically demonstrated. The analysis of indirect costs makes assumptions about the relationship between headache-attributed disability and lost productivity. Disability levels of zero and 100% would, presumably, be associated with the same levels of lost productivity, but there is emerging evidence that the relationship between these extremes is far from linear. This is depicted, for migraine, in Fig. 15.2, again showing population-based data from the Global Campaign, from Spain and Luxembourg. At *population level*, the relationship between disability and lost productivity is clearly complex, with R^2 indicating that a linear model explains <12% of the variation.

Actually this is not surprising, since many external factors are operating. People have a choice when they wake in the morning with headache, and work beckons. As well as "How ill do I feel?", personal but non-illness-related questions are brought into play, such as "Is my work important?", "Do I enjoy it?", "Can I make up the time later?", and "Do other people depend on me for their own work?", along with random factors such as "Is the weather bad?". All may be influential, but to very different degrees in different people. At *individual level*, on the other hand, most of these external factors are constant, or at least much less variable, so disability and

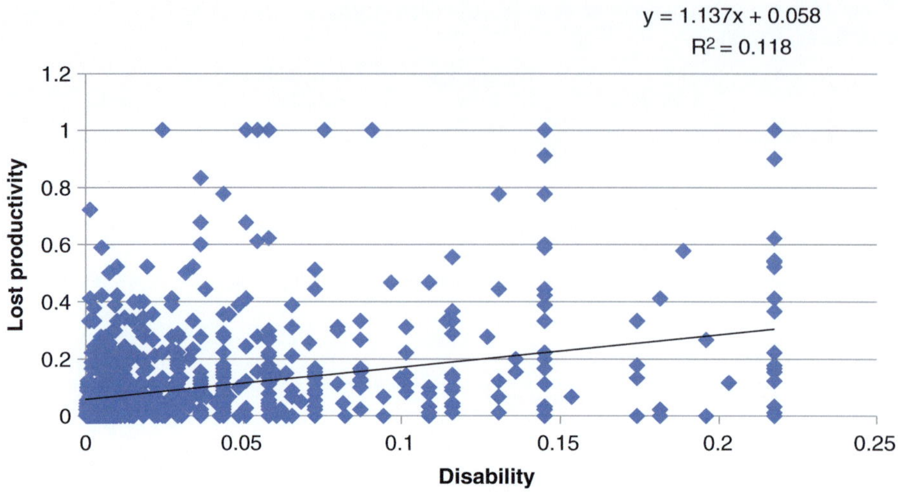

Fig. 15.2 The relationship between migraine-attributed disability (D) and lost productivity (LP) in population samples from Spain and Luxembourg. D is a proportion on a scale 0–1, calculated as the product of proportion of time in ictal state (attack frequency ∗ attack duration) and disability weight (DW) from GBD2016 ([5]; also, Chap. 9). LP is the proportion of time lost from work (also 0–1), estimated over 3 months from responses to the HALT-90 index [80]

lost productivity may show the high level of correlation expected. The empirical evidence for this, however, has still to be generated.

In the economic analyses including indirect costs (Table 15.9), structured headache services remain cost-saving *if only 4% of lost productivity, proportionately, is recovered by mitigating disability*.

15.6 Concluding Remarks

There are many problems with the current compartmentalized division of headache services between primary and secondary care. The model described seeks vertical integration while recognizing that headache services not only must but readily can be delivered for the most part in primary care. The size of the demand dictates this as the only way forward, but it is a perfectly good way forward in terms of effectiveness of care. The model is capable of adaptation to suit local cultures and healthcare systems. It is cost-effective, and almost certainly cost-saving in all economies.

In all countries, essentially the same need exists, differing only quantitatively. Wherever health-service reform is shifting resources from secondary to primary care, for which momentum is again developing [43, 46, 47], there is opportunity for change. At the same time, in low- and middle-income countries in particular, the growing shift of emphasis in health policy towards chronic non-communicable diseases [81] creates a fair climate for change. Economic (cost-effectiveness) analyses support change.

These arguments must be acknowledged if political will is to be fostered and harnessed and change made to happen. This is the greatest challenge.

References

1. World Health Organization. Headache disorders and public health. Education and management implications. Geneva: WHO (WHO/MSD/MBD/00.9); 2000.
2. World Health Organization. Headache disorders. Fact sheet no. 277. Geneva: WHO; 2003.
3. World Health Organization. Headache disorders. Ch 3.3 in: Neurological disorders: public health challenges. Geneva: WHO; 2007. p. 70–84.
4. World Health Organization and *Lifting The Burden*. Atlas of headache disorders and resources in the world 2011. Geneva: WHO; 2011. http://www.who.int/mental_health/management/atlas_headache_disorders/en/2011.
5. Vos T, Abajobir AA, Abate KH, Abbafati C, Abbas KM, Abd-Allah F, Abdulkader RS, Abdulle AM, Abebo TA, Abera SF, Aboyans V, Abu-Raddad LJ, Ackerman IN, Adamu AA, Adetokunboh O, Afarideh M, Afshin A, Agarwal SK, Aggarwal R, Agrawal A, Agrawal S, Ahmadieh H, Ahmed MB, Aichour MTE, Aichour AN, Aichour I, Aiyar S, Akinyemi RO, Akseer N, Al Lami FH, Alahdab F, Al-Aly Z, Alam K, Alam N, Alam T, et al. Global, regional, and national incidence, prevalence, and years lived with disability for 328 diseases and injuries for 195 countries, 1990–2016: a systematic analysis for the Global Burden of Disease Study 2016. Lancet. 2017;390:1211–59.
6. Steiner TJ, Stovner LJ, Vos T, Jensen R, Katsarava Z. Migraine is *first* cause of disability in under 50s: will health politicians now take notice? J Headache Pain. 2018;19:17.
7. GBD 2017 Disease and Injury Incidence and Prevalence Collaborators. Global, regional, and national incidence, prevalence, and years lived with disability for 354 diseases and injuries for 195 countries and territories, 1990–2017: a systematic analysis for the Global Burden of Disease Study 2017. Lancet. 2018;392:1789–858.
8. Headache Classification Committee of the International Headache Society. The International Classification of Headache Disorders, 3rd edition. Cephalalgia. 2018;38:1–211.
9. Steiner TJ, Gururaj G, Andrée C, Katsarava Z, Ayzenberg I, Yu SY, Al Jumah M, Tekle-Haimanot R, Birbeck GL, Herekar A, Linde M, Mbewe E, Manandhar K, Risal A, Jensen R, Queiroz LP, Scher AI, Wang SJ, Stovner LJ. Diagnosis, prevalence estimation and burden measurement in population surveys of headache: presenting the HARDSHIP questionnaire. J Headache Pain. 2014;15:3.
10. Hopkins A, Menken M, De Friese GA. A record of patient encounters in neurological practice in the United Kingdom. J Neurol Neurosurg Psychiatry. 1989;52:436–8.
11. Wiles CM, Lindsay M. General practice referrals to a department of neurology. J Roy Coll Physicians. 1996;30:426–31.
12. Laughey WF, Holmes WF, MacGregor AE, Sawyer JPC. Headache consultation and referral patterns in one UK general practice. Cephalalgia. 1999;19:328–9.
13. Rasmussen BK, Jensen R, Olesen J. Impact of headache on sickness absence and utilisation of medical services: a Danish population study. J Epidemiol Community Health. 1992;46:443–6.
14. Dowson A, Jagger S. The UK migraine patient survey: quality of life and treatment. Curr Med Res Opin. 1999;15:241–53.
15. Lipton RB, Scher AI, Steiner TJ, Kolodner K, Liberman J, Stewart WF. Patterns of health care utilization for migraine in England and in the United States. Neurology. 2003;60:441–8.
16. Takeshima T, Ishizaki K, Fukuhara Y, Ijiri T, Kusumi M, Wakutani Y, Mori M, Kawashima M, Kowa H, Adachi Y, Urakami K, Nakashima K. Population-based door-to-door survey of migraine in Japan: the Daisen study. Headache. 2004;44:8–19.
17. Radtke A, Neuhauser H. Prevalence and burden of headache and migraine in Germany. Headache. 2009;49:79–89.

18. Katsarava Z, Mania M, Lampl C, Herberhold J, Steiner TJ. Poor medical care for people with migraine in Europe—evidence from the Eurolight study. J Headache Pain. 2018;19:10.
19. Antonaci F, Valade D, Lanteri-Minet M, Láinez JM, Jensen J, Steiner TJ. Proposals for the organisation of headache services in Europe. Intern Emerg Med. 2008;3:S25–8.
20. Steiner TJ, Antonaci F, Jensen R, Lainez MJ, Lanteri-Minet M, Valade D. Recommendations for headache service organisation and delivery in Europe. J Headache Pain. 2011;12:419–26.
21. American Association for the Study of Headache, International Headache Society. Consensus statement on improving migraine management. Headache. 1998;38:736.
22. Andrée C, Stovner LJ, Steiner TJ, Barré J, Katsarava Z, Lainez JM, Lair M-L, Lanteri-Minet M, Mick G, Rastenyte D, Ruiz de la Torre E, Tassorelli C, Vriezen P, Lampl C. The Eurolight project: the impact of primary headache disorders in Europe. Description of methods. J Headache Pain. 2011;12:541–9.
23. Steiner TJ, Stovner LJ, Katsarava Z, Lainez JM, Lampl C, Lantéri-Minet M, Rastenyte D, Ruiz de la Torre E, Tassorelli C, Barré J, Andrée C. The impact of headache in Europe: principal results of the Eurolight project. J Headache Pain. 2014;15:31.
24. Ayzenberg I, Katsarava Z, Sborowski A, Chernysh M, Osipova V, Tabeeva G, Steiner TJ. Headache-attributed burden and its impact on productivity and quality of life in Russia: structured healthcare for headache is urgently needed. Eur J Neurol. 2014;21:758–65.
25. Ayzenberg I, Katsarava Z, Sborowski A, Obermann M, Chernysh M, Osipova V, Tabeeva G, Steiner TJ. Headache yesterday in Russia: its prevalence and impact, and their application in estimating the national burden attributable to headache disorders. J Headache Pain. 2015;16:7.
26. Braschinsky M, Haldre S, Kals M, Iofik A, Kivisild A, Korjas J, Koljal S, Katsarava Z, Steiner TJ. Structured education can improve primary-care management of headache: the first empirical evidence, from a controlled interventional study. J Headache Pain. 2016;17:24.
27. Manandhar K, Risal A, Linde M, Steiner TJ. Health-care utilization for headache disorders in Nepal: a population-based door-to-door survey. J Headache Pain. 2018;19:116.
28. Wang SJ, Fuh JL, Young YH, Lu SR, Shia BC. Frequency and predictors of physician consultations for headache. Cephalalgia. 2001;21:25–30.
29. Lampl C, Buzath A, Baumhackl U, Klingler D. One-year prevalence of migraine in Austria: a nation-wide survey. Cephalalgia. 2003;23:280–6.
30. Lipton RB, Scher AI, Kolodner K, Liberman J, Steiner TJ, Stewart WF. Migraine in the United States: epidemiology and patterns of health care use. Neurology. 2002;58:885–94.
31. Edmeads J, Findlay H, Tugwell P, Pryse-Phillips W, Nelson RF, Murray TJ. Impact of migraine and tension-type headache on life-style, consulting behaviour, and medication use: a Canadian population survey. Can J Neurol Sci. 1993;20:131–7.
32. Liu R, Yu S, He M, Zhao G, Yang X, Qiao X, Feng J, Fang Y, Cao X, Steiner TJ. Health-care utilization for primary headache disorders in China: a population-based door-to-door survey. J Headache Pain. 2013;14:47.
33. Manandhar K, Risal A, Linde M, Steiner TJ. The burden of headache disorders in Nepal: estimates from a population-based survey. J Headache Pain. 2016;17:3.
34. Linde M, Steiner TJ, Chisholm D. Cost-effectiveness analysis of interventions for migraine in four low- and middle-income countries. J Headache Pain. 2015;16:15.
35. World Bank. https://data.worldbank.org/indicator/SP.POP.1564.TO.ZS.
36. World Bank. https://data.worldbank.org/indicator/SP.POP.0014.TO.ZS.
37. Saylor D, Steiner TJ. The global burden of headache. Semin Neurol. 2018;38:182–90.
38. Lipton RB, Diamond S, Reed M, Diamond M, Stewart WF. Migraine diagnosis and treatment: results from the American migraine study II. Headache. 2001;41:638–45.
39. Salomon JA, Vos T, Hogan DR, Gagnon M, Naghavi M, Mokdad A, Begum N, Shah R, Karyana M, Kosen S, Farje MR, Moncada G, Dutta A, Sazawal S, Dyer A, Seiler J, Aboyans V, Baker L, Baxter A, Benjamin EJ, Bhalla K, Bin Abdulhak A, Blyth F, Bourne R, Braithwaite T, Brooks P, Brugha TS, Bryan-Hancock C, Buchbinder R, Burney P, Calabria B, Chen H, Chugh SS, Cooley R, Criqui MH, et al. Common values in assessing health outcomes from disease and injury: disability weights measurement study for the Global Burden of Disease Study 2010. Lancet. 2012;380:2129–43.

40. Westergaard ML, Hansen EH, Glumer C, Olesen J, Jensen RH. Definitions of medication-overuse headache in population-based studies and their implications on prevalence estimates: a systematic review. Cephalalgia. 2014;34:409–25.
41. Stovner LJ, Hagen K, Jensen R, Katsarava Z, Lipton R, Scher AI, Steiner TJ, Zwart J-A. The global burden of headache: a documentation of headache prevalence and disability worldwide. Cephalalgia. 2007;27:193–210.
42. Lyngberg AC, Rasmussen BK, Jørgensen T, Jensen R. Secular changes in health care utilization and work absence for migraine and tension-type headache: a population based study. Eur J Epidemiol. 2005;20:1007–14.
43. World Health Organization International Conference on Primary Health Care. Declaration of Alma-Ata. Geneva: WHO; 1978.
44. Tarino E, Webster EG. Primary health care concepts and challenges in a changing world. Alma-Ata revisited. Geneva: WHO; 1995.
45. Coulter A. Shifting the balance from secondary to primary care. BMJ. 1995;311:1447–8.
46. Walley J, Lawn JE, Tinker A, de Francisco A, Chopra M, Rudan I, Bhutta ZA, Black RE and the Lancet Alma-Ata Working Group. Primary health care: making Alma-Ata a reality. Lancet. 2008;372:1001–7.
47. World Health Organization and United Nations Children's Fund (UNICEF) Global Conference on Primary Health Care. Declaration of Astana. From Alma-Ata towards universal health coverage and the sustainable development goals. Astana, Kazakhstan: WHO/UNICEF; 2018.
48. Steiner TJ, Jensen R, Katsarava Z, Linde M, MacGregor EA, Osipova V, Paemeleire K, Olesen J, Peters M, Martelletti P on behalf of the European Headache Federation and *Lifting The Burden*: the Global Campaign against Headache. Aids to management of headache disorders in primary care (2nd edition). J Headache Pain. 2019;20:57.
49. Harpole LH, Samsa GP, Jurgelski AE, Shipley JL, Bernstein A, Matchar DB. Headache management program improves outcome for chronic headache. Headache. 2003;43:715–24.
50. Lake AE, Saper JR, Hamel RL. Comprehensive inpatient treatment of refractory chronic daily headache. Headache. 2009;49:555–62.
51. Göbel H, Heinze A, Heinze-Kuhn K, Henkel K, Roth A, Rüschmann HH. Development and implementation of integrated health care in pain medicine: the nationwide German headache treatment network. Schmerz. 2009;23:653–70.
52. Jensen R, Zeeberg P, Dehlendorff C, Olesen J. Predictors of outcome of the treatment programme in a multidisciplinary headache center. Cephalalgia. 2010;30:1214–24.
53. Diener H, Gaul C, Jensen R, Göbel H, Heinze A, Silberstein S. Integrated headache care. Cephalalgia. 2011;31:1039–47.
54. Saper JR, Lake AE, Madden SF, Kreeger C. Comprehensive tertiary care for headache: a 6-month outcome study. Headache. 1999;39:249–63.
55. Lemstra M, Stewart B, Olszynski WP. Effectiveness of multidisciplinary intervention in the treatment of migraine: a randomized clinical trial. Headache. 2002;42:845–54.
56. Rothrock JF, Parada VA, Sims C, Key K, Walters NS, Zweifler RM. The impact of intensive patient education on clinical outcome in a clinic-based migraine population. Headache. 2006;46:726–31.
57. Populationpyramid.net. https://www.populationpyramid.net/brazil/2010.
58. Masruha MR, Souza JA, Barreiros H, Piovesan EJ, Kowacs F, Queiroz LP, Ciciarelli MC, Peres MFP. Distribution of "Brazilian headache specialists". Analyses of Brazilian Headache Society members. Einstein. 2007;5:48–50.
59. Ferris TG, Chang Y, Blumenthal D, Pearson SD. Leaving gatekeeping behind—effects of opening access to specialists for adults in a health maintenance organization. NEJM. 2001;345:1312–7.
60. Jones R, Lamont T, Haines A. Setting priorities for research and development in the NHS: a case study on the interface between primary and secondary care. BMJ. 1995;311:1076–80.
61. Preston C, Cheater F, Baker R, Hearnshaw H. Left in limbo: patients views on care across the primary/secondary interface. Qual Health Care. 1999;8:16–21.
62. UK Department of Health. Guidelines for the appointment of general practitioners with special interests in the delivery of clinical services: headaches. London: Department of Health; 2003.

63. Hedenrud T, Jonsson P, Linde M. Beliefs about medicines and adherence among Swedish migraineurs. Ann Pharmacother. 2008;42:39–45.
64. Mulleners WM, Whitmarsh TE, Steiner TJ. Noncompliance may render migraine prophylaxis useless, but once-daily regimens are better. Cephalalgia. 1998;18:52–6.
65. Braschinsky M, Haldre S, Kals M, Arge M, Saar B, Niibek M, Katsarava Z, Steiner TJ. Structured education to improve primary-care management of headache: how long do the benefits last? A follow-up observational study. Eur J Neurol. 2018;25:497–502.
66. Linde M, Gustavsson A, Stovner LJ, Steiner TJ, Barré J, Katsarava Z, Lainez JM, Lampl C, Lantéri-Minet M, Rastenyte D, Ruiz de la Torre E, Tassorelli C, Andrée C. The cost of headache disorders in Europe: the Eurolight project. Eur J Neurol. 2012;19:703–11.
67. Hu XH, Markson LE, Lipton RB, Stewart WF, Berger ML. Burden of migraine in the United States: disability and economic costs. Arch Intern Med. 1999;159:813–8.
68. Yu S, Liu R, Zhao G, Yang X, Qiao X, Feng J, Fang Y, Cao X, He M, Steiner T. The prevalence and burden of primary headaches in China: a population-based door-to-door survey. Headache. 2012;52:582–91.
69. Selekler MH, Gökmen G, Steiner TJ. Productivity impact of headache on a heavy-manufacturing workforce in Turkey. J Headache Pain. 2013;14:88.
70. Selekler HM, Gökmen G, Alvur TM, Steiner TJ. Productivity losses attributable to headache, and their attempted recovery, in a heavy-manufacturing workforce in Turkey: implications for employers and politicians. J Headache Pain. 2015;16:96.
71. Mbewe E, Zairemthiama P, Paul R, Birbeck GL, Steiner TJ. The burden of primary headache disorders in Zambia: national estimates from a population-based door-to-door survey. J Headache Pain. 2015;16:36.
72. Steiner TJ, Rao GN, Kulkarni GB, Gururaj G, Stovner LJ. Headache yesterday in Karnataka state, India: prevalence, impact and cost. J Headache Pain. 2016;17:74.
73. Zebenigus M, Tekle-Haimanot R, Worku DK, Thomas H, Steiner TJ. The burden of headache disorders in Ethiopia: national estimates from a population-based door-to-door survey. J Headache Pain. 2017;18:58.
74. Vos T, Flaxman AD, Naghavi M, Lozano R, Michaud C, Ezzati M, Shibuya K, Salomon JA, Abdalla S, Aboyans V, Abraham J, Ackerman I, Aggarwal R, Ahn SY, Ali MK, Alvarado M, Anderson HR, Anderson LM, Andrews KG, Atkinson C, Baddour LM, Bahalim AN, Barker-Collo S, Barrero LH, Bartels DH, Basáñez MG, Baxter A, Bell ML, Benjamin EJ, Bennett D, Bernabé E, Bhalla K, Bhandari B, Bikbov B, Bin Abdulhak A, et al. Years lived with disability (YLD) for 1160 sequelae of 289 diseases and injuries 1990–2010: a systematic analysis for the Global Burden of Disease Study 2010. Lancet. 2012;380:2163–96.
75. Kulkarni GB, Rao GN, Gururaj G, Stovner LJ, Steiner TJ. Headache disorders and public ill-health in India: prevalence estimates in Karnataka state. J Headache Pain. 2015;16:67.
76. Rao GN, Kulkarni GB, Gururaj G, Stovner LJ, Steiner TJ. The burden attributable to headache disorders in India: estimates from a community-based study in Karnataka state. J Headache Pain. 2015;16:94.
77. Ayzenberg I, Katsarava Z, Sborowski A, Chernysh M, Osipova V, Tabeeva G, Yakhno N, Steiner TJ. The prevalence of primary headache disorders in Russia: a countrywide survey. Cephalalgia. 2012;32:373–81.
78. Mbewe E, Zairemthiama P, Yeh H-H, Paul R, Birbeck GL, Steiner TJ. The epidemiology of primary headache disorders in Zambia: a population-based door-to-door survey. J Headache Pain. 2015;16:30.
79. World Health Organization. Cost effectiveness and strategic planning (WHO-CHOICE). http://www.who.int/choice/cost-effectiveness/en/.
80. Steiner TJ, Lipton RB on behalf of *Lifting The Burden*: The Global Campaign against Headache. The Headache-Attributed Lost Time (HALT) indices: measures of burden for clinical management and population-based research. J Headache Pain. 2018;19:12.
81. World Health Organization. Noncommunicable diseases. 2018. http://www.who.int/news-room/fact-sheets/detail/noncommunicable-diseases.

Chapter 16
Evaluation: Quality in Headache Services

Timothy J. Steiner, Rigmor Jensen, Raquel Gil-Gouveia, and Zaza Katsarava

16.1 Introduction

Measuring the effect of interventions, when these involve policy, service or structured programmes of care rather than single technologies (drugs, devices, surgical procedures), is methodologically challenging. Ideally it is done in terms of intended final outcomes (e.g. reduction in population burden attributable to headache), but this is especially difficult.

In theory, measurement of effect is the essential next step after any intervention, to be followed, if evaluation indicates the need, by revision and modified intervention

T. J. Steiner (✉)
Department of Neuromedicine and Movement Science, NTNU Norwegian University of Science and Technology, Trondheim, Norway

Division of Brain Sciences, Imperial College London, London, UK
e-mail: t.steiner@imperial.ac.uk

R. Jensen
Department of Neurology, Danish Headache Centre, University of Copenhagen, Rigshospitalet Glostrup, Glostrup, Denmark
e-mail: rigmor.jensen@regionh.dk

R. Gil-Gouveia
Hospital da Luz Headache Center, Lisbon, Portugal
e-mail: rgouveia@hospitaldaluz.pt

Z. Katsarava
Evangelical Hospital Unna, Unna, Germany

Department of Neurology, University of Duisburg-Essen, Essen, Germany

EVEX Medical Corporation, Tbilisi, Georgia

IM Sechenov First Moscow State Medical University (Sechenov University), Moscow, Russian Federation
e-mail: zaza.katsarava@uk-essen.de

T. J. Steiner, L. J. Stovner (eds.), *Societal Impact of Headache*, Headache,
https://doi.org/10.1007/978-3-030-24728-7_16

in plan-do-study-act (PDSA) cycles (Fig. 16.1). This is standard methodology in change management [1]. The reality reflects the difficulty of the requirement (although political expediency is, perhaps, a more potent factor). As the UK National Health Service ACT Academy admits: "This approach [PDSA] has been unusual in a healthcare setting … new ideas are often introduced without sufficient testing" [2].

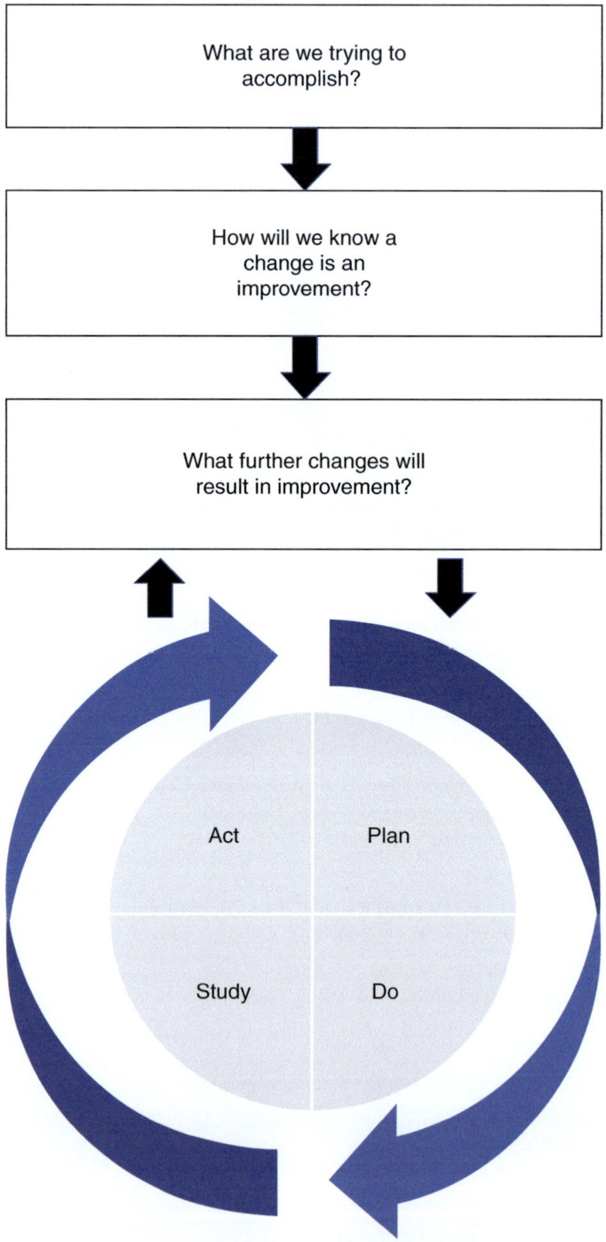

Fig. 16.1 The model for improvement (plan-do-study-act cycle) (adapted from [1])

It is axiomatic, nonetheless, that healthcare systems should aspire to high *quality of care*. All such systems must therefore measure and monitor quality. Evaluation of healthcare quality underpins optimal care, efficient use of resources, avoidance of medical errors, service advancement, professional development and accountability of health professionals and managers [3, 4], and is central to meeting patients' expectations and needs [5].

But, before quality can be assessed, it must be defined; and methods for assessing it are required.

Different *definitions of quality* are both possible and legitimate. Quality is multidimensional, with many and varied elements [6]. Different stakeholders—patients, health professionals and managers—may disagree over what the dimensions are or place different values on them [7–9]. And there is commonly a tension between dimensions: it is rarely possible to deliver care that is optimal on all of them simultaneously.

16.1.1 Quality Assessment; Quality Indicators

Quality indicators are specific, explicitly defined and employed to assess measurable elements of practice that can be changed in order to improve healthcare [3, 9, 10]. Based either on current evidence or on expert consensus, they define *standards of care* that are realistic and achievable in the specific circumstances (setting, resources or patient acceptability).

Quality indicators are statements, used retrospectively, about the structure, process or outcome of care or services provided to patients [11]. *Process indicators* (e.g. the proportion of headache patients who receive a timely appointment) are, typically, direct measures of quality of care. *Outcome indicators* (such as the proportion of patients treated for migraine who report specified reductions in headache frequency after 1 year) are indirect measures. Both have a role, and each has advantages and disadvantages [12].

Process indicators, because they are direct, are more sensitive to differences in quality of care and intuitively easy to interpret. However, many care processes are not routinely monitored, and it may not be easy to do so. To know how many patients with migraine are offered triptans, for example, requires additional contemporaneous recording or, later, time-consuming chart review. Furthermore, objective standards are needed, themselves based in quality (in the example, this knowledge is useful only if it can be stipulated, taking due account of case mix, how many *should* be offered triptans) [12].

Outcomes on the other hand commonly *are* measured routinely—indeed they should be, as a matter of course: for headache, many outcome measures have been validated [13]. Information thereby provided is usable for quality evaluation with relatively little effort, particularly when records are computerized [14] (although accuracy and completeness often vary). Outcome indicators—when they are both valid for purpose and appropriately chosen—reflect the summary results of all aspects of care, even those that are otherwise difficult to measure such as technical expertise [12]. But they have major disadvantages. Being indirect, outcome measures are influenced by many factors, not all dependent on quality of care. Changes that may be observed are always much smaller than any changes in the processes that led to them. Larger amounts of data are usually required for analysis: for example, the sample size needed to show a significant improvement in HALT scores ([15]; also, Chap. 7) is much greater than to show an increase in the number of patients prescribed triptans. Additionally, a clear causal link between processes and outcomes can be difficult to establish.

Since healthcare is complex, one method of quality assessment alone is unlikely to show how quality can be improved; rather, different methods, each tailored appropriately, should be employed together.

16.2 Quality in Headache Care

Worldwide, care for headache disorders is less than optimal, so that high levels of ill health, disability and lost productivity persist, with huge costs to society ([16]; also, Chaps. 4 and 8). Improving the quality of headache care goes beyond better diagnosis and treatment of *patients*, since large numbers of people with headache do not consult doctors, do not become patients, and will not benefit from improvements in care processes. While there are significant barriers obstructing access to care ([16–18]; also, Chap. 13), dismantling them is high on the agenda for headache-service improvement, and *service quality* is not achieved unless this is done.

16.2.1 Definition and Indicators of "Quality" in Headache Care

Only three initiatives have sought to develop quality indicators for headache. In two of these, one in the USA [19, 20] and one in the UK [21], headache was only one of many conditions for which this was attempted. The 21 US headache indicators covered three main domains: symptoms, examinations and medications (acute and prophylactic) [20]. In the UK, 11 quality indicators for headache care in primary care covered diagnosis, referral and treatment. There is no published evidence that the UK indicators were ever used, but the US indicators showed, on average, that adult patients consulting physicians for headache received only 45% of the recommended care processes, well below the mean (55%) for all conditions studied [20].

Both these sets of indicators have multiple limitations. They focus on diagnosis and treatment, taking no account of other dimensions of quality. They are specific to single countries and single settings within each country's healthcare system—primary care in the UK and the health-plan level in the USA. Developed in wealthy countries with sophisticated medical infrastructures, they are of unclear relevance in resource-poor areas of the world.

The third initiative, a collaborative project of European Headache Federation (EHF) and *Lifting The Burden* (LTB) within the Global Campaign against Headache [22–24], found there was a prior need to define "quality" in headache care, since no accepted definition existed. Only then could quality indicators be formulated, both to identify deficiencies in existing services and to guide the development of structured headache services in countries that lacked them ([25–29]; also, Chap. 15).

In the service model described in Chap. 15, headache care spans three care levels, from primary to specialist, requiring that quality indicators be relevant regardless of who delivers the care (in terms of level of care or type of health professional). For the purposes of the Global Campaign [22–24], they need also to be applicable across countries and cultures. Since healthcare quality indicators are not easily transferred between different countries [9], the multinational development group undertook worldwide consultation [25, 26]. There were three distinct steps to the project, briefly described below.

The first, a *structured literature review*, found four articles reporting either development or use of indicators to assess quality, one review article identifying measures that could be so used and 28 original research articles assessing at least one aspect of headache care [25]. The second step was a *qualitative study* with representatives of the three stakeholder groups considered to be of key importance: physicians and nurses, who deliver headache care, and people with headache, who are the recipients of care. Three focus groups, one with each stakeholder group, explored how these stakeholders defined and described "good" quality care for headache.

The aim of these steps was to extract elements of headache care that might be regarded as part of quality. An initial long list, 160 putative indicators in 14 domains, was reviewed, refined and shortened through *wide consultation*, the third step. Initial consultation with 18 stakeholder representatives from 16 countries (neurologists, GPs with special interest in headache, specialist nurses, headache researchers, patient association representatives and people with headache) informed the second, worldwide consultation. Invited into this were all members of the International Headache Society, along with a large list of people, with professional or personal interests in headache, who had initially been recruited by the World Health Organization (WHO) and LTB as contributors to their *Atlas of Headache Disorders* ([16]; also, Chap. 5). A total of 157 responded, from 45 countries representing all six WHO world regions.

From these steps, a multidimensional definition of *quality of headache care* emerged, identifying nine domains (Table 16.1), all essential and none claiming especial importance [26]:

> "Good quality headache care achieves accurate diagnosis and individualized management, has appropriate referral pathways, educates patients about their headaches and their management, is convenient and comfortable, satisfies patients, is efficient and equitable, assesses outcomes and is safe."

At the same time, 30 indicators also emerged (Table 16.1) [26].

Table 16.1 The nine domains of quality of headache care and 30 quality indicators that address them (from [26])

Domain A: Accurate diagnosis is essential for optimal headache care	
A1	Patients are asked about onset of their headaches
A2	Diagnosis is according to current ICHD criteria
A3	A working diagnosis is made at the first visit
A4	A definitive diagnosis is made at first or subsequent visit
A5	Diagnosis is reviewed during later follow-up
A6	Diaries are used to support or confirm diagnosis
Domain B: Individualized management is essential for optimal headache care	
B1	Waiting-list times for appointments are related to urgency of need
B2	Sufficient time is allocated to each visit for the purpose of good management
B3	Patients are asked about the temporal profile of their headaches
B4	Treatment plans follow evidence-based guidelines, reflecting diagnosis
B5	Treatment plans include psychological approaches to therapy when appropriate
B6	Treatment plans reflect disability assessment
B7	Patients are followed up to ascertain optimal outcome
Domain C: Appropriate referral pathways are essential for optimal headache care	
C1	Referral pathway is available from primary to specialist care
C2	Urgent referral pathway is available when necessary
Domain D: Education of patients about their headaches and their management is essential for optimal headache care	
D1	Patients are given the information they need to understand their headache and its management
D2	Patients are given appropriate reassurance
Domain E: Convenience and comfort are part of optimal headache care	
E1	The service environment is clean and comfortable
E2	The service is welcoming
E3	Waiting times in the clinic are acceptable
Domain F: Achieving patient satisfaction is part of optimal headache care	
F1	Patients are satisfied with their management
Domain G: Optimal headache care is efficient and equitable	
G1	Procedures are followed to ensure resources are not wasted
G2	Patients are not over-investigated
G3	Costs of the service are measured as part of a cost-effectiveness policy
G4	There is equal access to headache services for all who need it
Domain H: Outcome assessment is essential in optimal headache care	
H1	Outcome measures are based on self-reported symptom burden (headache frequency, duration and intensity)
H2	Outcome measures are based on self-reported disability burden
H3	Outcome measures are based on self-reported quality of life
Domain I: Optimal headache care is safe	
I1	Patients are not over-treated
I2	Systems are in place to be aware of serious adverse events

16.2.2 Implementation

Three studies have since tested the implementation of these indicators in specialist care [27–29], finding them workable. Although it was not its primary purpose, one study demonstrated common trends among the 14 participating centres, producing evidence of what is majority practice [28]. While this might be a means of setting benchmarks against which service quality is judged, it should not be assumed that majority practice sets an appropriate standard. The three studies all uncovered deficiencies that might or ought to be remedied in order to improve quality [27–29]. There is more work to be done to establish benchmarks.

Meanwhile, the next step, and the next phase in EHF/LTB's service quality evaluation project [27, 28], is to take the process into non-specialist care (service levels 1 and 2) (see Chap. 15). Evaluation in primary care (the principal target for the indicators) is ongoing. Detailed methodology has been developed for this also (Table 16.2), along with the requisite questionnaires.

Table 16.2 Methods of implementation of quality indicators (from [28])

	Indicator	Measure	Application
Domain A: Accurate diagnosis is essential for optimal headache care			
A1	Patients are asked about the temporal profile of their headaches	(a) Duration of presenting complaint is recorded in patient's record (yes/no) (b) Frequency or days/month of symptoms is recorded in patient's record (yes/no)	Review of relevant fields in records of retrospective (random or consecutive) sample of patients ($n = 50$)
A2	Diagnosis is according to current ICHD criteria	(a) Diagnosis is recorded in patient's record (yes/no) (b) Diagnostic record uses ICHD terminology (yes/no)	
A3	A working diagnosis is made at the first visit	Working diagnosis at first visit is recorded in patient's record (yes/no)	
A4	A definitive diagnosis is made at first or subsequent visit	Definitive diagnosis is recorded in patient's record, or, if not, an appointment for review has been given (yes/no)	
A5	Diagnosis is reviewed during later follow-up	Diagnostic review during follow-up is routinely undertaken (yes/no)	Enquiry of doctors
A6	Diaries are used to support or confirm diagnosis	The service has a diagnostic diary available, and doctors are aware of its availability (yes/no)	Enquiry of service manager and doctors into availability
Domain B: Individualized management is essential for optimal headache care			
B1	Waiting-list times for appointments are related to urgency of need	(a) A formal triage system exists (yes/no) (b) ... to expedite appointments in cases of perceived urgency (yes/no)	Enquiry of doctors, service manager and appointments administrator

(continued)

Table 16.2 (continued)

	Indicator	Measure	Application
B2	Sufficient time is allocated to each visit for the purpose of good management	(a) Actual time (minutes) per visit is recorded by patient in exit questionnaire (b) Satisfaction (yes/no) with actual time is recorded by patient in exit questionnaire (c) HCPs express overall satisfaction (yes/no)	(a/b) Review of questionnaires from prospective consecutive sample of patients ($n = 50$) (c) Enquiry of HCPs
B4	Treatment plans include psychological approaches to therapy when appropriate	Access route to psychological therapies exists, and doctors are aware of its availability (yes/no/not applicable)	Enquiry of service manager and doctors into availability
B5	Treatment plans reflect disability assessment	An instrument for disability assessment is available, and HCPs are aware of its availability (yes/no)	
B6	Patients are followed up to ascertain optimal outcome	(a) The service permits follow-up as needed (yes/no) (b) A follow-up diary and/or calendar is available (yes/no)	Enquiry of service manager and HCPs
Domain C: Appropriate referral pathways are essential for optimal headache care			
C1	Referral pathway is available from primary to specialist care	A usable pathway exists, and doctors and appointments administrator are aware of its existence (yes/no)	Enquiry of service manager, doctors and appointments administrator into availability
C2	Urgent referral pathway is available when necessary	A usable pathway exists and doctors and appointments administrator are aware of its existence (yes/no)	
Domain D: Education of patients about their headaches and their management is essential for optimal headache care			
D1	Patients are given the information they need to understand their headache and its management	(a) Information leaflets are available (yes/no), and doctors and appointments administrator are aware of their existence (yes/no) (b) Doctors provide patients with information (yes/no) (c) Information was understandable (yes/no) (d) Amount of information was about right (yes/no)	(a) Enquiry of service manager, doctors and appointments administrator into availability (b) Review of questionnaires from prospective consecutive sample of patients ($n = 50$) (c/d) Review of questionnaires from prospective consecutive sample of patients ($n = 50$)
D2	Patients are given appropriate reassurance	Satisfaction (yes/no) with reassurance given is recorded by patient in exit questionnaire	Review of questionnaires from prospective consecutive sample of patients ($n = 50$)
Domain E: Convenience and comfort are part of optimal headache care			
E1	The service environment is clean and comfortable	(a) Satisfaction (yes/no) with cleanliness and comfort is recorded by patient in exit questionnaire (b) HCPs are satisfied with cleanliness and comfort (yes/no)	(a) Review of questionnaires from prospective consecutive sample of patients ($n = 50$) (b) Enquiry of HCPs

Table 16.2 (continued)

	Indicator	Measure	Application
E2	The service is welcoming	Satisfaction (yes/no) with welcome is recorded by patient in exit questionnaire	Review of questionnaires from prospective consecutive sample of patients ($n = 50$)
E3	Waiting times in the clinic are acceptable	(a) Actual waiting time (minutes) per visit is recorded by patient in exit questionnaire (b) Satisfaction (yes/no) with waiting time is recorded by patient in exit questionnaire (c) HCPs are satisfied with waiting times (yes/no)	(a/b) Review of questionnaires from prospective consecutive sample of patients ($n = 50$) (c) Enquiry of HCPs
Domain F: Achieving patient satisfaction is part of optimal headache care			
F1	Patients are satisfied with their management	Satisfaction (yes/no) with overall management is recorded by patient in exit questionnaire	Review of questionnaires from prospective consecutive sample of patients ($n = 50$)
Domain G: Optimal headache care is efficient and equitable			
G1	Procedures are followed to ensure resources are not wasted	A protocol to limit wastage exists (yes/no)	Enquiry of service manager
G2	Costs of the service are measured as part of a cost-effectiveness policy	A record of input costs exists (yes/no)	
G3	There is equal access to headache services for all who need it	A policy to ensure equal access exists (yes/no)	Enquiry of service manager and HCPs
Domain H: Outcome assessment is essential in optimal headache care			
H1	Outcome measures are based on self-reported symptom burden (headache frequency, duration and intensity)	An outcome measure (HURT or similar) is available, and HCPs are aware of its existence (yes/no)	Enquiry of service manager and HCPs
H2	Outcome measures are based on self-reported disability burden	An outcome measure (HALT or similar) is available, and HCPs are aware of its existence (yes/no)	
H3	Outcome measures are based on self-reported quality of life	An outcome measure (WHOQoL or similar) is available, and HCPs are aware of its existence (yes/no)	
Domain I: Optimal headache care is safe			
I1	Systems are in place to be aware of serious adverse events[a]	A system or protocol exists, and HCPs are aware of its existence (yes/no)	Enquiry of service manager and HCPs

HCPs healthcare providers, *ICHD* International classification of headache disorders, *HURT* headache under-response to treatment questionnaire [13, 30], *HALT* headache-attributed lost time index [15], *WHOQoL* World Health Organization Quality of Life questionnaire [31]

[a]Serious adverse events are those that cause death, are life-threatening, terminate or put at risk a pregnancy or cause hospitalization, prolonged illness, disability and/or malignancy

16.3 Concluding Remarks

This chapter sets out a multidimensional definition of *quality* in the context of headache care, along with a related set of quality indicators. Both were developed for the purposes, *inter alia*, of guiding implementation of headache services in countries that lack them and improving them elsewhere. Chapter 15 described structured headache services as the healthcare solution to the public-health emergency that is headache. Insofar as evaluation (followed by modification when indicated) is the final step in intervention, here is methodology for the purpose.

It will be observed that the domains of quality, and indicators, relate to structure and process: they include outcome assessment, but, other than patient satisfaction, not outcomes themselves. As noted earlier, outcome indicators can summarize all aspects of care [12]; while this seems a desirable attribute, for this very reason they may offer little or no guidance as to what needs improving when deficiency is revealed. This would not be helpful. Also noted earlier, outcome measures are influenced by many factors [12], not all dependent on quality of care. Most challengingly, outcome measures, if used to evaluate quality of care, require objective standards (what outcomes were expected?), which cannot be set independently of circumstances, setting and patient mix. These difficulties might not be insoluble, but the development group opted to sidestep them [25, 26]. Quality assured in structure and process is, for now, the best available guarantor of quality in outcome.

References

1. Shewhart WA. Statistical method from the viewpoint of quality control. Mineola, NY: Dover Publications; 1939.
2. ACT Academy, NHS Improvement Plan, Do, Study, Act (PDSA) cycles and the model for improvement. https://improvement.nhs.uk/documents/2142/plan-do-study-act.pdf.
3. Lawrence M, Olesen F, for the EQuiP Working Party on Indicators. Indicators of quality in health care. Eur J Gen Pract. 1997;3:103–8.
4. Grol R, Baker R, Moss F. Quality improvement research: the science of change in health care. In: Grol R, Baker R, Moss F, editors. Quality improvement research. Understanding the science of change in health care. London: BMJ Books; 2004. p. 1–5.
5. Campbell SM, Braspenning J, Hutchinson A, Marshall MN. Research methods used in developing and applying quality indicators in primary care. BMJ. 2003;326:816–9.
6. Donabedian A. The quality of care. How can it be assessed. JAMA. 1988;260:1743–8.
7. Donabedian A. The seven pillars of quality. Arch Pathol Lab Med. 1990;114:1115–8.
8. Institute of Medicine, Committee to Design a Strategy for Quality Review and Assurance in Medicare. Medicare: a strategy for quality assurance, vol. 1. Washington, DC: National Academies Press; 1990.
9. Marshall M, Campbell S. Introduction to quality assessment in general practice. In: Marshall M, Campbell S, Hacker J, Roland M, editors. Quality indicators for general practice. A practical guide to clinical quality indicators for primary care health professionals and managers. London: Royal Society of Medicine Press; 2002. p. 1–6.

10. Campbell S, Braspenning J, Hutchinson A, Marshall M. Research methods used in developing and applying quality indicators in primary care. In: Grol R, Baker R, Moss F, editors. Quality improvement research. Understanding the science of change in health care. London: BMJ Books; 2001. p. 6–28.
11. McGlynn EA, Asch SM. Developing a clinical performance measure. Am J Prev Med. 1998;14(3 Suppl):14–21.
12. Mant J. Process versus outcome indicators in the assessment of quality of health care. Int J Qual Health Care. 2001;13:475–80.
13. Buse DC, Sollars CM, Steiner TJ, Jensen RH, Al Jumah MA, Lipton RB. Why HURT? A review of clinical instruments for headache management. Curr Pain Headache Rep. 2012;16:237–54.
14. Powell A, Davies H, Thomson R. Using routine comparative data to assess the quality of health care: understanding and avoiding common pitfalls. In: Grol R, Baker R, Moss F, editors. Quality improvement research. Understanding the science of change in health care. London: BMJ Books; 2004. p. 29–50.
15. Steiner TJ, Lipton RB on behalf of *Lifting The Burden*: The Global Campaign against Headache. The headache-attributed lost time (HALT) indices: measures of burden for clinical management and population-based research. J Headache Pain. 2018;19:12.
16. World Health Organization and *Lifting The Burden*. Atlas of headache disorders and resources in the world 2011. Geneva: WHO; 2011. http://www.who.int/mental_health/management/atlas_headache_disorders/en/2011.
17. Sheftell FD, Tepper SJ, Bigal ME. Migraine: barriers for care. Neurol Sci. 2005;26(Suppl 2):s140–2.
18. Ravishankar K. Barriers to headache care in India and efforts to improve the situation. Lancet Neurol. 2004;3:564–7.
19. McGlynn EA, Asch SM, Adams J, Keesey J, Hicks J, DeCristofaro A, Kerr EA. The quality of health care delivered to adults in the United States. NEJM. 2003;348:2635–45.
20. Loder EW, Sheftell F. The quality of headache treatment in the United States: review and analysis of recent data. Headache. 2005;45:939–46.
21. O'Flynn N, Ridsdale L. Headache. In: Marshall M, Campbell S, Hacker J, Roland M, editors. Quality indicators in general practice. A practical guide to clinical quality indicators for primary health care professionals and managers. London: Royal Society of Medicine Press; 2002. p. 112–20.
22. Steiner TJ. *Lifting The Burden*: the global campaign against headache. Lancet Neurol. 2004;3:204–5.
23. Steiner TJ. *Lifting The Burden*: the global campaign to reduce the burden of headache worldwide. J Headache Pain. 2005;6:373–7.
24. *Lifting The Burden*. The Global Campaign against Headache. http://www.l-t-b.org.
25. Peters M, Perera S, Loder E, Jenkinson C, Gil Gouveia R, Jensen R, Katsarava Z, Steiner TJ. Quality in the provision of headache care. 1: systematic review of the literature and commentary. J Headache Pain. 2012;13:437–47.
26. Peters M, Jenkinson C, Perera S, Loder E, Jensen R, Katsarava Z, Gil Gouveia R, Broner S, Steiner T. Quality in the provision of headache care. 2: defining quality and its indicators. J Headache Pain. 2012;13:449–57.
27. Katsarava Z, Gil Gouveia R, Jensen R, Gaul C, Schramm S, Schoppe A, Steiner TJ. Evaluation of headache service quality indicators: pilot implementation in two specialist-care centres. J Headache Pain. 2015;16:53.
28. Schramm S, Uluduz D, Gil Gouveia R, Jensen R, Siva A, Uygunoglu U, Gvantsa G, Mania M, Braschinsky M, Filatova E, Latysheva N, Osipova V, Skorobogatykh K, Azimova J, Straube A, Emre Eren O, Martelletti P, De Angelis V, Negro A, Linde M, Hagen K, Radojicic A, Zidverc-Trajkovic J, Podgorac A, Paemeleire K, De Pue A, Lampl C, Steiner TJ, Katsarava Z. Headache service quality: evaluation of quality indicators in 14 specialist-care centres. J Headache Pain. 2016;17:111.

29. Pellesi L, Benemei S, Favoni V, Lupi C, Mampreso E, Negro A, Paolucci M, Steiner TJ, Ulivi M, Cevoli S, Guerzoni S. Quality indicators in headache care: an implementation study in six Italian specialist-care centres. J Headache Pain. 2017;18:55.
30. Steiner TJ, Buse DC, Al Jumah M, Westergaard ML, Jensen RH, Reed ML, Prilipko L, Mennini FS, Láinez MJA, Ravishankar K, Sakai F, Yu S-Y, Fontebasso M, Al Khathami A, MacGregor EA, Antonaci F, Tassorelli C, Lipton RB on behalf of *Lifting The Burden*: The Global Campaign against Headache. The headache under-response to treatment (HURT) questionnaire, an outcome measure to guide follow-up in primary care: development, psychometric evaluation and assessment of utility. J Headache Pain. 2018;19:15.
31. Schmidt S, Mühlan H, Power M. The EUROHIS-QOL 8-item index: psychometric results of a cross-cultural field study. Eur J Pub Health. 2005;16:420–8.

Part IV
Conclusions

Chapter 17
The Way Forward

Timothy J. Steiner and Lars Jacob Stovner

17.1 Introduction

Earlier chapters have portrayed a world in which headache-attributed burden is high but neglected. Abundant research attests not only the existence of the barriers to care described in Chap. 13 but also the global public ill health these barriers so trenchantly sustain (see Chaps. 4, 8 and 9). The research needed now, above all else, is that which will find, implement and test solutions.

The healthcare solution elaborated in Chap. 15 is incomplete. Its basis and the details of its essential but flexible elements are described in that chapter, along with various supports, and both Chaps. 15 and 16 set out methods of evaluation to justify implementation. Yet to be established are the *methods of implementation*, which are not self-evident. Both the *status quo* and the desired destination are discerned, but the path between them, and how best to negotiate it, are not.

What key purpose(s) should headache research now serve? And what, especially, must be done?

T. J. Steiner (✉)
Department of Neuromedicine and Movement Science, NTNU Norwegian University of Science and Technology, Trondheim, Norway

Division of Brain Sciences, Imperial College London, London, UK
e-mail: t.steiner@imperial.ac.uk

L. J. Stovner
Department of Neuromedicine and Movement Science, NTNU Norwegian University of Science and Technology, Trondheim, Norway

Norwegian Advisory Unit on Headaches, Department of Neurology and Clinical Neurophysiology, St Olavs University Hospital, Trondheim, Norway
e-mail: lars.stovner@ntnu.no

T. J. Steiner, L. J. Stovner (eds.), *Societal Impact of Headache*, Headache,
https://doi.org/10.1007/978-3-030-24728-7_17

17.2 Five Research Fronts

To answer the first question simply: headache research, in our view, has a single, clear purpose—to produce knowledge and generate understanding that will translate into better care and, thereby, into less headache.

Within this purpose, five research fronts each have the potential, by different means, to bring benefits; but the crucial word in all of them is *translate*. If the Global Campaign against Headache [1–3] were required to summarize its purpose and activities by a single keyword, it would be *translation*.

17.2.1 Basic Research

This is the first front, focused on elucidating disease mechanisms, particularly those with a genetic basis.

Basic research guides the development of new treatments. Efficacious therapies exist, but with deficiencies so apparent, especially for non-migraine headache disorders, that research on this front remains an essential and worthwhile effort. But there is a proviso, made apparent later.

17.2.2 Pharmaceutical Research

This is second. Clinical trials, which support the translation of new discoveries into better treatments for people with headache, are necessarily complementary to the first research front and similarly essential—as opportunities arise.

But again there is a proviso: are they always worthwhile? About 5 years ago, expounding a 5-year forward view, one of us berated big pharma for abjectly failing to deliver benefits that might substantially have reduced the global burden of headache [4]:

> "Within the [pharmaceutical] industry, a 20-year period of unprecedented investment in headache has not been without benefit to patients … But it has to be said that, after sumatriptan, the return on big pharma's huge investments has been rather limited for patients. Largely this is because companies and their drugs have competed, head-to-head, for the same small (wealthy) sector of the market instead of working together to expand it."

A new wave of pharma investment is being rewarded with the launch of new drug classes for migraine therapy, including, at long last, a number of preventative drugs—the first to be developed specifically for migraine. CGRP antagonists are entering the markets of the USA and Europe at high cost. Will history repeat itself? In 20 years' time, shall we be reporting, again, "that people in low-income countries have derived no benefit from the drug developments of the last two decades that so excited the West" [4]?

Probably, regrettably, the answer is yes.

17.2.3 Epidemiological Research

On the third front, epidemiological research establishes the scope and scale of headache-related burden of illness and reveals, in ways that no other research can, the public-health importance of headache disorders (see Chaps. 8 and 9).

Poor understanding of headache burden based on poor epidemiological data has, historically, encouraged the persistence of inadequate healthcare for headache, inadequate education for care providers, inadequate or wrong treatments and high individual and societal burdens—all for want of priority ([5]; also, Chap. 13). Unless policy makers are persuaded by indisputable evidence to alter their views on priority and recognize the damage to public health caused by headache, there will never be an appropriate allocation of healthcare resources to bring new, or existing, headache treatments to those who need them. Below the various horizons described in Chap. 13, much headache will continue to be underdiagnosed and undertreated.

In 2001, prior to the launch of the Global Campaign against Headache [1, 2] and thanks to the Global Burden of Disease 2000 (GBD2000) study ([6]; also, Chap. 9), we "knew", and could show politicians if they would listen, that migraine accounted for 1.4% of all disability in the world [6]. *Lifting The Burden* (LTB) believed this was a very substantial underestimate and predicted that future iterations of GBD, informed by better epidemiological evidence, would show this. Indeed they did: headache disorders are now recognized as the second-highest cause of disability worldwide ([7–9]; also, Chaps. 4 and 9).

Epidemiological research may do more. By identifying preventable risk factors for headache, if they exist, it can underpin preventative measures that are able, more efficiently than reactive therapy, to mitigate the burden of headache (see Chap. 10).

17.2.4 Outcomes Research

Fourth is research that determines the effectiveness, or not, of specific actions taken to meet healthcare needs. Outcomes research makes no prior assumptions about *how* effectiveness is measured: this question is a key part of its enquiry. Outcomes research identifies the treatment objectives that are most important to achieve.

Outcomes research thus has the potential to guide optimal, patient-centred healthcare and its delivery within organized health services (see Chap. 15).

In the headache field, outcomes research is a young science, mostly focused until now on short-term outcomes, despite that headache disorders are chronic: 24–48 h after acute treatment and 3–6 months for prophylaxis. And it has mostly measured outcomes within the limited confines of symptoms. It needs to extend itself beyond narrow measures of *efficacy* to broadly-defined indices of *utility*: health and wellbeing, disability and its consequences of lost time and productivity, functional impact in relation to the environment (see Chap. 11) and quality of life (which is not measured over 24 h, as has been suggested [10]). This research will consider comorbidity, and other uses of healthcare resources by people with headache, always including assessments of costs (see Chaps. 12 and 15). All of these are long-term measures, technically difficult to apply because of losses to follow-up, non-adherence and a range of extraneous factors, which indicates that further methodological research is needed first.

17.2.5 Health-Services Research

This is the fifth, last and perhaps most important front, since it tests the "final common pathway". Health-services research is the means of assessing effectiveness in achieving desired outcomes of treatments *actually delivered* by health services.

It is a woefully neglected infant in the field of headache.

High prevalence of illness, even illness that causes demonstrable and costly disability, is not sufficient to establish a priority call upon healthcare resources (see Chap. 15). In a world where these are scarce, none should be allocated to treatments unless they measurably reduce the adverse consequences of disease. But where, until now, has there been any clear demonstration that the provision of good headache care reduces the burden of headache?

The Institute for Health Metrics and Evaluation (IHME), which leads the GBD studies, is beginning to relate disease burdens to the health services in place to relieve them. Maybe, in a not too distant future, this initiative will confirm that poor headache services are, indeed, an important determinant of headache burden. In a more distant but still foreseeable future, hopefully, GBD will report improvements in headache burden in countries over time as, under the guidance of evidence, better headache services are implemented.

17.3 Ways Forward

Given these facts and arguments, *health-services research*, among the five fronts of headache research, promises the most profitable future. If health-services research is ignored, as historically it has been, what might be the value of everything before it—the apparently important achievements of research on the four preceding fronts, available to a select few but otherwise left to decay because nothing has demonstrated the worth of implementing them widely? Backed by health-economic studies, health-services research is likely to show that the reallocation of resources towards better healthcare delivery, making more effective use of treatments already available, has far greater potential to benefit people with headache than the search for new drugs. Furthermore, reallocation of resources does *not* imply additional investment; this would almost certainly also be worthwhile (see Chap. 15), but judicious reallocation makes achievements possible without it.

In time, pharmaceutical research and clinical trials *will* employ outcome measures that reflect what patients want and value, identified by outcomes research that is still to be done but eventually will be. They will build in pharmacoeconomic analysis to justify the opportunity cost of introducing new and invariably more expensive treatments. Regulators will demand these things—generally, not just for headache.

Health-services research will evaluate not headache treatment, or even headache care, but headache *services*, their provision (whether in primary or secondary care or by doctor, clinical officer, nurse or other healthcare provider), access to them and their effectiveness in terms of improved public health. Health-services research will review the role, alongside headache services, of over-the-counter medications and other means of self-management (or mismanagement). It will not assess single treatments but seek to understand the value of a management "package", of which diagnosis, impact assessment, information and advice, medication and other therapeutic interventions, follow-up and outcome assessment are all essential components, tied together. Such a package not only exists but is already partly evaluated (see Chap. 15). Health-services research will show how to put it in place and whether it does what it should.

This needs to be done throughout the world, not just in rich countries and, conversely, not just in poor countries. Headache disorders manifestly trouble the people of wealthy industrialized nations, but they are not uniquely their problem (see Chaps. 4, 5, 8 and 9). The pain and disability, the lifestyle compromises, the damaged relationships and the lost opportunities described in Chap. 4, which are headache's much-unwanted gifts, may be less evident in developing countries but weigh no less heavily for that. The poverty of low-income countries, and its consequences of poor sanitation and infectious diseases, may seem of overwhelming priority, but why should these burdens of headache be any less disagreeable in the presence of hunger and other illness?

17.4 Concluding Remarks

While headache is undertreated everywhere [5], it *is* a fact that all the therapeutic advances of the last 30 years have not touched the lives of more than 90% of people in the world with headache. This must change.

If the *sole* purpose of headache research is to produce knowledge and generate understanding that will translate into better care and less headache, as we fervently believe, there is far greater utility gain to be had from finding ways to take these advances to some of the more than 90% than from striving to do a little better in the fewer than 10% who are relatively well-served already.

This is the challenge of the future.

References

1. Steiner TJ. *Lifting The Burden*: the global campaign to reduce the burden of headache worldwide. J Headache Pain. 2005;6:373–7.
2. Steiner TJ, Birbeck GL, Jensen R, Katsarava Z, Martelletti P, Stovner LJ. *Lifting The Burden*: the first 7 years. J Headache Pain. 2010;11:451–5.

3. Steiner TJ, Birbeck GL, Jensen R, Katsarava Z, Martelletti P, Stovner LJ. The global campaign, World Health Organization and *Lifting The Burden*: collaboration in action. J Headache Pain. 2011;12:273–4.
4. Steiner TJ. Headache in the world: public health and research priorities. Expert Rev Pharmacoecon Outcomes Res. 2013;13:51–7.
5. World Health Organization, *Lifting The Burden*. Atlas of Headache Disorders and Resources in the World 2011. Geneva: WHO; 2011.
6. World Health Organization. World Health Report 2001. Geneva: WHO; 2001.
7. Vos T, Abajobir AA, Abate KH, Abbafati C, Abbas KM, Abd-Allah F, Abdulkader RS, Abdulle AM, Abebo TA, Abera SF, Aboyans V, Abu-Raddad LJ, Ackerman IN, Adamu AA, Adetokunboh O, Afarideh M, Afshin A, Agarwal SK, Aggarwal R, Agrawal A, Agrawal S, Ahmadieh H, Ahmed MB, Aichour MTE, Aichour AN, Aichour I, Aiyar S, Akinyemi RO, Akseer N, Al Lami FH, Alahdab F, Al-Aly Z, Alam K, Alam N, Alam T, et al. Global, regional, and national incidence, prevalence, and years lived with disability for 328 diseases and injuries for 195 countries, 1990–2016: a systematic analysis for the Global Burden of Disease Study 2016. Lancet. 2017;390:1211–59.
8. Steiner TJ, Stovner LJ, Vos T, Jensen R, Katsarava Z. Migraine is *first* cause of disability in under 50s: will health politicians now take notice? J Headache Pain. 2018;19:17.
9. GBD 2017 Disease and Injury Incidence and Prevalence Collaborators. Global, regional, and national incidence, prevalence, and years lived with disability for 354 diseases and injuries for 195 countries and territories, 1990–2017: a systematic analysis for the Global Burden of Disease Study 2017. Lancet. 2018;392:1789–858.
10. Steiner TJ. Please don't hijack "quality of life". Cephalalgia. 1998;18:227.

MIX
Papier aus verantwortungsvollen Quellen
Paper from responsible sources
FSC® C105338

If you have any concerns about our products,
you can contact us on
ProductSafety@springernature.com

In case Publisher is established outside the EU,
the EU authorized representative is:
Springer Nature Customer Service Center GmbH
Europaplatz 3, 69115 Heidelberg, Germany

Printed by Libri Plureos GmbH
in Hamburg, Germany